The *Thesaurus of Medical Terms* is designed to enable the reader to find the more technical terms that apply to a variety of health-related subjects. By locating the Key Word that applies to a particular subject and reading across the page, the pertinent adjective, study, specialist, and major disorders may be found. For example, if one wants to know the technical term for an eye doctor, one looks under the Key Word column for *eye,* and under Specialist, finds the words *ophthalmologist* and *oculist.* If one cannot recall the name of a common heart disease, one looks under *heart* in the Key Word column and finds, under Major Disorders, *angina* and other conditions listed. These disorders may in turn be looked up in the glossary following for definitions and in the index for page references to the text.

SPECIALIST	MAJOR DISORDERS
allergist, allergologist	respiratory and skin disorders, e.g. asthma and contact dermatitis
anesthesiologist	
hematologist	anemia, leukemia, hemophilia
vascular surgeon	varicose veins, phlebitis
orthopedist, orthopedic surgeon, orthopod	back disorders, fractures, trauma
etiologist	
thoracic surgeon	lung cancer, tuberculosis, emphysema
pediatrician	all diseases children are subject to
proctologist	hemorrhoids, cancer of the rectum or colon
nutritionist	malnutrition, obesity
gastroenterologist	digestive difficulties, ulcers, gallstones, inguinal hernia
pathologist	
otologist	hearing or equilibrium disorders
otolaryngologist, ENT specialist	hearing or equilibrium disorders, laryngitis, upper respiratory infections
epidemiologist	forms of cancer, cholera, influenza
ophthalmologist, oculist	glaucoma, cataract, detached retina
podiatrist, chiropodist	arch troubles, bunions, ingrown toenails
general practitioner (GP)	

The New Complete
MEDICAL
and HEALTH
ENCYCLOPEDIA

EDITED BY
Richard J. Wagman, M.D., F.A.C.P.
Assistant Clinical Professor of Medicine
Downstate Medical Center
New York, New York

AND BY
the J. G. Ferguson Editorial Staff,
Sidney I. Landau, Managing Editor

Volume 4

J. G. FERGUSON PUBLISHING COMPANY / CHICAGO

Contents

Volume 4

Color Illustrations

Illustrations of Emergency Procedures

Medical Emergencies

Anyone attempting to deal with a medical emergency will do so with considerably more confidence if he has a clear notion of the order of importance of various problems. Over and above all technical knowledge about such things as tourniquets or cardiac massage is the ability of the rescuer to keep a cool head so that he can make the right decisions and delegate tasks to others who wish to be helpful.

Cessation of Breathing

The medical emergency which requires prompt attention before any others is cessation of breathing. No matter what other injuries are involved, artificial respiration must be administered immediately to anyone suffering from respiratory arrest.

To determine whether a person is breathing naturally, place your cheek as near as possible to the victim's mouth and nose. While you are feeling and listening for evidence of respiration, watch the victim's chest and upper abdomen to see if they rise and fall. If respiratory arrest is indicated, begin artificial respiration immediately.

Time is critical; a human body has only about a four-minute reserve supply of oxygen in its tissues, although some persons have been revived after being submerged in water for 10 minutes or more. Do not waste time moving the victim to a more comfortable location unless his position is life-threatening.

If more than one person is available, the second person should summon a doctor. A second rescuer can also assist in preparing the victim for artificial respiration by helping to loosen clothing around the neck, chest, and waist, and by inspecting the mouth for false teeth, chewing gum, or other objects that could block the flow of air. The victim's tongue must be pulled forward before artificial respiration begins.

Normal breathing should start after not more than 15 minutes of artificial respiration. If it doesn't, you should continue the procedure for at least two hours, alternating, if possible, with other persons to maintain maximum efficiency. Medical experts have defined normal breathing as 8 or more breaths per minute; if breathing resumes but slackens to a rate of fewer than 8 breaths per minute, or if breathing stops suddenly for more than 30 seconds, continue artificial respiration.

Mouth-to-Mouth and Mouth-to-Nose Artificial Respiration

Following is a description of the techniques used to provide mouth-to-mouth or mouth-to-nose artificial respiration. These are the preferred methods of artificial respiration because they move a greater volume of air into a victim's lungs than any alternative method.

After quickly clearing the victim's mouth and throat of obstacles, tilt the victim's head back as far as possible, with the chin up and neck stretched to insure an open passage of air to the lungs. If mouth-to-mouth breathing is employed, pull the lower jaw of the victim open with one hand, inserting your thumb between the victim's teeth, and pinch the nostrils with the other to prevent air leakage through the nose. If using the mouth-to-nose technique, hold one hand over the mouth to seal it against air leakage.

Next, open your own mouth and take a deep breath. Then blow forcefully into the victim's mouth (or nose) until you can see the chest rise. Quickly remove your mouth and listen for normal exhalation sounds from the victim. If you hear gurgling sounds, try to move the jaw higher because the throat may not be stretched open properly. Continue blowing forcefully into the victim's mouth (or nose) at a rate of once every three or four seconds. (For infants, do not blow forcefully; blow only small puffs of air from your cheeks.)

If the victim's stomach becomes distended, it may be a sign that air is being blown into the stomach; press firmly with one hand on the upper abdomen to push the air out of the stomach.

If you are hesitant about direct physical contact of the lips, make a ring with the index finger and thumb of the hand being used to hold the

MOUTH-TO-MOUTH RESPIRATION

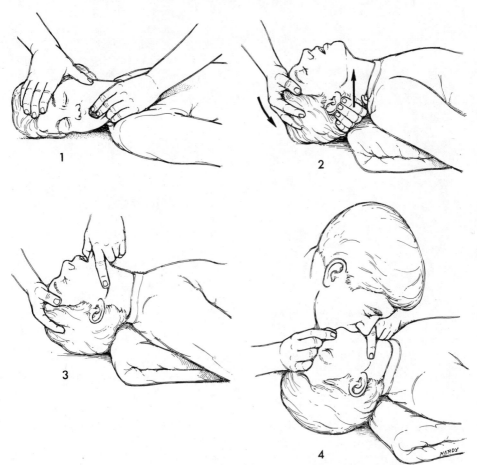

(1) Clear the victim's mouth and throat of obstructions. (2) Tilt the head back as far as possible, with the chin up and neck stretched taut. (3) Insert your thumb between the victim's teeth to pull his lower jaw open. Keep his head pushed back. (4) Pinch the nostrils shut. Open your mouth, take a deep breath, and, placing your mouth firmly against the victim's, blow forcefully. Repeat every 3 or 4 seconds.

victim's chin in position. Place the ring of fingers firmly about the victim's mouth; the outside of the thumb may at the same time be positioned to seal the nose against air leakage. Then blow the air into the victim's mouth through the finger-thumb ring. Direct lip-to-lip contact can also be avoided by placing a piece of gauze or other clean porous cloth over the victim's mouth.

Severe Bleeding

If the victim is not suffering from respiration failure or if breathing has been restored, severe bleeding is the second most serious emergency to attend to. Such bleeding occurs when either an artery or a vein has been severed. Arterial blood is bright red and spurts rather than flows from the body, sometimes in

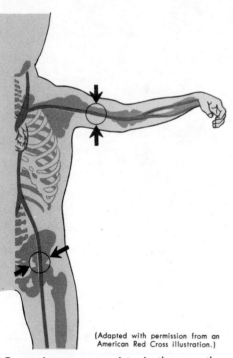

(Adapted with permission from an
American Red Cross illustration.)

**Two major pressure points: in the arm, the
brachial artery; in the leg, the femoral artery.
Continue to apply direct pressure and elevate
the wounded part while utilizing pressure
points to stop blood flow.**

very large amounts. It is also more
difficult to control than blood from a
vein, which can be recognized by its
dark red color and steady flow.

EMERGENCY TREATMENT: The quickest and most effective way to stop
bleeding is by direct pressure on the
wound. If heavy layers of sterile
gauze are not available, use a clean
handkerchief, or a clean piece of
material torn from a shirt, slip, or
sheet to cover the wound. Then
place the fingers or the palm of the
hand directly over the bleeding area.
The pressure must be *firm and constant* and should be interrupted only
when the blood has soaked through
the dressing. *Do not remove the
soaked dressing*. Cover it as quickly
as possible with additional new

layers. When the blood stops seep-
ing through to the surface of the
dressing, secure it with strips of cloth
until the victim can receive medical
attention. This procedure is almost
always successful in stopping blood
flow from a vein.

If direct pressure doesn't stop arterial bleeding, two alternatives are
possible: pressure by finger or hand
on the pressure point nearest the
wound, or the application of a tourniquet. No matter what the source of
the bleeding, if the wound is on an
arm or leg, elevation of the limb as
high as is comfortable will reduce
the blood flow.

TOURNIQUETS: A tourniquet improperly applied can be an extremely
dangerous device, and should only
be considered for a hemorrhage that
can't be controlled in any other way.

It must be remembered that arterial blood flows away from the heart,
and that venous blood flows toward
the heart. Therefore, while a tourniquet placed on a limb between the
site of a wound and the heart may
slow or stop arterial bleeding, it may
actually increase venous bleeding. By obstructing blood flow in
the veins beyond the wound site,
the venous blood flowing toward the
heart will have to exit from the
wound. Thus, the proper application
of a tourniquet depends upon an understanding and differentiation of
arterial from venous bleeding. Arterial bleeding can be recognized by
the pumping action of the blood and
by the bright red color of the blood.

Once a tourniquet is applied, it
should not be left in place for an excessive period of time, since the tissues in the limb beyond the site of
the wound need to be supplied with
blood.

Shock

In any acute medical emergency, the possibility of the onset of shock must always be taken into account, especially following the fracture of a large bone, extensive burns, or serious wounds. If untreated, or if treated too late, shock can be fatal.

Shock is an emergency condition in which the circulation of the blood is so disrupted that all bodily functions are affected. It occurs when

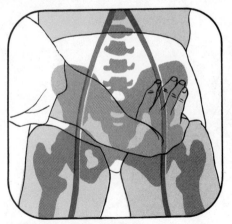

(Top) Use the femoral artery for control of severe bleeding from an open leg wound. Place the victim flat on his back, and put the heel of your hand directly over the pressure point. Apply pressure by forcing the artery against the pelvic bone. *(Bottom)* Use the brachial artery for control of severe bleeding from an open arm wound. Apply pressure by forcing the artery against the arm bone. Continue to apply direct pressure over the wound, and keep the wounded part elevated.

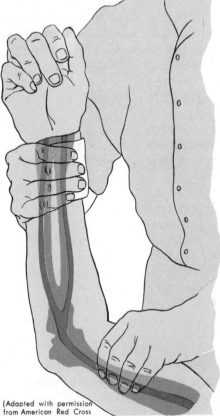

(Adapted with permission from American Red Cross illustrations.)

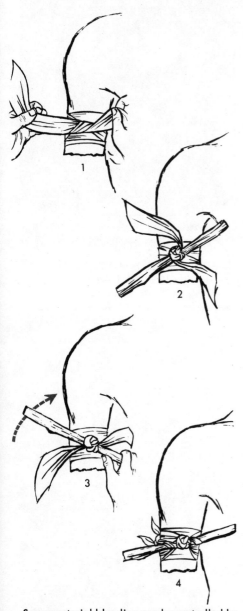

Severe arterial bleeding can be controlled by the correct application of a tourniquet. (1) A long strip of gauze or other material is wrapped twice around the arm or leg above the wound and tied in a half-knot. (2) A stick, called a windlass, is placed over the knot, and the knot is completed. (3) The windlass is turned to tighten the knot and finally, (4) the windlass is secured with the tails of the tourniquet. Improper use of a tourniquet can be very dangerous.

blood pressure is so low that insufficient blood supply reaches the vital tissues.

Types of Circulatory Shock and Their Causes

• *Low-volume shock* is a condition brought about by so great a loss of blood or blood plasma that the remaining blood is insufficient to fill the whole circulatory system. The blood loss may occur outside the body, as in a hemorrhage caused by injury to an artery or vein, or the loss may be internal because of the blood loss at the site of a major fracture, burn, or bleeding ulcer. Professional treatment involves replacement of blood loss by transfusion.

• *Neurogenic shock,* manifested by *fainting,* occurs when the regulating capacity of the nervous system is impaired by severe pain, profound fright, or overwhelming stimulus. This type of shock is usually relieved by having the victim lie down with his head lower than the rest of his body.

• *Allergic shock*, also called *anaphylactic shock*, occurs when the functioning of the blood vessels is disturbed by a person's sensitivity to the injection of a particular foreign substance, as in the case of an insect sting or certain medicines.

• *Septic shock* is brought on by infection from certain bacteria that release a poison which affects the proper functioning of the blood vessels.

• *Cardiac shock* can be caused by any circumstance that affects the pumping action of the heart.

SYMPTOMS: Shock caused by blood loss makes the victim feel restless, thirsty, and cold. He may perspire a great deal, and although his pulse is fast, it is also very weak. His breathing becomes labored and his lips turn blue.

EMERGENCY TREATMENT: A doctor should be called immediately if the onset of shock is suspected. Until medical help is obtained, the following procedures can alleviate some of the symptoms:

1. With a minimum amount of disturbance, arrange the victim so that he is lying on his back with his head somewhat lower than his feet. (*Exception:* If the victim's breathing is difficult, or if he has suffered a head injury or a stroke, keep his body flat but place a pillow or similar cushioning material under his head.) Loosen any clothing that may cause constriction, such as a belt, tie, waistband, shoes. Cover him warmly against possible chill, but see that he isn't too hot.

2. If his breathing is weak and shallow, begin mouth-to-mouth respiration.

3. If he is hemorrhaging, try to control bleeding.

4. When appropriate help and transportation facilities are available, quickly move the victim to the nearest hospital or health facility in order to begin resuscitative measures.

5. *Do not* try to force any food or stimulant into the victim's mouth.

Cardiac Arrest

Cardiac arrest is a condition in which the heart has stopped beating altogether or is beating so weakly or so irregularly that it cannot maintain proper blood circulation.

Common causes of cardiac arrest are heart attack, electric shock, hemorrhage, suffocation, and other forms of respiratory arrest. Symp-

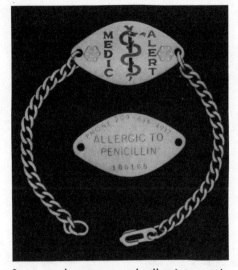

Some people are so severely allergic to certain medications that exposure to them can produce unconsciousness and, if not treated promptly, even death. To alert others, emblems identifying the allergy are available for a slight charge from the nonprofit Medic Alert Foundation, Turlock, California 95380.

toms of cardiac arrest are unconsciousness, the absence of respiration and pulse, and the lack of a heartbeat or a heartbeat that is very weak or irregular.

Cardiac Massage

If the victim of a medical emergency manifests signs of cardiac arrest, he should be given cardiac massage at the same time that another rescuer is administering mouth-to-mouth resuscitation. Both procedures can be carried on in the moving vehicle taking him to the hospital.

It is assumed that he is lying down with his mouth clear and his air passage unobstructed. The massage is given in the following way:

1. The heel of one hand with the heel of the other crossed over it should be placed on the bottom third of the breastbone and pressed firmly

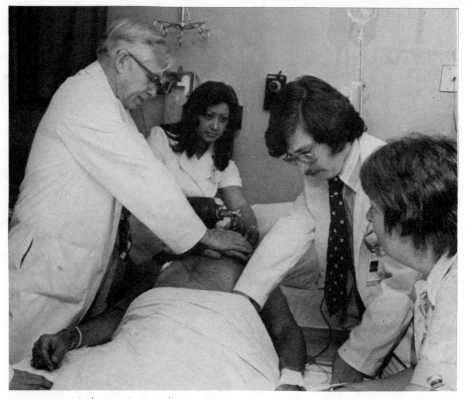

A doctor gives cardiac massage to a patient in a hospital who has suffered cardiac arrest, while a nurse administers oxygen.

down with a force of about 80 pounds so that the breastbone moves about two inches toward the spine. Pressure should not be applied directly on the ribs by the fingers.

2. The hands are then relaxed to allow the chest to expand.

3. If one person is doing both the cardiac massage and the mouth-to-mouth respiration, he should stop the massage after every 15 chest compressions and administer two very quick lung inflations to the victim.

4. The rescuer should try to make the rate of cardiac massage simulate restoration of the pulse rate. This is not always easily accomplished, but compression should reach 60 times per minute.

The techniques for administering cardiac massage to children are the same as those used for adults, except that much less pressure should be applied to a child's chest, and, in the case of babies or young children, the pressure should be exerted with the tips of the fingers rather than with the heel of the hand.

CAUTION: Cardiac massage can be damaging if applied improperly. Courses in emergency medical care offered by the American Red Cross and other groups are well worth taking. In an emergency in which cardiac massage is called for, an untrained person should seek the immediate aid of someone trained in the technique before attempting it himself.

Obstruction in the Windpipe

Many people die each year from choking on food; children incur an additional hazard in swallowing foreign objects. Most of these victims could be saved through quick action by nearly any other person, and without special equipment.

Food choking usually occurs because a bite of food becomes lodged at the back of the throat or at the opening of the trachea, or windpipe. The victim cannot breathe or speak. He may become pale or turn blue before collapsing. Death can occur within four or five minutes. But the lungs of an average person may contain at least one quart of air, inhaled before the start of choking, and that air can be used to unblock the windpipe and save the victim's life.

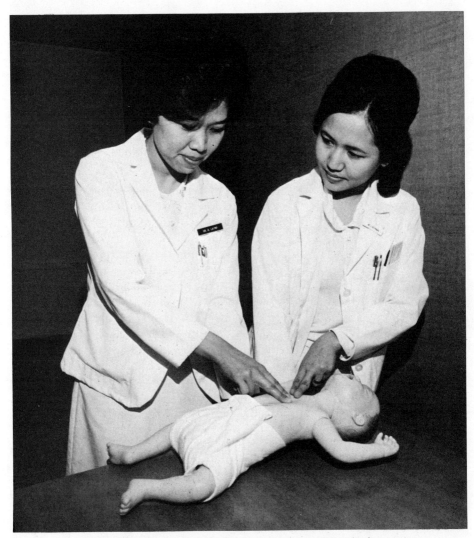

Doctors demonstrate on a doll how cardiac massage is applied to an infant. Only someone trained in the procedure should attempt it.

Finger Probe

If the object can be seen, a quick attempt can be made to remove it by probing with a finger. Use a hooking motion to dislodge the object. Under no circumstances should this method be pursued if it appears that the object is being pushed farther downward rather than being released and brought up.

BACK BLOWS FOR TREATMENT OF STRANGULATION

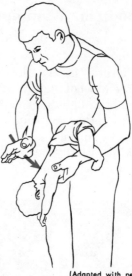

(Adapted with permission from an American Red Cross illustration.)

An infant should be held firmly upside down by the torso, as shown, and struck much more lightly than an adult.

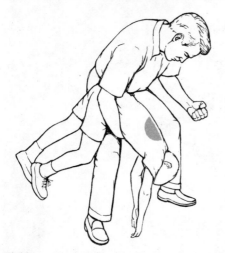

Children may be placed over the knee and struck sharply between the shoulders.

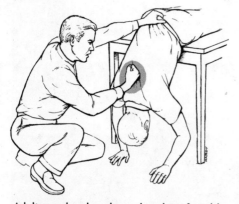

Adults may be placed over the edge of a table, supported by grasping the waist, and struck sharply between the shoulders with the fist.

Back Blows

Give the victim four quick, hard blows with the fist on his back between the shoulder blades. The blows should be given in rapid succession. If the victim is a child, he can be held over the knee while being struck; an adult should lie face down on a bed or table, with the upper half of his body suspended in the direction of the floor so that he can receive the same type of blows. A very small child or infant should be held upside down by the torso or legs and struck much more lightly than an adult.

The Heimlich Maneuver

If the back blows fail to dislodge the obstruction, the Heimlich maneuver should be given without delay. (Back blows may loosen the object even if they fail to dislodge it completely; that is why they are given first.) The lifesaving technique

THE HEIMLICH MANEUVER

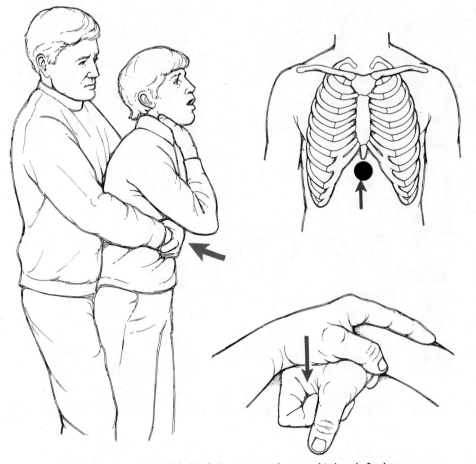

(Left) The rescuer stands behind the victim and grasps his hands firmly over the victim's abdomen just below the rib cage *(top right)*. The position of the rescuer's hands and the direction of thrust are shown at the bottom right.

known as the *Heimlich maneuver* (named for Dr. Henry J. Heimlich) works simply by squeezing the volume of air trapped in the victim's lungs. The piece of food literally pops out of the throat as if it were ejected from a squeezed balloon.

To perform the Heimlich maneuver, the rescuer stands behind the victim and grasps his hands firmly over the victim's abdomen, just below the victim's rib cage. The rescuer makes a fist with one hand and places his other hand over the clenched fist. Then, the rescuer forces his fist sharply inward and upward against the victim's diaphragm. This action compresses the lungs within the rib cage. If the food does not pop out on the first try, the maneuver should be repeated until the air passage is unblocked.

When the victim is unable to stand, he should be rolled over on his back on the floor. The rescuer then kneels astride the victim and per-

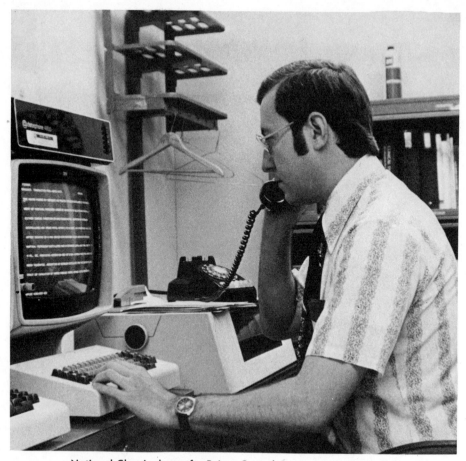

National Clearinghouse for Poison Control Centers uses a computer terminal for quick viewing of information about a particular product.

forms a variation of the Heimlich maneuver by placing the heel of one open hand, rather than a clenched fist, just below the victim's rib cage. The second hand is placed over the first. Then the rescuer presses upward (toward the victim's head) quickly to compress the lungs, repeating several times if necessary.

The Heimlich maneuver has been used successfully by persons who were alone when they choked on food; some pressed their own fist into their abdomen, others forced the edge of a chair or sink against their abdomen.

Poisoning

In all cases of poisoning, it is imperative to get professional assistance as soon as possible.

Listed below are telephone numbers for Poison Control Centers throughout the United States. These health service organizations are accessible 24 hours a day to provide information on how best to counteract the effects of toxic substances.

In the event of known or suspected poisoning, call the center nearest you immediately. Give the staff
(continued on p. 1083)

TELEPHONE NUMBERS OF POISON CONTROL CENTERS*

ALABAMA

Anniston
  205   237-5421

Auburn
  205   826-4037;
  Night: 887-6778,
  3235

Birmingham
  205   933-4050

Dothan
  205   794-3131

Florence
  205   764-8321

Gadsden
  205   492-1240

Mobile
  205   473-3325

Opelika
  205   745-4611

ALASKA

Anchorage
  907   277-6671

Fairbanks
  907   456-6655

Juneau
  907   586-2611

Ketchikan
  907   225-5171

Sitka-Mt.
Edgecumbe
  907   966-2411

ARIZONA

Douglas
  602   364-8473

Flagstaff
  602   744-5233

Ganado
  602   755-3411

Kingman
  602   757-2101

Nogales
  602   287-2771

Phoenix
  602   252-6611;
  267-5011; 252-
  5911; 277-6611;
  258-7373

Prescott
  602   445-2700

Tucson
  602   624-2721;

622-5833; 327-
5461; 882-6300

Winslow
  602   289-4691

Yuma
  602   344-2000

ARKANSAS

El Dorado
  501   863-2266

Fort Smith
  501   782-3071;
  441-4381

Harrison
  501   365-6141

Helena
  501   338-6411

Little Rock
  501   664-5000

Osceola
  501   563-2611

Pine Bluff
  501   535-6800

CALIFORNIA

Fresno
  209   233-0911

Los Angeles
  213   664-2121

Oakland
  415   652-8171;
  654-5600

Orange
  714   633-9393;
  997-2722

Sacramento
  916   453-3692,
  3797

San Diego
  714   294-6000

San Francisco
  415   553-1574;
  558-3881

San Jose
  408   393-0262

CANAL ZONE

Balboa Heights
  2-2600

COLORADO

Denver
  303   893-7771

CONNECTICUT

Bridgeport
  203   334-3566,
  1081

Danbury
  203   774-2300

Hartford
  203   566-3456

Middletown
  203   347-9471

New Britain
  203   224-5672

New Haven
  203   772-3900;
  436-1960

Norwalk
  203   838-3611

Waterbury
  203   756-8351

DELAWARE

Wilmington
  302   655-3389

DISTRICT OF COLUMBIA

Washington, DC
  202   835-4080,
  4081

FLORIDA

Apalachicola
  904   653-3311

Bartow
  813   533-1111

Bradenton
  813   746-5111

Daytona Beach
  904   255-0161

Ft. Lauderdale
  305   525-5411

Fort Myers
  813   334-5286

Ft. Walton Beach
  904   242-1111

Gainesville
  904   372-4321;
  392-3261

Jacksonville
  904   389-7751

Key West
  305   294-5531

Lakeland
  813   683-0411

Leesburg
  904   787-7222

Melbourne
  305   727-7000

Miami
  305   325-7429

Miami Beach
  305   674-2121,
  2200

Naples
  813   649-3131

Ocala
  904   732-1111

Orlando
  305   841-8411

Panama City
  904   769-1511

Pensacola
  904   434-4011

Plant City
  813   752-1188

Pompano
  305   941-8300

Punta Gorda
  813   639-3131

Rockledge
  305   636-2211

St. Petersburg
  813   894-1161

Sarasota
  813   955-1111

Tallahassee
  904   599-5100

Tampa
  813   253-0711

Titusville
  305   269-1100

West Palm Beach
  306   655-5511

Winter Haven
  813   293-1121

GEORGIA

Albany
  912   883-1800

Athens
  404   549-9977

Atlanta
  404   659-1212

*From the *National Clearinghouse for Poison Control Centers* Bulletin, July–August, 1976, U.S. Department of Health, Education, and Welfare

Augusta
404   724-7171

Columbus
404   324-4711

Macon
912   742-1122

Rome
404   232-1541

Savannah
912   355-3200

Thomasville
912   226-4121

Valdosta
912   242-3450

Waycross
912   283-3030

GUAM

Agana
746-9171

HAWAII

Honolulu
808   537-1831

IDAHO

Boise
208   376-1211

Idaho Falls
208   522-3620

Pocatello
208   232-2733

ILLINOIS

Alton
618   462-8851

Aurora
312   897-6021;
896-3911

Belleville
618   233-7750

Belvidere
815   547-5441

Berwyn
312   797-3159

Bloomington
309   828-5241;
662-3311

Cairo
618   734-2400

Canton
309   647-5240

Carbondale
618   549-0721

Carthage
217   357-3131

Centralia
618   532-6731

Champaign
217   337-2533

Chanute AFB
217   495-3133

Chester
618   826-4581

Chicago
312   942-5969;
649-4161; 633-
6542, 6543,
6544; 567-2017;
791-2810; 542-
2030; 774-8000;
770-2419; 978-
2000; 996-6885,
6886; 947-6231

Danville
217   443-5221;
442-6300

Decatur
217   877-8121;
429-2966

Des Plaines
312   297-1800

East St. Louis
618   874-7076;
274-1900

Effingham
217   342-2121

Elgin
312   695-3200;
742-9800

Elmhurst
312   833-1400

Evanston
312   492-6460,
2440

Evergreen Park
312   445-6000

Fairbury
815   692-2346

Freeport
815   235-4131

Galesburg
309   343-8131,
3161

Granite City
618   876-2020

Harvey
312   333-2300

Highland
618   654-2171

Highland Park
312   432-8000

Hinsdale
312   887-2600

Hoopeston
217   283-5531

Jacksonville
217   245-9541

Joliet
815   725-7133;
729-7563, 7565

Kankakee
815   933-1671;
939-4111

Kewanee
309   853-3361

Lake Forest
312   234-5600

La Salle
815   223-0607

Lincoln
217   732-2161

Macomb
309   833-4101

Mattoon
217   234-8881

Maywood
312   531-3000

McHenry
815   385-2200

Melrose Park
312   681-3000

Mendota
815   539-7461

Moline
309   762-3651

Monmouth
309   734-3141

Mt. Carmel
618   263-3112

Mt. Vernon
618   242-4600

Naperville
312   355-0450

Normal
309   829-7685

Oak Lawn
312   425-8000

Oak Park
312   383-6200

Olney
618   395-2131

Ottawa
815   433-3100

Park Ridge
312   696-5151

Pekin
309   347-1151

Peoria
309   672-5500,
4950; 691-4702;
672-2109, 2110,
2111

Peru
815   223-3300

Pittsfield
217   285-2113

Princeton
815   875-2811

Quincy
217   223-5811,
1200

Rockford
815   968-6861;
226-2041; 968-
6898

Rock Island
309   793-1000

St. Charles
312   584-3300

Scott Air Force
Base
618   256-7595

Springfield
217   528-2041;
544-6464

Spring Valley
815   663-2611

Streator
815   673-2311

Urbana
217   337-3311,
2131

Waukegan
312   688-4181,
6181

Winfield
312   653-6900

Woodstock
815   338-2500

Zion
312   872-4561

INDIANA

Anderson
317   649-2511

Angola
219   665-2141,
2166

Crown Point
219   738-2100

East Chicago
219   392-1700,
7203

Elkhart
219   294-2621

Evansville
812   426-3405;
477-6261;
426-8000

Fort Wayne
 219   484-6636;
 423-2614

Frankfort
 317   654-4451

Gary
 219   886-4710

Goshen
 219   533-2141

Hammond
 219   932-2300

Huntington
 219   356-3000

Indianapolis
 317   924-8355;
 639-6671

Kokomo
 217   453-0702

Lafayette
 317   742-0221

La Grange
 219   463-2144

La Porte
 219   362-7541

Lebanon
 317   482-2700

Madison
 812   265-5211

Marion
 317   662-4694

Mishawaka
 219   259-2431

Muncie
 317   747-3241

Portland
 317   726-7131

Richmond
 317   692-7010

Shelbyville
 317   392-3211

South Bend
 219   284-7458;
 234-2151

Terre Haute
 812   232-0361

Vincennes
 812   885-3348

IOWA

Des Moines
 515   283-6212

Dubuque
 319   588-8210

Fort Dodge
 515   573-3101

Iowa City
 319   356-1616

KANSAS

Atchison
 913   367-2131

Dodge City
 316   227-8133

Emporia
 316   342-7120

Fort Riley
 913   239-2323

Fort Scott
 316   223-2200;
 Night: 223-0476

Great Bend
 316   793-3523;
 Night: 792-2511

Hays
 913   628-8251

Kansas City
 913   831-6633;
 287-8881

Lawrence
 913   843-3680

Parsons
 316   421-4880

Salina
 913   827-5591

Topeka
 913   234-9961

Wichita
 316   685-2151

KENTUCKY

Ashland
 606   325-7755

Berea
 606   986-3061

Fort Thomas
 606   292-3215

Lexington
 606   278-3411;
 233-5320

Louisville
 502   589-8222

Murray
 502   753-7588

Owensboro
 502   683-3511

Paducah
 502   444-6361

Whitesburg
 606   633-2160

LOUISIANA

Bogalusa
 504   735-1322

Lake Charles
 318   478-1310

Monroe
 318   325-6454;
 Night: 325-2611

New Orleans
 504   524-3617,
 3618, 3619

Shreveport
 318   222-0709

MAINE

Portland
 207   871-0111

MARYLAND

Baltimore
 301   955-5000;
 528-7701;
 800   494-2414

Bethesda
 301   530-3880

Cumberland
 301   722-6677

Easton
 301   822-5555

Hagerstown
 301   797-2400

MASSACHUSETTS

Boston
 617   232-2120

Fall River
 617   674-5789

New Bedford
 617   997-1515

Springfield
 413   788-7321;
 787-3200

Webster
 617   943-2600

Worcester
 617   756-1551

MICHIGAN

Adrian
 517   263-2412

Ann Arbor
 313   764-5102

Battle Creek
 616   963-5521

Bay City
 517   895-8511

Berrien Center
 616   471-7761

Coldwater
 517   278-2359

Detroit
 313   494-5711;
 864-5400

Eloise
 313   722-3748,
 3749; Night:
 274-3000, 6232

Flint
 313   766-0111

Grand Rapids
 616   774-1774;
 247-7123; 774-
 6794, 7854

Hancock
 906   482-1122

Holland
 616   396-4661

Jackson
 517   783-2771

Kalamazoo
 616   383-7333,
 6401

Lansing
 517   372-5112

Marquette
 906   228-9440

Midland
 517   631-7700

Monroe
 313   241-6509

Petoskey
 616   347-7373

Pontiac
 313   858-3000

Port Huron
 313   987-5555

Saginaw
 517   755-1111

Traverse City
 616   947-6140

MINNESOTA

Bemidji
 218   751-5430

Brainerd
 218   829-2861

Crookston
 218   281-4682

Duluth
 218   727-6636,
 4551

Edina
 612   920-4400

Fergus Falls
 218   736-5475

Fridley
 612   786-2200

Mankato
 507   387-4031

Marshall
 507   532-9661

Minneapolis
612 332-0282;
347-3141; 296-
5276; 588-0616;
874-4233

Morris
612 589-1313

Rochester
507 285-5123;
282-4461

St. Cloud
612 251-2700

St. Paul
612 224-9121;
227-6521; 228-
3132; 291-3348,
3139; 298-8201;
222-4260

Virginia
218 741-3340

Willmar
612 235-4543

Worthington
507 372-2941

MISSISSIPPI

Brandon
601 825-2811

Columbia
601 736-6303

Greenwood
601 453-9751

Hattiesburg
601 544-7000

Jackson
601 968-1704;
982-0121; 354-
6650

Keesler AFB
Biloxi
601 377-2516,
6555, 6556

Laurel
601 649-4000

Meridian
601 483-6211

Pascagoula
601 762-6121

University
601 234-1522

Vicksburg
601 636-2131

MISSOURI

Cape Girardeau
314 334-4461

Columbia
314 882-8091

Hannibal
314 221-0414

Joplin
417 781-2727

Kansas City
816 471-0626;
421-8060

Kirksville
816 665-4611

Poplar Bluff
314 785-7721

Rolla
314 364-3100

St. Joseph
816 232-8461

St. Louis
314 865-4000;
367-6880

Springfield
417 836-3193;
881-8811

West Plains
417 256-3141

MONTANA

Bozeman
406 586-5431

Great Falls
406 761-1200

Helena
406 442-2480

NEBRASKA

Lincoln
402 483-3244

Omaha
402 553-5400

NEVADA

Las Vegas
702 385-1277

Reno
702 785-4129;
Night: 785-4140

NEW
HAMPSHIRE

Hanover
603 643-4000

NEW JERSEY

Atlantic City
609 344-4081

Belleville
201 751-1000

Boonton
201 334-5000

Bridgeton
609 451-6600

Camden
609 795-5554

Denville
201 627-3000

East Orange
201 672-8400

Elizabeth
201 527-5059

Englewood
201 568-3400

Flemington
201 782-2121

Livingston
201 992-5161

Long Branch
201 222-2210

Montclair
201 746-6000

Morristown
201 538-0900

Mount Holly
609 267-7877

Neptune
201 988-1818

Newark
201 926-7240,
7241, 7242, 7243

New Brunswick
201 828-3000;
545-8000

Newton
201 383-2121

Orange
201 678-1100

Passaic
201 473-1000

Perth Amboy
201 442-3700

Phillipsburg
201 859-1500

Point Pleasant
201 892-1100

Princeton
609 921-7700

Saddle Brook
201 843-6700

Somers Point
609 927-3501

Somerville
201 725-4000

Summit
201 522-2232

Teaneck
201 837-3070

Trenton
609 396-1077

Union
201 687-1900

Wayne
201 684-6900

NEW MEXICO

Alamogordo
505 437-3770

Albuquerque
505 843-2551

Carlsbad
505 887-3521

Clovis
505 763-4493

Las Cruces
505 522-8641

Roswell
505 622-8170

NEW YORK

Albany
518 445-3131

Binghamton
607 772-1100;
729-6521

Buffalo
716 878-7000

Dunkirk
716 366-1111

East Meadow
516 542-2323,
2324, 2325

Elmira
607 737-4194;
733-6541

Endicott
607 754-7171

Glens Falls
518 792-3151

Ithaca
607 274-4011,
4383, 4411

Jamestown
716 487-0141

Johnson City
607 773-6611

Kingston
914 331-3131

New York
212 340-4495

Niagara Falls
716 278-4511

Nyack
914 358-6200

Oswego
315 343-1920

Rochester
716 275-5151

Syracuse
315 476-3166;
473-5831

Watertown
315 788-8700

NORTH CAROLINA

Asheville
704 255-4660

Charlotte
704 372-5100

Durham
919 684-8111

Greensboro
919 379-4109

Hendersonville
704 693-6522

Hickory
704 328-2191

Jacksonville
919 353-1234

Wilmington
919 763-9021

NORTH DAKOTA

Bismarck
701 223-4700

Dickinson
701 225-6771

Fargo
701 237-8115

Grand Forks
701 775-4241

Jamestown
701 252-1050

Minot
701 838-0341

Williston
701 572-7661

OHIO

Akron
216 379-8562

Canton
216 452-9911

Cincinnati
513 872-5111

Cleveland
216 231-4455

Columbus
614 228-1323

Dayton
513 461-4790;
878-6623

Lorain
216 282-2220

Mansfield
419 522-3411

Springfield
513 325-0531

Toledo
419 382-7971

Youngstown
216 746-2222

Zanesville
614 '454-4000

OKLAHOMA

Ada
405 332-2323

Ardmore
405 223-5400

Lawton
405 355-8620

McAlester
918 426-1800

Oklahoma City
405 271-5454

Ponca City
405 765-3321

Tulsa
918 584-1351

OREGON

Portland
503 225-8500

PENNSYLVANIA

Allentown
215 433-2311;
821-3252

Altoona
814 944-1681

Bethlehem
215 691-4141

Bloomsburg
717 784-7121

Bradford
814 368-4143

Bryn Mawr
215 527-0600

Carlisle
717 249-1212

Chambersburg
717 264-5171

Chester
215 494-0721

Clearfield
814 765-5341

Coaldale
717 645-2131

Coudersport
814 274-9300

Danville
717 275-6116

Doylestown
215 345-2281

Drexel Hill
215 259-3800

Du Bois
814 371-2200

East Stroudsburg
717 421-3194

Easton
215 258-6221

Erie
814 455-3961;
864-4031;
455-6711; 459-
4000

Gettysburg
717 334-2121

Greensburg
412 837-0100

Hanover
717 637-3711

Harrisburg
717 782-3639,
4141

Hershey
717 534-6111

Indiana
412 463-0261

Jeannette
412 527-3551,
1511

Jersey Shore
717 398-0100

Johnstown
814 536-6671;
535-7541; 536-
5353

Kittanning
814 542-5011

Lancaster
717 299-5511,
4546

Lansdale
215 368-2100

Latrobe
412 539-9711

Lebanon
717 272-7611

Lehighton
215 377-1300

Lewistown
717 248-5411

Muncy
717 546-8282

Nanticoke
717 735-5000

Oil City
814 644-1211

Paoli
215 647-2200

Philadelphia
215 823-8460

Philipsburg
814 342-3320

Pittsburgh
412 681-6669;
766-8300

Pittston
717 654-3341

Pottstown
215 327-1000

Pottsville
717 622-3400

Reading
215 376-4881;
378-6218

Sayre
717 888-6666

Scranton
717 346-3801;
961-4205; 343-
5566

Sellersville
215 257-3611

Sewickley
412 741-6600

Sharon
412 981-1700

Somerset
814 443-2626

State College
814 238-4351

Titusville
814 827-1851

Tunkhannock
717 836-2161

Uniontown
412 437-4531

Washington
412 225-7000

Wellsboro
717 724-1631

Wilkes-Barre
717 823-1121

Williamsport
717 322-7861

York
717 843-8623

PUERTO RICO

Arecibo
809 878-3535

Fajardo
809   863-0505

Mayaguez
809   832-8686

Ponce
809   842-8354,
2080

Rio Piedras
809   764-3515

RHODE ISLAND

Kingston
401   792-2775,
2762

Pawtucket
401   724-1230

Providence
401   277-4000;
521-5055

**SOUTH
CAROLINA**

Charleston
803   792-4201

Columbia
803   765-7359

SOUTH DAKOTA

Aberdeen
605   225-5110

Sioux Falls
605   336-3894

TENNESSEE

Chattanooga
615   755-6100

Columbia
615   388-2320

Cookeville
615   528-2541

Jackson
901   424-0424

Johnson City
615   926-1131

Knoxville
615   971-3261

Memphis
901   522-3000

Nashville
615   322-3391

TEXAS

Abilene
915   677-3551

Amarillo
806   376-4431

Austin
512   478-4490

Beaumont
713   833-7409

Corpus Christi
512   884-4511

El Paso
915   544-1200

Fort Worth
817   336-5521,
6611

Galveston
713   765-1420,
1561

Grand Prairie
214   641-1313

Harlingen
512   423-1224

Laredo
512   722-2431

Lubbock
806   792-1011

Midland
915   684-8257

Odessa
915   337-7311

Plainview
806   296-9601

San Angelo
915   653-6741

San Antonio
512   223-1481

Tyler
214   597-0351

Waco
817   753-1412;
756-6111

Wharton
713   532-2440;
Night: 532-1440

Wichita Falls
817   322-6771

UTAH

Salt Lake City
801   581-3711

**VIRGIN
ISLANDS**

St. Croix
809   773-1212,
1311; 772-0260,
0212

St. John
809   776-1469

St. Thomas
809   774-1321

VIRGINIA

Alexandria
703   370-9000

Arlington
703   558-6161

Blacksburg
804   951-1111

Charlottesville
804   296-9888

Danville
804   799-2100

Falls Church
703   698-3600,
3111

Hampton
804   722-1131

Harrisonburg
804   434-4421

Lexington
804   463-9141

Lynchburg
804   846-6511

Nassawadox
804   442-8000

Norfolk
804   489-5111

Petersburg
804   732-7220

Portsmouth
804   397-6541

Richmond
804   770-5123

Roanoke
703   981-7336

Staunton
703   885-0361

Waynesboro
703   942-8355

Williamsburg
804   229-1120

WASHINGTON

Aberdeen
206   533-0450

Bellingham
206   676-8400

Longview
206   636-5252

Madigan
206   967-6972

Olympia
206   491-0222

Richland
509   943-1283

Seattle
206   634-5252

Spokane
509   747-1077

Tacoma
206   272-1281

Vancouver
206   256-2064

Yakima
509   248-4400

WEST VIRGINIA

Beckley
304   252-6431

Belle
304   949-4314

Charleston
304   348-4211

Clarksburg
304   623-3177

Huntington
304   696-6160,
2224, 2573

Martinsburg
304   267-8981

Morgantown
304   293-5341

Parkersburg
304   424-2212,
4251

Pt. Pleasant
304   675-4340

Ronceverte
304   647-4411,
4412, 4413

Weirton
304   748-3232

Welch
304   436-3161

Weston
304   269-3000

Wheeling
304   243-3281

WISCONSIN

Eau Claire
715   835-1511

Green Bay
414   432-8621

Kenosha
414   656-2201

Madison
608   262-3702

Milwaukee
414   344-7100

WYOMING

Casper
307   577-7201

Cheyenne
307   634-3341

member to whom you speak as much information as possible: the name or nature of the poison ingested, if you know; if not, the symptoms manifested by the victim.

If for any reason it is impossible to telephone or get to a Poison Control Center (or a doctor or hospital), follow these two general rules:

1. If a strong acid or alkali or a petroleum product has been ingested, dilute the poison by administering large quantities of milk or water. Do not induce vomiting.

2. For methanol or related products such as window cleaners, antifreeze, paint removers, and shoe polish, induce vomiting—preferably with syrup of ipecac.

Calling for Help

Every household should have a card close by the telephone—if possible attached to an adjacent wall—that contains the numbers of various emergency services. In most communities, it is possible to simply dial the operator and ask for the police or fire department. In many large cities, there is a special three-digit number that can be dialed for reaching the police directly.

An ambulance can be summoned either by asking for a police ambulance, by calling the nearest hospital, or by having on hand the telephone numbers of whatever private ambulance services are locally available.

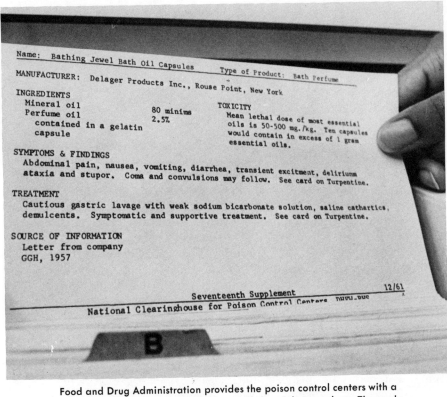

Food and Drug Administration provides the poison control centers with a card file that lists the contents of potentially hazardous products. The card lists ingredients, toxicity, symptoms, and recommended treatment.

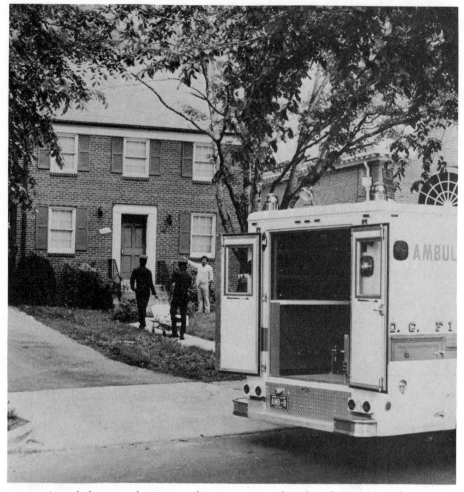

An ambulance can be summoned in an emergency by asking for a police ambulance or by calling the nearest hospital. Private ambulances are also available.

Such services are listed in the classified pages of the telephone directory.

Practically all hospitals have emergency rooms for the prompt treatment of accident cases. If the victim is in good enough physical condition, he can be placed in a prone position in a family station wagon for removal to a hospital. However, under no circumstances should a person who has sustained major injuries or who has collapsed be made to sit upright in a car. First aid must be administered to him on the spot until a suitable conveyance arrives.

Every family should find out the telephone number of the nearest Poison Control Center (see p. 1077) and note it on the emergency number card.

Reaching a Doctor

Emergencies are usually best handled in a hospital since they are likely to require oxygen, blood transfusions, or other services only a hospital can provide. However, there are many situations in which a doctor's guidance on the phone can be extremely helpful and reassuring.

Since there are times when the family physician may not be available by phone, it's a good idea to ask for the names and phone numbers of doctors who can be called when your own doctor can't be reached. In many communities, it is also possible to get the services of a physician by calling the County Medical Society.

A family on vacation in a remote area or on a cross-country trip by car can be directed to the nearest medical services by calling the telephone operator. If the operator can't provide adequate information promptly, ask to be connected with the nearest headquarters of the State Police.

Emergency Transport

In the majority of situations, the transfer of an injured person should be handled only by experienced rescue personnel. If you yourself must move a victim to a doctor's office or hospital emergency room, here are a few important rules to remember:

1. Give all necessary first aid before attempting to move the victim. Do everything to reduce pain and to make the patient comfortable.

2. If you improvise a stretcher, be sure it is strong enough to carry the victim and that you have enough people to carry it. Shutters, doors, boards, and even ladders may be used as stretchers. Just be sure that the stretcher is padded underneath to protect the victim and that a blanket or coat is available to cover him and protect him from exposure.

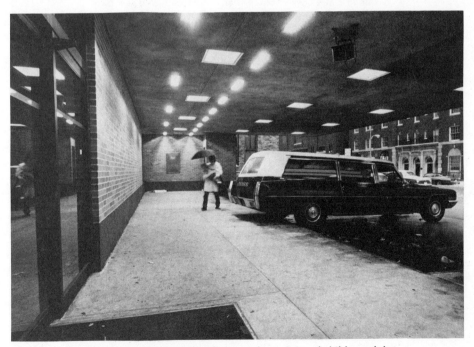

In an emergency, it is much wiser to take an injured child or adult to a hospital equipped to handle emergencies than to a doctor's office.

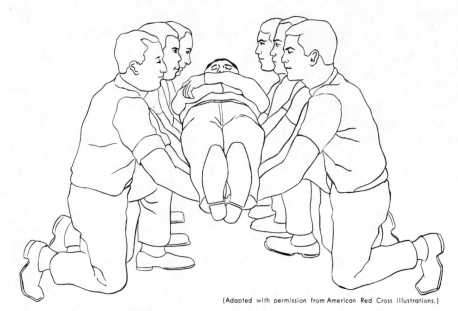

(Adapted with permission from American Red Cross illustrations.)

How to lift an injured or unconscious person to place him on a
stretcher. Three bearers on each side of the victim kneel on the
knee closer to the victim's feet. The bearers work their hands and
forearms gently under the victim to about the midline of the
back. On signal, they lift together as shown; on a following signal, they stand as a unit, if that is necessary. In lowering the
victim to a stretcher or other litter, the procedure is reversed.

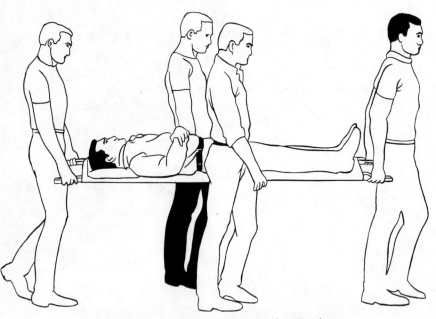

The proper way to carry a victim on a stretcher. One bear-
er is at the head, one at the foot, and one at either side
of the stretcher. The victim should be carried feet first.

3. Bring the stretcher to the victim, not the victim to the stretcher. Slide him onto the stretcher by grasping his clothing or lift him—if enough bearers are available—as shown in the illustration.

4. Secure the victim to the stretcher so he won't fall off. You may want to tie his feet together to minimize his movements.

5. Unless specific injuries prevent it, the victim should be lying on his back while he is being moved. However, a person who is having difficulty breathing because of a chest injury might be more comfortable if his head and shoulders are raised slightly. A person with a severe injury to the back of his head should be kept lying on his side. In any case, place the patient in a comfortable position that will protect him from further injury.

6. Try to transport the patient feet first.

7. Unless absolutely necessary, don't try to put a stretcher into a passenger car. It's almost impossible to get the stretcher or injured person into a passenger car without further injuring him. If there is no ambulance, a station wagon or truck makes a good substitute.

8. When you turn the patient over to a doctor or take him to an emergency room of a hospital, give a complete account of the situation to the person taking charge. Tell the doctor what you've done for the patient and what you suspect might cause further problems or complications.

ALPHABETIC GUIDE TO MEDICAL EMERGENCIES

Abdominal wound

Abdominal wounds can result from gunshots during hunting or working with firearms, from falling on a knife or sharp object at home or work, or from a variety of other mishaps ranging from automobile accidents to a mugging attack. Such a wound can be a major emergency requiring surgery and other professional care. Call a doctor or arrange for quick transportation to a hospital as quickly as possible.

EMERGENCY TREATMENT: If there is severe bleeding, try to control it with pressure. Keep the victim lying on his back with the knees bent; place a pillow, coat, or a similar soft object under the knees to help hold them in the bent position. If abdominal organs are exposed, do not touch them for any reason. Cover the wound with a sterile dressing. Keep the dressing moistened with sterile water or the cleanest water available. Boiled water can be used to moisten the dressing, but be sure it has cooled before applying.

If the victim is to be moved to a hospital or doctor's office, be sure the dressing over the wound is large enough and is held in place with a bandage. In addition to pain, you can expect the victim to experience nausea and vomiting, muscle spasms, and severe shock. Make the victim as comfortable as possible under the circumstances; if he complains of thirst, moisten his mouth with a few drops of water, but do not permit him to swallow the liquid.

Abrasions

EMERGENCY TREATMENT: Wash the area in which the skin is scraped or rubbed off with soap and water, using clean gauze or cotton. Allow the abrasion to air-dry, and then cover it with a loose sterile dressing held in place with a bandage. If a sterile dressing is not available, use a clean handerchief.

Change the dressing after the first 24 hours, using household hydrogen peroxide to ease its removal if it sticks to the abrasion because of clotted blood. If the skinned area appears to be accompanied by swelling, or is painful or tender to the touch, consult a doctor.

Acid burns

Among acids likely to be encountered at work and around the home are sulphuric, nitric, and hydrochloric acids. Wet-cell batteries, such as automobile batteries, contain acid powerful enough to cause chemical destruction of body tissues, and some metal cleaners contain powerful acids.

EMERGENCY TREATMENT: Wash off the acid immediately, using large amounts of clean, fresh, cool water. Strip off or cut off any clothing that may have absorbed any of the acid. If possible, put the victim in a shower bath; if a shower is not available, flood the affected skin areas with as much water as possible. However, do not apply water forcefully since this could aggravate damage already done to skin or other tissues.

After as much of the acid as possible has been eliminated by flooding with water, apply a mild solution of sodium bicarbonate or another mild alkali such as lime water. However,

caution should be exercised in neutralizing an acid burn because the chemical reaction between an acid and an alkali can produce intense heat that would aggravate the injury; also, not all acids are effectively neutralized by alkalis—carbolic acid burns, for example, should be neutralized with alcohol.

Wash the affected areas once more with fresh water, then dry gently with sterile gauze; be careful not to break the skin or to open blisters. Extensive acid burns will cause extreme pain and shock; have the victim lie down with the head and chest a little lower than the rest of the body. As soon as possible, summon a physician or rush the victim to the emergency room of a hospital.

Aerosol sprays

Although aerosol sprays generally are regarded as safe when handled according to directions, they can be directed accidentally toward the face with resulting contamination of the eyes or inhalation of the fumes. The pressurized containers may also contain products or propellants that are highly flammable, producing burns when used near an open flame. When stored near heat, in direct sunlight, or in a closed auto, the containers may explode violently.

EMERGENCY TREATMENT: If eyes are contaminated by spray particles, flush the eye surfaces with water to remove any particles of the powder mist. Then carefully examine eye surfaces to determine if chemicals appear to be imbedded in the surface of the cornea. If aerosol spray is inhaled, move the patient to a well-ventilated area; keep him lying down, warm, and quiet. If breathing fails, administer artificial respiration. Victims of exploding containers or burning contents of aerosol containers should be given appropriate emergency treatment for bleeding, burns, and shock.

The redness and irritation of eye injuries should subside within a short time. If they do not, or if particles of spray seem to be imbedded in the surface of the eyes, take the victim to an ophthalmologist. A doctor should also be summoned if a victim fails to recover quickly from the effects of inhaling an aerosol spray, particularly if the victim suffers from asthma or a similar lung disorder or from an abnormal heart condition.

Alkali burns

Alkalis are used in the manufacture of soap and cleaners and in certain household cleaning products. They combine with fats to form soaps and may produce a painful injury when in contact with body surfaces.

EMERGENCY TREATMENT: Flood the burned area with copious amounts of clean, cool, fresh water. Put the victim under a shower if possible, or otherwise pour running water over the area for as long as is necessary to dilute and weaken the corrosive chemical. Do not apply the water with such force that skin or other tissues are damaged. Remove clothing contaminated by the chemical.

Neutralize the remaining alkali with diluted vinegar, lemon juice, or a similar mild acid. Then wash the affected areas again with fresh water. Dry carefully with sterile gauze, being careful not to open blisters or otherwise cause skin breaks that could result in infection. Summon professional medical care as soon as possible. Meanwhile, treat the victim for shock.

Angina pectoris

Angina pectoris is a condition that causes acute chest pain because of interference with the supply of oxygen to the heart. Although the pain is sometimes confused with ulcer or acute indigestion symptoms, it has a distinct characteristic of its own, producing a feeling of heaviness, strangling, tightness, or suffocation. Angina is a symptom rather than a disease, and may be a chronic condition with those over 50. It is usually treated by placing a nitroglycerine tablet under the tongue.

An attack of acute angina can be brought on by emotional stress, overeating, strenuous exercise, or by any activity that makes excessive demands on heart function.

EMERGENCY TREATMENT: An attack usually subsides in about ten minutes, during which the patient appears to be gasping for breath. He should be kept in a semireclining position rather than made to lie flat, and should be moved carefully only in order to place pillows under his head and chest so that he can breathe more easily. A doctor should be called promptly after the onset of an attack.

Animal bites/rabies

Wild animals, particularly bats, serve as a natural reservoir of rabies, a disease that is almost always fatal unless promptly and properly treated. But the virus may be present in the saliva of any warm-blooded animal. Domestic animals should be immunized against rabies by vaccines injected by a veterinarian.

Rabies is transmitted to humans by an animal bite or through a cut or scratch already in the skin. The in-

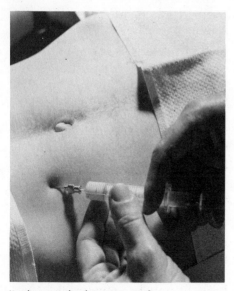

In the standard treatment for exposure to rabies, daily injections of vaccine are given in the abdomen for 14 to 21 days.

fected saliva may enter through any opening, including the membranes lining the nose or mouth. After an incubation period of about ten days, a person infected by a rabid animal experiences pain at the site of infection, extreme sensitivity of the skin to temperature changes, and painful spasms of the larynx that make it almost impossible to drink. Saliva thickens and the patient becomes restless and easily excitable. By the time symptoms develop, death may be imminent. Obviously, professional medical attention should begin promptly after having been exposed to the possibility of infection.

EMERGENCY TREATMENT: The area around the wound should be washed thoroughly and repeatedly with soap and water, using a sterile gauze dressing to wipe fluid away from—not toward—the wound. Another sterile dressing is used to dry the wound and a third to cover it while the patient is taken to a hospital or doctor's office. A tetanus injection is also indicated, and police and health authorities should be promptly notified of the biting incident.

If at all possible the biting animal should be identified—if a wild animal, captured alive—and held for observation for a period of 10 to 15 days. If it can be determined during that period that the animal is not rabid, further treatment may not be required. If the animal is rabid, however, or if it cannot be located and impounded, the patient may have to undergo a series of daily rabies vaccine injections lasting from 14 days for a case of mild exposure to 21 days for severe exposure (a bite near the head, for example), plus several booster shots. Because of the sensitivity of some individuals to the rabies vaccines used, the treatment itself can be quite dangerous.

Recent research, however, has established that a new vaccine called HDCV (human diploid cell vaccine), which requires only six or fewer injections, is immunologically effective and is not usually accompanied by any side effects. The new vaccine has been used successfully on people of all ages who had been bitten by animals known to be rabid.

Appendicitis

The common signal for approaching appendicitis is a period of several days of indigestion and constipation, culminating in pain and tenderness on the lower right side of the abdomen. Besides these symptoms, appendicitis may be accompanied by nausea and a slight fever. Call a doctor immediately and describe the symptoms in detail; delay may result in a ruptured appendix.

EMERGENCY TREATMENT: While awaiting medical care, the victim may find some relief from the pain and discomfort by having an ice bag placed over the abdomen. Do not apply heat and give nothing by mouth. A laxative should not be offered.

Asphyxiation

See GAS POISONING.

Asthma attack

EMERGENCY TREATMENT: Make the patient comfortable and offer reassurance. If he has been examined by a doctor and properly diagnosed, the patient probably has an inhalant device or other forms of medication on his person or nearby.

The coughing and wheezing spell may have been triggered by the presence of an allergenic substance such as animal hair, feathers, or kapok in pillows or cushions. Such items should be removed from the presence of the patient. In addition, placing the patient in a room with high humidity, such as a bathroom with the shower turned on, may be helpful.

Asthma attacks are rarely fatal in young people, but elderly persons should be watched carefully because of possible heart strain. In a severe attack, professional medical care including oxygen equipment may be required.

Back injuries

In the event of any serious back injury, call a doctor or arrange for immediate professional transfer of the victim to a hospital.

EMERGENCY TREATMENT: Until determined otherwise by a physician, treat the injured person as a victim of a fractured spine. If he complains that he cannot move his head, feet, or toes, the chances are that the back is fractured. But even if he can move his feet or legs, it does not necessarily mean that he can be moved safely, since the back can be fractured without immediate injury to the spinal cord.

If the victim shows symptoms of shock, do not attempt to lower his head or move his body into the usual position for shock control. If it is absolutely essential to move the victim because of immediate danger to his life, make a rigid stretcher from a wide piece of solid lumber such as a door and cover the stretcher with a blanket for padding. Then carefully slide or pull the victim onto the stretcher, using his clothing to hold him. Tie the body onto the stretcher with strips of cloth.

Back pain

See SCIATICA.

Black eye

Although a black eye is frequently regarded as a minor medical problem, it can result in serious visual problems, including cataract or glaucoma.

EMERGENCY TREATMENT: Inspect the area about the eye for possible damage to the eye itself, such as hemorrhage, rupture of the eyeball, or dislocated lens. Check also for cuts around the eye that may require professional medical care. Then treat the bruised area by putting the victim to bed, covering the eye with a bandage, and applying an ice bag to the area.

If vision appears to be distorted or lacerations need stitching and antibiotic treatment, take the victim to

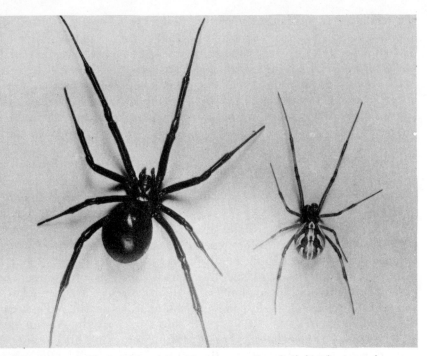

Male and female black widow spiders. The venomous female *(left)* is larger and has a distinctive reddish hourglass shape on the underside of its abdomen.

a doctor's office. A doctor should also be consulted about continued pain and swelling about the eye.

Black widow spider bites

EMERGENCY TREATMENT: Make the victim lie still. If the bite is on the arm or leg, position the victim so that the bite is lower than the level of the heart. Apply a rubber band or similar tourniquet between the bite and the heart to retard venom flow toward the heart. The bite usually is marked by two puncture points. Apply ice packs to the bite. Summon a doctor or carry the patient to the nearest hospital.

Loosen the tourniquet or constriction band for a few seconds every 15 minutes while awaiting help; you should be able to feel a pulse beyond the tourniquet if it is not too tight. Do not let the victim move about. Do not permit him to drink alcoholic beverages. He probably will feel weakness, tremor, and severe pain, but reassure him that he will recover. Medications, usually available only to a physician, should be administered promptly.

Bleeding, internal

Internal bleeding is always a very serious condition; it requires immediate professional medical attention.

In cases of internal bleeding, blood is sometimes brought to the outside of the body by coughing from the lungs, by vomiting from the stomach, by trickling from the ear or nose, or by passing in the urine or bowel movement.

Often, however, internal bleeding is concealed, and the only symptom may be the swelling that appears around the site of broken bones. A person can lose three or four pints of blood inside the body without a trace of blood appearing outside the body.

SOME SYMPTOMS OF INTERNAL BLEEDING: The victim will appear ill and pale. His skin will be colder than normal, especially the hands and feet; often the skin looks clammy because of sweating. The pulse usually will be rapid (over 90 beats a minute) and feeble.

EMERGENCY TREATMENT: Serious internal bleeding is beyond the scope of first aid. If necessary treat the victim for respiratory and cardiac arrest and for shock while waiting for medical aid.

Bleeding, minor

Bleeding from minor cuts, scrapes, and bruises usually stops by itself, but even small injuries of this kind should receive attention to prevent infection.

EMERGENCY TREATMENT: The injured area should be washed thoroughly with soap and water, or if possible, held under running water. The surface should then be covered with a sterile bandage.

The type of wound known as a puncture wound may bleed very little, but is potentially extremely dangerous because of the possibility of tetanus infection. Anyone who steps on a rusty nail or thumbtack or has a similar accident involving a pointed object that penetrates deep under the skin surface should consult a physician about the need for anti-tetanus inoculation or a booster shot.

Blisters

EMERGENCY TREATMENT: If the blister is on a hand or foot or other easily accessible part of the body, wash the area around the blister thoroughly with soap and water. After carefully drying the skin around the blister, apply an antiseptic to the same area. Then sterilize the point and a substantial part of a needle by heating it in an open flame. When the needle has been thoroughly sterilized, use the point to puncture the blister along the margin of the blister. Carefully squeeze the fluid from the blister by pressing it with a sterile gauze dressing; the dressing should soak up most of the fluid. Next, place a fresh sterile dressing over the blister and fasten it in place with a bandage. If a blister forms in a tender area or in a place that is not easily accessible, such as under the arm, do not open it yourself; consult your doctor.

The danger from any break in the skin is that germs or dirt can slip through the natural barrier to produce an infection or inflammation. Continue to apply an antiseptic each day to the puncture area until it has healed. If it appears that an infection has developed or healing is unusually slow, consult a doctor. Persons with diabetes or circulatory problems may have to be more cautious about healing of skin breaks than other individuals.

Blood blisters

Blood blisters, sometimes called hematomas, usually are caused by a sharp blow to the body surface such as hitting a finger with a hammer while pounding nails.

EMERGENCY TREATMENT: Wash the area of the blood blister thoroughly with soap and water. Do not open it. If it is a small blood blister, cover it with a protective bandage; in many cases, the tiny pool of blood under the skin will be absorbed by the surrounding tissues if there is no further pressure at that point.

If the blood blister fails to heal quickly or becomes infected, consult a physician. Because the pool of blood has resulted from damage to a blood vessel, a blood blister usually is more vulnerable to infection or inflammation than an ordinary blister.

Boils

Boils frequently are an early sign of diabetes or another illness and should be watched carefully if they occur often. In general, they result from germs or dirt being rubbed into the skin by tight-fitting clothing, scratching, or through tiny cuts made during shaving.

EMERGENCY TREATMENT: If the boil is above the lip, do not squeeze it or apply any pressure. The infection in that area of the face may drain into the brain because of the pattern of blood circulation on the face. Let a doctor treat any boil on the face. If the boil is on the surface of another part of the body, apply moist hot packs, but do not squeeze or press on the boil because that action can force the infection into the circulatory system. A wet compress can be made by soaking a wash cloth or towel in warm water.

If the boil erupts, carefully wipe away the pus with a sterile dressing, and then cover it with another sterile dressing. If the boil is large or slow to erupt, or if it is slow to heal, consult a doctor.

Bone bruises

EMERGENCY TREATMENT: Make sure the bone is not broken. If the injury is limited to the thin layer of tissue surrounding the bone, and the function of the limb is normal though painful, apply a compression dressing and an ice pack. Limit use of the injured limb for the next day or two.

As the pain and swelling recede, cover the injured area with a foam-rubber pad held in place with an elastic bandage. Because the part of the limb that is likely to receive a bone bruise lacks a layer of muscle and fat, it will be particularly sensitive to any pressure until recovery is complete.

Botulism

The bacteria that produce the lethal toxin of botulism are commonly present on unwashed farm vegetables and thrive in containers that are improperly sealed against the damaging effects of air. Home-canned vegetables, particularly string beans, are a likely source of botulism, but the toxin can be found in fruits, meats, and other foods. It can also appear in food that has been properly prepared but allowed to cool before being served. Examples are cold soups and marinated vegetables.

EMERGENCY TREATMENT: As soon as acute symptoms—nausea, diarrhea, and abdominal distress—appear, try to induce vomiting. Vomiting usually can be started by touching the back of the victim's throat with a finger or the handle of a spoon, which should be smooth and blunt, or by offering him a glass of water in which two tablespoons of salt have been dissolved. Call a doctor; describe all of the symptoms, which also may include, after several hours, double vision, muscular weakness, and difficulty in swallowing and breathing. Save samples of the food suspected of contamination for analysis.

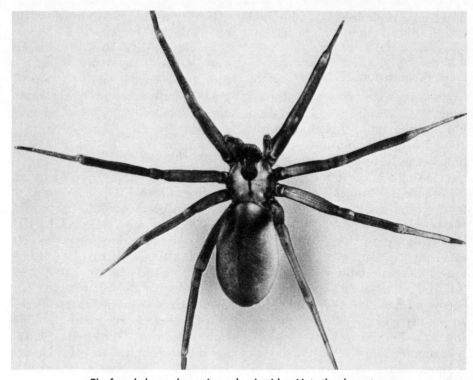

The female brown house (or recluse) spider. Note the characteristic dark fiddle-shapped area on the front half of its back.

Prompt hospitalization and injection of antitoxin are needed to save most cases of botulism poisoning. Additional emergency measures may include artificial respiration if regular breathing fails because of paralysis of respiratory muscles. Continue artificial respiration until professional medical care is provided. If other individuals have eaten the contaminated food, they should receive treatment for botulism even if they show no symptoms of the toxin's effects, since symptoms may be delayed several days.

Brown house (or recluse) spider bites

EMERGENCY TREATMENT: Apply an ice bag or cold pack to the wound area. Aspirin and antihistamines may be offered to help relieve any pain or feeling of irritation. Keep the victim lying down and quiet. Call a doctor as quickly as possible and describe the situation; the doctor will advise what further action should be taken at this point.

The effects of a brown spider bite frequently last much longer than the pain of the bite, which may be comparatively mild for an insect bite or sting. But the poison from the bite can gradually destroy the surrounding tissues, leaving at first an ulcer and eventually a disfiguring scar. A physician's treatment is needed to control the loss of tissue; he probably will prescribe drugs and recommend continued use of cold compresses. The victim, meanwhile, will feel numbness and muscular weakness, requiring a prolonged period of bed rest in addition to the medical treatments.

Bruises/contusions

EMERGENCY TREATMENT: Bruises or contusions result usually from a blow to the body that is powerful enough to damage muscles, tendons, blood vessels, or other tissues without causing a break in the skin.

Because the bruised area will be tender, protect it from further injury. If possible, immobilize the injured body part with a sling, bandage, or other device that makes the victim feel more comfortable; pillows, folded blankets, or similar soft materials can be used to elevate an arm or leg. Apply an ice bag or cold water dressing to the injured area.

A simple bruise usually will heal without extensive treatment. The swelling and discoloration are due to blood oozing from damaged tissues. However, severe bruising can be quite serious and requires medical attention. Keep the victim quiet and watch for symptoms of shock. Give aspirin for pain.

Bullet wounds

Bullet wounds, whether accidental or purposely inflicted, can range from those that are superficial and external to those that involve internal bleeding and extensive tissue damage.

EMERGENCY TREATMENT: A surface bullet wound accompanied by bleeding should be covered promptly with sterile gauze to prevent further infection. The flow of blood should be controlled as described on p. 1067. Don't try to clean the wound with soap or water.

If the wound is internal, keep the patient lying down and wrap him with coats or blankets placed over and under his body. If respiration has ceased or is impaired, give mouth-to-mouth respiration and treat him for shock. Get medical aid promptly.

Burns, thermal

Burns are generally described according to the depth or area of skin damage involved. First-degree burns are the most superficial. They are marked by reddening of the skin and swelling, increased warmth, tenderness and pain. Second-degree burns, deeper than first-degree, are in effect open wounds, characterized by blisters and severe pain in addition to redness. Third-degree burns are deep enough to involve damage to muscles and bones. The skin is charred and there may be no pain because nerve endings have been destroyed. However, the area of the burn generally is more important than the degree of burn; a first or second-degree burn covering a large area of the body is more likely to be fatal than a small third-degree burn.

EMERGENCY TREATMENT: You will want to get professional medical help for treatment of a severe burn, but there are a number of things you can do until such help is obtained. If burns are minor, apply ice or ice water until pain subsides. Then wash the area with soap and water. Cover with a sterile dressing. Give the victim one or two aspirin tablets to help relieve discomfort. A sterile gauze pad soaked in a solution of two tablespoons of baking soda (sodium bicarbonate) per quart of lukewarm water may be applied.

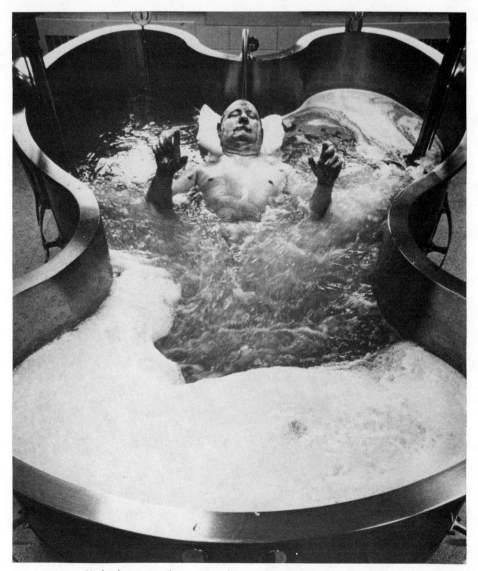

Hydrotherapy—therapy involving the use of water, as in this whirlpool bath—is one of the methods of treating burn patients.

For more extensive or severe burns, there are three first-aid objectives: (1) relieve pain, (2) prevent shock, (3) prevent infection. To relieve pain, exclude air by applying a thick dressing of four to six layers plus additional coverings of clean, tightly-woven material; for extensive burns, use clean sheets or towels. Clothing should be cut away —never pulled—from burned areas; where fabric is stuck to the wound, leave it for a doctor to remove later. Do not apply any ointment, grease, powder, salve, or other medication; the doctor simply will

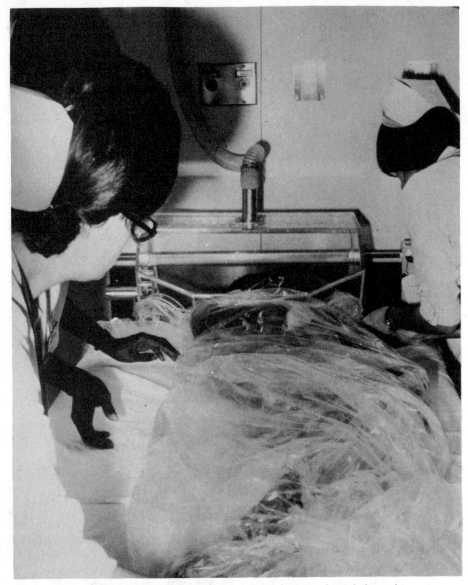

Wrapping the injured parts of a burn victim's body in plastic helps stabi-
lize his internal body temperature and enables him to conserve energy.

have to remove such material before he can begin professional treatment of the burns.

To prevent shock, make sure the victim's head is lower than his feet. Be sure that the victim is covered sufficiently to keep him warm, but not enough to make him overheated; exposure to cold can make the effects of shock more severe. Provide the victim with plenty of nonalcoholic liquids such as sweetened water, tea, or fruit juices, so long as he is conscious and able to swallow.

To prevent infection, do not permit absorbent cotton or adhesive tape to touch the wound caused by a burn. Do not apply iodine or any other antiseptic to the burn. Do not open any blisters. Do not permit any unsterile matter to contact the burn area. If possible, prevent other persons from coughing, sneezing, or even breathing toward the wound resulting from a burn. Serious infections frequently develop in burn victims from contamination by microorganisms of the mouth and nose.

See also CHEMICAL BURNS OF THE EYE.

Carbuncles

Carbuncles are quite similar to boils except that they usually develop around multiple hair follicles and commonly appear on the neck or face. Personal hygiene is one factor involved in the development of carbuncles; persons apparently susceptible to the pustular inflammations must exercise special care in cleansing areas in which carbuncles occur, particularly if they suffer from diabetes or circulatory ailments.

EMERGENCY TREATMENT: Apply moist hot packs to the boil-like swelling. Change the moist hot packs frequently, or place a hot-water bottle on the moist dressing to maintain the moist heat application. Do not handle the carbuncle beyond whatever contact is necessary to apply or maintain the moist heat. The carbuncle should eventually rupture or reach a point where it can be opened with a sterile sharp instrument. After the carbuncle has ruptured and drained, and the fluid from the growth has been carefully cleaned away, apply a sterile dressing.

Frequently, carbuncles, must be opened and drained by a physician.

Cat scratch fever

Although the scratch or bite of a house cat or alley cat may appear at first to be only a mild injury, the wound can become the site of entry for a disease virus transmitted by apparently healthy cats. The inflammation, accompanied by fever, generally affects the lymph nodes and produces some aches and pains as well as fatigue. Although the disease is seldom fatal, an untreated case can spread to brain tissues and lead to other complications.

EMERGENCY TREATMENT: Wash the scratch thoroughly with water and either soap or a mild detergent. Apply a mild antiseptic such as hydrogen peroxide. Cover with a sterile dressing.

Watch the area of the scratch carefully for the next week or two. If redness or swelling develop, even after the scratch appears healed, consult your doctor. The inflammation of the scratch area may be accompanied by mild fever and symptoms similar to those of influenza; in small children, the symptoms may be quite serious. Bed rest and antibiotics usually are prescribed.

Charley horse

A charley horse occurs because a small number of muscle fibers have been torn or ruptured by overstraining the muscle, or by the force of a blow to the muscle.

EMERGENCY TREATMENT: Rest the injured muscle and apply an ice pack if there is swelling. A compression dressing can be applied to support the muscle. Avoid movement that stretches the muscle, and restrict other movements that make the victim uncomfortable. If pain and swelling persist, call a doctor.

During the recovery period, which may not begin for a day or two, apply local heat with a hot water bottle or an electric heating pad, being careful not to burn the victim. A return to active use of the muscle can begin gradually as pain permits.

Chemical burns of the eye

EMERGENCY TREATMENT: Flush the victim's eye immediately with large quantities of fresh, clean water; a drinking fountain can be used to provide a steady stream of water. If a drinking fountain is not available, lay the victim on the floor or ground with his head turned slightly to one side and pour water into the eye from a cup or glass. Always direct the stream of water so that it enters the eye surface at the inside corner and flows across the eye to the outside corner. If the victim is unable, because of intense pain, to open his eyes, it may be necessary to hold the lids apart while water pours across the eye. Continue flushing the eye for at least 15 minutes. (An alternate method is to immerse the victim's face in a pan or basin or bucket of water while he opens and closes his eyes repeatedly; continue the process for at least 15 minutes.)

When the chemical has been flushed from the victim's eye, the eye should be covered with a small, thick compress held in place with a bandage that covers both eyes, if possible; the bandage can be tied around the victim's head. NOTE: Apply nothing but water to the eye; do not attempt to neutralize a chemical burn of the eye and do not apply oil, ointment, salve, or other medications. Rush the victim to a doctor as soon as possible, preferably to an ophthalmologist.

Chemicals on skin

Many household and industrial chemicals, such as ammonia, lye, iodine, creosote, and a wide range of insecticides can cause serious injury if accidentally spilled on the skin.

EMERGENCY TREATMENT: Wash the body surface which has been affected by the chemical with large amounts of water. Do not try to neutralize the chemical with another substance; the reaction may aggravate the injury. If blisters appear, apply a sterile dressing. If the chemical is a refrigerant, such as Freon, or carbon dioxide under pressure, treat for frostbite.

If the chemical has splashed into the eyes or produces serious injury to the affected body surface, call a doctor. The victim should be watched closely for possible poisoning effects if the chemical is a pesticide, since such substances may be absorbed through the skin to produce internal toxic reactions. If there is any question about the toxicity of a chemical, ask your doctor or call the nearest poison control center.

Chigger bites

EMERGENCY TREATMENT: Apply ice water or rub ice over the area afflicted by bites of the tiny red insects. Bathing the area with alcohol, ammonia water or a solution of baking soda also will provide some relief from the itching.

Wash thoroughly with soap, using a scrub brush to prevent further infestation by the chiggers in other areas of the body. Rub alcohol over the surrounding areas and apply sulfur ointment as protection against mites that may not have attached themselves to the skin. Continue applications of ice water or alcohol to skin areas invaded by the insects. Clothing that was worn should be laundered immediately.

Chilblains

EMERGENCY TREATMENT: Move the victim to a moderately warm place and remove wet or tight clothing. Soak the affected body area in warm —but not hot—water for about 10 minutes. Then carefully blot the skin dry, but do not rub the skin. Replace the clothing with garments that are warm, soft, and dry.

Give the victim a stimulant such as tea or coffee, or an alcoholic beverage, and put him to bed with only light blankets; avoid the pressure of heavy blankets or heavy, tight garments on the sensitive skin areas. The victim should move the affected body areas gently to help restore normal circulation. If complications develop, such as marked discoloration of the skin, pain, or blistering and splitting of the skin, call a doctor.

Cold sores/fever blisters

EMERGENCY TREATMENT: Apply a soothing ointment or a medication such as camphor ice. Avoid squeezing or otherwise handling the blisters; moisture can aggravate the sores and hinder their healing. Repeated appearances of cold sores or fever blisters, which are caused by the herpes simplex virus, may require treatment by a physician.

Concussion

See HEAD INJURIES.

Contusions

See BRUISES.

Convulsions

EMERGENCY TREATMENT: Protect the victim from injury by moving him to a safe place; loosen any constricting clothing such as a tie or belt; put a pillow or coat under his head; if his mouth is open, place a folded cloth between his teeth to keep him from biting his tongue. Do not force anything into his mouth. Keep the patient warm but do not disturb him; do not try to restrain his convulsive movements.

Send for a doctor as quickly as possible. Watch the patient's breathing and begin artificial respiration if breathing stops for more than one minute. Be sure that breathing actually has stopped; the patient may be sleeping or unconscious after an attack but breathing normally.

Convulsions in a small child may signal the onset of an infectious disease and may be accompanied by a high fever. The same general precautions should be taken to prevent self-injury on the part of the child. If placed in a bed, the child should be protected against falling onto the floor. Place him on his side—not on his back or stomach—if he vomits. Cold compresses or ice packs on the back of the neck and the head may help relieve symptoms. Immediate professional medical care is vital because brain damage can result if treatment is delayed.

See also EPILEPTIC SEIZURES.

Cramps

See MUSCLE CRAMPS.

Croup

Croup is a breathing disorder usually caused by a virus infection and less often by bacteria or allergy. It is a common condition during childhood, and in some cases, may require brief hospitalization for proper treatment.

The onset of a croup attack is likely to occur during the night with a sudden hoarse or barking cough accompanied by difficulty in breathing. The coughing is usually followed by choking spasms that sound as though the child is strangling. There may also be a mild fever. A doctor should be called immediately when these symptoms appear.

EMERGENCY TREATMENT: The most effective treatment for croup is cool moist air. Cool water vaporizers are available as well as warm steam vaporizers. Another alternative is to take the child into the bathroom, close the door and windows, and let the hot water run from the shower and sink taps until the room is filled with steam.

It is also possible to improvise a croup tent by boiling water in a kettle on a portable hot plate and arranging a blanket over the back of a chair so that it encloses the child and an adult as well as the steaming kettle. A child should never be left alone even for an instant in such a makeshift arrangement.

If the symptoms do not subside in about 20 minutes with any of the above procedures, or if there is mounting fever, and if the doctor is not on his way, the child should be rushed to the closest hospital. Cold moist night air, rather than being a danger, may actually make the symptoms subside temporarily.

Diabetic coma and insulin shock

Diabetics should always carry an identification tag or card to alert others of their condition in the event of a diabetic coma—which is due to a lack of insulin. They also should advise friends or family members of their diabetic condition and the proper emergency measures that can be taken in the event of an onset of diabetic coma. A bottle of rapid-acting insulin should be kept on hand for such an emergency.

EMERGENCY TREATMENT: If the victim is being treated for diabetes, he probably will have nearby a supply of insulin and a hypodermic apparatus for injecting it. Find the insulin, hypodermic syringe, and needle; clean a spot on the upper arm or thigh, and inject about 50 units of insulin. Call a doctor without delay, and describe the patient's symptoms and your treatment. The patient usually will respond without ill effects, but may be quite thirsty. Give him plenty of fluids, as needed.

If the victim does not respond to the insulin, or if you cannot find the insulin and hypodermic syringe, rush the victim to the nearest doctor's office.

Insulin shock—which is due to a reaction to too much insulin and not enough sugar in the blood—can be treated in an emergency by offering a sugar-rich fluid such as a cola beverage or orange juice. Diabetics frequently carry a lump of sugar or candy which can be placed in their mouth in case of an insulin shock reaction. It should be tucked between the teeth and cheek so the victim will not choke on it.

If you find a diabetic in a coma and do not know the cause, assume the cause is an insulin reaction and treat him with sugar. This will give immediate relief to an insulin reaction but will not affect diabetic coma.

Diarrhea

EMERGENCY TREATMENT: Give the victim an antidiarrheal agent; all drugstores carry medications composed of kaolin and pectin that are useful for this purpose. Certain bismuth compounds also are recommended for diarrhea control.

Put the victim in bed for a period of at least 12 hours and withhold food and drink for that length of time. Do not let the victim become dehydrated; if he is thirsty, let him suck on pieces of ice. If the diarrhea appears to be subsiding, let him sip a mild beverage like tea or ginger ale; cola syrup is also recommended.

Later on the patient can try eating bland foods such as dry toast, crackers, gelatin desserts, or jellied consomme. Avoid feeding rich, fatty, or spicy foods. If the diarrhea fails to subside or is complicated by colic or vomiting, call a physician.

Dizziness/vertigo

Emotional upsets, allergies, and improper eating and drinking habits— too much food, too little food, or foods that are too rich—can precipitate symptoms of dizziness. The cause also can be a physical disorder such as abnormal functioning of the inner ear or a circulatory problem. Smoking tobacco, certain drugs such as quinine, and fumes of some chemicals also can produce dizziness.

EMERGENCY TREATMENT: Have the victim lie down with the eyes closed. In many cases, a period of simple bed rest will alleviate the symptoms. Keep the victim quiet and comfortable. If the feeling of dizziness continues, becomes worse, or is accompanied by nausea and vomiting, call a physician.

Severe or persistent dizziness or vertigo requires a longer period of bed rest and the use of medicines prescribed by a doctor. While recovering, the victim should avoid sudden changes in body position or turning the head rapidly. In some types of vertigo, surgery is required to cure the disorder.

Drowning

Victims of drowning seldom die because of water in the lungs or stomach. They die because of lack of air.

EMERGENCY TREATMENT: If the victim's breathing has been impaired, start artificial respiration immediately. If there is evidence of cardiac arrest, administer cardiac massage. When the victim is able to breathe for himself, treat him for shock and get medical help.

Drug overdose (barbiturates)

Barbiturates are used in a number of drugs prescribed as sedatives, although many are also available through illegal channels. Because the drugs can affect the judgment of the user, he may not remember having taken a dose and so may take additional pills, thus producing overdose effects.

EMERGENCY TREATMENT: If the drug was taken orally, try to induce vomiting in the victim. Have him drink a glass of water containing two tablespoons of salt. Or touch the back of his throat gently with a finger or a smooth blunt object like the handle of a spoon. Then give the victim plenty of warm water to drink. It is important to rid the stomach of as much of the drug as possible and to dilute the substance remaining in the gastrointestinal tract.

As soon as possible, call a doctor or get the victim to the nearest hospital or doctor's office. If breathing fails, administer artificial respiration.

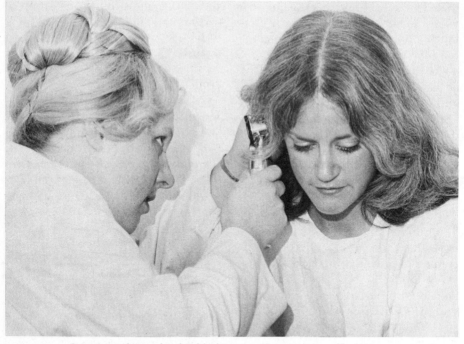

Symptoms of earache should always receive prompt medical attention. An ear infection can spread to the mastoid bone or to the brain.

Drug overdose (stimulants)

Although most of the powerful stimulant drugs, or pep pills, are available only through a doctor's prescription, the same medications are available through illicit sources. When taken without direction of a supervising physician, the stimulants can produce a variety of adverse side effects, and when used frequently over a period of time can result in physical and psychological problems that require hospital treatment.

EMERGENCY TREATMENT: Give the victim a solution of one tablespoon of activated charcoal mixed with a small amount of water, or give him a glass of milk, to dilute the effects of the medication in the stomach. Then induce vomiting by pressing gently on the back of the throat with a finger or the smooth blunt edge of a spoon handle. Vomiting also may be induced with a solution made of one teaspoonful of mustard in a half glass of water. Do not give syrup of ipecac to a victim who has been taking stimulants.

As soon as possible call a doctor or get the victim to the nearest hospital or doctor's office. If breathing fails, administer artificial respiration.

Earaches

An earache may be associated with a wide variety of ailments ranging from the common cold or influenza to impacted molars or tonsillitis. An earache also may be involved in certain infectious diseases such as measles or scarlet fever. Because of the relationship of ear structures to other parts of the head and throat, an infection involving the symptoms of earache can easily spread to the brain tissues or the spongy mastoid bone behind the ear. Call a doctor and describe all of the symptoms, including temperature, any discharge, pain, ringing in the ear, or deafness. Delay in reporting an earache to a doctor can result in complications that require hospital treatment.

EMERGENCY TREATMENT: This may include a few drops of warm olive oil or sweet oil held in the ear by a small wad of cotton. Aspirin can be given to help relieve any pain. Professional medical treatment may include the use of antibiotics.

Ear, foreign body in

EMERGENCY TREATMENT: Do not insert a hairpin, stick, or other object in the ear in an effort to remove a foreign object; you are likely to force the object farther into the ear canal. Instead, have the victim tilt his head to one side, with the ear containing the foreign object facing upward. While pulling gently on the lobe of the ear to straighten the canal, pour a little warmed olive oil or mineral oil into the ear. Then have the victim tilt that ear downward so the oil will run out quickly; it should dislodge the foreign object.

Wipe the ear canal gently with a cotton-tipped matchstick, or a similar device that will not irritate the lining of the ear canal, after the foreign body has been removed. If the emergency treatment is not successful, call a doctor.

Electric shocks

An electric shock from the usual 110-volt current in most homes can be a serious emergency, especially if the person's skin or clothing is wet. Under these circumstances, the shock may paralyze the part of the brain that controls breathing and stop the heart completely or disorder its pumping action.

EMERGENCY TREATMENT: It is of the utmost importance to break the electrical contact *immediately* by unplugging the wire of the appliance involved or by shutting off the house current switch. *Do not touch the victim of the shock while he is still acting as an electrical conductor.*

If the shock has come from a faulty wire out of doors and the source of the electrical current can't be reached easily, make a lasso of dry rope on a long sturdy dry stick. Catch the victim's hand or foot in the loop and drag him away from the wire. Another way to break the contact is to cut the wire with a dry axe.

If the victim of the shock is unconscious, or if his pulse is very weak, administer mouth-to-mouth respiration and cardiac massage until he can get to a hospital.

Epileptic seizures

Epilepsy is a disorder of the nervous system that produces convulsive seizures. In a major seizure or *grand mal,* the epileptic usually falls to the ground. Indeed, falling is in most cases one of the principal dangers of the disease. Then the epileptic's body begins to twitch or jerk spasmodically. His breathing may be labored, and saliva may appear on his lips. His face may become pale or bluish. Although the scene can be frightening, it is not truly a medical emergency; the afflicted person is in no danger of losing his life.

EMERGENCY TREATMENT: Make the person suffering the seizure as comfortable as possible. If he is on a hard surface, put something soft under his head, and move any hard or dangerous objects away from him. *Make no attempt to restrain his movements, and do not force anything into his mouth.* Just leave him alone until the attack is over, as it should be in a few minutes. If his mouth is already open, you might put something soft, such as a folded handerchief, between his side teeth. This will help to prevent him from biting his tongue or lips. If he seems to go into another seizure after coming out of the first, or if the seizure lasts more than ten minutes, call a doctor. If his lower jaw sags and begins to obstruct his breathing, support of the lower jaw may be helpful in improving his breathing.

When the seizure is over, the patient should be allowed to rest quietly. Some people sleep heavily after a seizure. Others awake at once but are disoriented or confused for a while. Treat the episode in a matter-of-fact way. If it is the first seizure the person is aware of having had, advise him to see his physician promptly.

Eye, foreign body in

EMERGENCY TREATMENT: Do not rub the eye or touch it with unwashed hands. The foreign body usually becomes lodged on the inner surface of the upper eyelid. Pull the upper eyelid down over the lower lid to help work the object loose. Tears or clean water can help wash out the dirt or other object. If the bit of irritating material can be seen on the surface of the eyeball, try very carefully to flick it out with the tip of a clean, moistened handkerchief or a piece of moistened cotton. Never touch the surface of the eye with dry materials. Sometimes a foreign body can be removed by carefully rolling the upper lid over a pencil or wooden matchstick to expose the object.

After the foreign object has been removed, the eye should be washed with clean water or with a solution made from one teaspoon of salt dissolved in a pint of water. This will help remove any remaining particles of the foreign body as well as any traces of irritating chemicals that might have been a part of it. Iron particles, for example, may leave traces of rust on the eye's surface unless washed away.

If the object cannot be located and removed without difficulty, a small patch of gauze or a folded handkerchief should be taped over the eye and the victim taken to a doctor's office—preferably the office of an ophthalmologist. A doctor also should be consulted if a feeling of irritation in the eye continues after the foreign body has been removed.

Fever

EMERGENCY TREATMENT: If the fever is mild, around 100° F. by mouth, have the victim rest in bed and provide him with a light diet. Watch closely for other symptoms, such as a rash, and any further increase in body temperature. Aspirin usually can be given.

If the temperature rises to 101° or higher, is accompanied by pain, headache, delirium, confused behavior, coughing, vomiting, or other indications of a severe illness, call a doctor. Describe all of the symptoms in detail, including the appearance of any rash and when it began.

Fever blisters

See COLD SORES.

Finger dislocation

EMERGENCY TREATMENT: Call a doctor and arrange for inspection and treatment of the injury. If a doctor is not immediately available, the finger dislocation may be reduced (put back in proper alignment) by grasping it firmly and carefully pulling it into normal position. Pull very slowly and avoid rough handling that might complicate the injury by damaging a tendon. If the dislocation cannot be reduced after the first try, go through the procedure once more. But do not try it more than twice.

Whether or not you are successful in reducing the finger dislocation, the finger should be immobilized after your efforts until a doctor can examine it. A clean flat wooden stick can be strapped along the palm side of the finger with adhesive tape or strips of bandage to hold it in place.

Fingernail injuries/hangnails

EMERGENCY TREATMENT: Wash the injured nail area thoroughly with warm water and soap. Trim off any torn bits of nail. Cover with a small adhesive dressing or bandage.

Apply petroleum jelly or cold cream to the injured nail area twice a day, morning and night, until it is healed. If redness or irritation develops in the adjoining skin area, indicating an infection, consult your doctor.

Fish poisoning

EMERGENCY TREATMENT: Induce vomiting in the victim to remove the bits of poisonous fish from the stomach. Vomiting usually can be started by pressing on the back of the throat with a finger or a spoon handle that is blunt and smooth, or by having the victim drink a solution of two tablespoons of salt in a glass of water.

Call a doctor as soon as possible. Describe the type of fish eaten and the symptoms, which may include nausea, diarrhea, abdominal pain, muscular weakness, and a numbness or tingling sensation that begins about the face and spreads to the extremities.

If breathing fails, administer mouth-to-mouth artificial respiration; a substance commonly found in poisonous fish causes respiratory failure. Also, be prepared to provide emergency treatment for convulsions.

Food poisoning

EMERGENCY TREATMENT: If the victim is not already vomiting, try to induce it to clear the stomach. Vomiting can be started in most cases by pressing gently on the back of the throat with a finger or a blunt smooth spoon handle, or by having the patient drink a glass of water containing two tablespoons of salt. If the victim has vomited, put him to bed.

Call a doctor and describe the food ingested and the symptoms which developed. If symptoms are severe, professional medical treatment with antibiotics and medications for cramps may be required. Special medications also may be needed for diarrhea caused by bacterial food poisoning.

Fractures

Any break in a bone is called a fracture. The break is called an *open* or *compound fracture* if one or both ends of the broken bone pierce the skin. A *closed* or *simple fracture* is one in which the broken bone doesn't come through the skin.

It is sometimes difficult to distinguish a strained muscle or a sprained ligament from a broken bone, since sprains and strains can be extremely painful even though they are less serious than breaks. However, when there is any doubt, the injury should be treated as though it were a simple fracture.

EMERGENCY TREATMENT: Don't try to help the injured person move around or get up unless he has slowly tested out the injured part of his body and is sure that nothing has been broken. If he is in extreme pain, or if the injured part has begun to swell, or if by running the finger lightly along the affected bone a break can be felt, *do not* move him. Under no circumstances should he be crowded into a car if his legs, hip, ribs, or back are involved in the accident. Call for an ambulance immediately, and until it arrives, treat the person for shock.

SPLINTING: In a situation where it is imperative to move someone who may have a fracture, the first step is to apply a splint so that the broken bone ends are immobilized.

Splints can be improvised from anything rigid enough and of the right length to support the fractured part of the body: a metal rod, board, long cardboard tube, tightly rolled newspaper or blanket. If the object being used has to be padded for softness, use a small blanket or any other soft material, such as a jacket.

The splint should be long enough so that it can be tied with a bandage, torn sheet, or neckties beyond the joint above and below the fracture as well as at the site of the break. If a leg is involved, it should be elevated with pillows or any other firm support after the splint has been applied. If the victim has to wait a considerable length of time before receiving professional attention, the splint bandaging should be checked from time to time to make sure it isn't too tight.

In the case of an open or compound fracture, additional steps must be taken. Remove that part of the victim's clothing which is covering the wound. Do not wash or probe into the wound, but control bleeding by applying pressure over the wound through a sterile or clean dressing.

Frostbite

EMERGENCY TREATMENT: Begin rapid rewarming of the affected tissues as soon as possible. If possible, immerse the victim in a warm bath, but avoid scalding. (The temperature should be between 102° and 105° F.) Warm wet towels also will help if changed frequently and applied gently. Do not massage, rub, or even touch the frostbitten flesh. If warm water or a warming fire is not available, place the patient in a sleeping bag or cover him with coats and blankets. Hot liquids can be offered if available to help raise the body temperature.

For any true frostbite case, prompt medical attention is important. The depth and degree of the frozen tissue cannot be determined without a careful examination by a physician.

Gall bladder attacks

Although gallstones can affect a wide variety of individuals, the most common victims are overweight persons who enjoy rich foods. The actual attack of spasms caused by gallstones passing through the duct leading from the gall bladder to the digestive tract usually is preceded by periods of stomach distress including belching. X rays usually will reveal the presence of gallstones when the early warning signs are noted, and measures can be taken to reduce the threat of a gall-bladder attack.

EMERGENCY TREATMENT: Call a doctor and describe in detail the symptoms, which may include colic high in the abdomen and pain extending to the right shoulder; the pain may be accompanied by nausea, vomiting, and sweating. Hot water bottles may be applied to the abdomen to help relieve distress while waiting for professional medical care. If the doctor permits, the victim may be allowed to sip certain fluids such as fruit juices, but do not offer him solid food.

Gas poisoning

Before attempting to revive someone overcome by toxic gas poisoning, the most important thing to do is to remove him to the fresh air. If this isn't feasible, all windows and doors should be opened to let in as much fresh air as possible.

Any interior with a dangerous concentration of carbon monoxide or other toxic gases is apt to be highly explosive. Therefore, gas and electricity should be shut off as quickly as possible. *Under no circumstances should any matches be lighted in an interior where there are noxious fumes.*

The rescuer needn't waste time covering his face with a handkerchief or other cloth. He should hold his breath instead, or take only a few quick, shallow breaths while bringing the victim to the out-of-doors or to an open window.

EMERGENCY TREATMENT: Administer artificial respiration if the victim is suffering respiratory arrest. Arrange for medical help as soon as possible, requesting that oxygen be brought to the scene.

Head injuries

Accidents involving the head can result in concussion, skull fracture, or brain injury. Symptoms of head injury include loss of consciousness, discharge of a watery or blood-tinged fluid from the ears, nose, or mouth, and a difference in size of the pupils of the eyes. Head injuries must be thought of as serious; they demand immediate medical assistance.

EMERGENCY TREATMENT: Place the victim in a supine position, and, if there is no evidence of injury to his neck, arrange for a slight elevation of his head *and* shoulders. Make certain that he has a clear airway and administer artificial respiration if necessary. If vomitus, blood, or other fluids appear to flow from the victim's mouth, turn his head gently to one side. Control bleeding and treat for shock. Do not administer stimulants or fluids of any kind.

Heart attack

A heart attack is caused by interference with the blood supply to the heart muscle. When the attack is brought on because of a blood clot in the coronary artery, it is known as *coronary occlusion* or *coronary thrombosis*.

The most dramatic symptom of a serious heart attack is a crushing chest pain that usually travels down the left arm into the hand or into the neck and back. The pain may bring on dizziness, cold sweat, complete

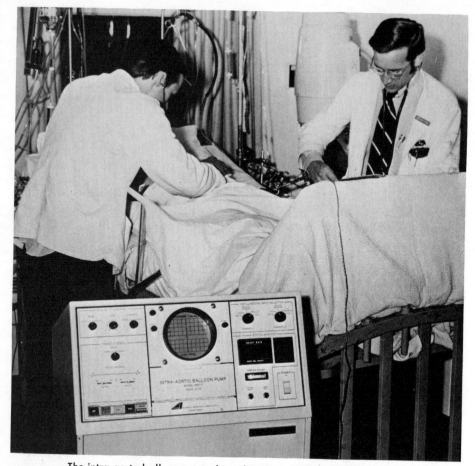

The intra-aorta balloon pump shown here is a device used to take over the major pumping action of the heart following an acute heart attack.

collapse, and loss of consciousness. The face has an ashen pallor, and there may be vomiting.

EMERGENCY TREATMENT: The victim *must not be moved* unless he has fallen in a dangerous place. If no doctor is immediately available, an ambulance should be called at once. No attempt should be made to get the victim of a heart attack into an automobile.

Until help arrives, give the victim every reassurance that he will get prompt treatment, and keep him as calm and quiet as possible. Don't give him any medicine or stimulants.

If oxygen is available, start administering it to the victim immediately, either by mask or nasal catheter, depending on which is available.

If the victim is suffering from respiratory arrest, begin artificial respiration. If he is suffering from cardiac arrest, begin cardiac massage.

Heat exhaustion

Heat exhaustion occurs when the body is exposed to high temperatures and large amounts of blood accumulate in the skin as a way of cooling it. As a result, there is a marked decrease in the amount of blood that circulates through the heart and to the brain. The victim becomes markedly pale and is covered with cold perspiration. Breathing is increasingly shallow and the pulse weakens. In acute cases, fainting occurs. Medical aid should be summoned for anyone suffering from heat exhaustion.

EMERGENCY TREATMENT: Place the victim in a reclining position with his feet raised about 10 inches above his body. Loosen or remove his clothing, and apply cold, wet cloths to his wrists and forehead. If he has fainted and doesn't recover promptly, smelling salts or spirits of ammonia should be placed under his nose. When the victim is conscious, give him sips of salt water (approximately one teaspoon of salt per glass of water), the total intake to be about two glasses in an hour's time. If the victim vomits, discontinue the salt solution.

Heatstroke/sunstroke

Heatstroke is characterized by an acutely high body temperature caused by the cessation of perspiration. The victim's skin becomes hot, dry, and flushed, and he may suffer collapse. Should the skin turn ashen gray, a physician must be called immediately. Prompt hospital treatment is recommended for anyone showing signs of sunstroke who has previously had any kind of heart damage.

EMERGENCY TREATMENT: The following measures are designed to reduce the victim's body temperature as quickly as possible and prevent damage to the internal organs:

Place him in a tub of very cold water, or, if this is not possible, spray or sponge his body repeatedly with cold water or rubbing alcohol. Take his temperature by mouth, and when it has dropped to about 100° F., remove him to a bed and wrap him in cold, wet sheets. If possible, expose him to an electric fan or an air conditioner.

Hiccups

EMERGENCY TREATMENT: Have the victim slowly drink a large glass of water. If cold water is not effective, have him drink warm water containing a teaspoonful of baking soda. Milk also can be employed. For babies and small children, offer sips of warm water. Do not offer carbonated beverages.

Another helpful measure is breathing into a large paper bag a number of times to raise the carbon dioxide level in the lungs. Rest and relaxation are recommended; have the victim lie down to read or watch television.

If the hiccups fail to go away, and continued spastic contractions of the diaphragm interfere with eating and sleeping, call your doctor.

Insect stings

Honeybees, wasps, hornets, and yellow jackets are the most common stinging insects and are most likely to attack on a hot summer day. Strongly scented perfumes or cosmetics and brightly colored, rough-finished clothing attract bees and should be avoided by persons working or playing in garden areas. It should also be noted that many commercial repellents do not protect against stinging insects.

EMERGENCY TREATMENT: If one is stung, the insect's stinger should be scraped gently but quickly from the skin; don't squeeze it. Apply Epsom

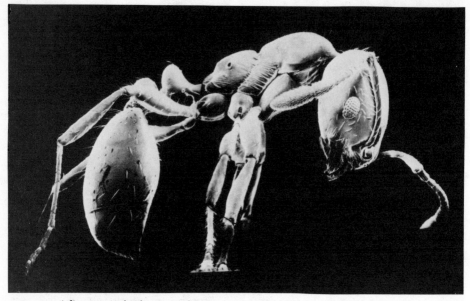

A fire ant. Multiple stings of venemous insects are serious and require medical attention. For allergic individuals a single sting can be dangerous.

salt solution to the sting area. Antihistamines are often helpful in reducing the patient's discomfort. If a severe reaction develops, call a doctor.

There are a few people who are critically allergic to the sting of wasps, bees, yellow jackets, or fire ants. This sensitivity causes the vocal cord tissue to swell to the point where breathing may become impossible. A single sting to a sensitive person may result in a dangerous drop in blood pressure, thus producing shock. Anyone with such a severe allergy who is stung should be rushed to a hospital immediately.

A person who becomes aware of having this type of allergy should consult with a physician about the kind of medicine to carry for use in a crisis.

Insulin shock

See DIABETIC COMA AND INSULIN SHOCK.

Jaw dislocation

The jaw can be dislocated during a physical attack or fight; from a blow on the jaw during sports activities; or from overextension of the joint during yawning, laughing, or attempting to eat a large mouthful of food. The jaw becomes literally locked open so the victim cannot explain his predicament.

EMERGENCY TREATMENT: Reducing a dislocated jaw will require that you insert your thumbs between the teeth of the victim. The jaw can be expected to snap into place quickly, and there is a danger that the teeth will clamp down on the thumbs when this happens, so the thumbs should be adequately padded with handkerchiefs or bandages. Once the thumbs are protected, insert them in the mouth and over the lower molars, as far back on the lower jaw as possible. While pressing down with the thumbs, lift the chin with the fingers outside the mouth. As the jaw begins to slip into normal position when it is pushed downward and backward with the chin lifted upward, quickly remove the thumbs from between the jaws.

Once the jaw is back in normal position, the mouth should remain closed for several hours while the ligaments recover from their displaced condition. If necessary, put a cravat bandage over the head to hold the mouth closed. If difficulty is experienced in reducing a jaw dislocation, the victim should be taken to a hospital where an anesthetic can be applied. A dislocated jaw can be extremely painful.

Jellyfish stings

EMERGENCY TREATMENT: Wash the area of the sting thoroughly with alcohol or fresh water. Be sure that any pieces of jellyfish tentacles have been removed from the skin. Aspirin or antihistamines can be administered to relieve pain and itching, but curtail the use of antihistamines if the victim has consumed alcoholic beverages. The leg or arm that received the sting can be soaked in hot water if the pain continues. Otherwise, apply calamine lotion.

If the victim appears to suffer a severe reaction from the sting, summon a doctor. The victim may experience shock, muscle cramps, convulsions, or loss of consciousness. Artificial respiration may be required while awaiting arrival of a doctor. The physician can administer drugs to relieve muscle cramps and provide sedatives or analgesics.

Kidney stones

EMERGENCY TREATMENT: Call a doctor if the victim experiences the agonizing cramps or colic associated with kidney stones. Discuss the symptoms in detail with the doctor to make sure the pain is caused by kidney stones rather than appendicitis.

Comforting heat may be applied to the back and the abdomen of the side affected by the spasms. Paregoric can be administered, if available, while waiting for medical care; about two teaspoonsful of paregoric in a half glass of water may help relieve symptoms.

Knee injuries

EMERGENCY TREATMENT: If the injury appears to be severe, including possible fracture of the kneecap, immobilize the knee. To immobilize the knee, place the injured leg on a board that is about four inches wide and three to four feet in length. Place padding between the board and the knee, and between the board and the back of the ankle. Then use four strips of bandage to fasten the leg to the padded board—one at the ankle, one at the thigh, and one each above and below the knee.

Summon a doctor or move the patient to a doctor's office. Keep the knee protected against cold or exposure to the elements, but otherwise do not apply a bandage or any type of pressure to the knee itself; any rapid swelling would be aggravated by unnecessary pressure in that area. Be prepared to treat the patient for shock.

Laryngitis

Laryngitis is associated with colds and influenza and may be accompanied by a fever. The ailment can be aggravated by smoking, and it is possible that the vocal cords can be damaged if the victim tries to force the use of his voice while the larynx is swollen by the infection.

EMERGENCY TREATMENT: Have the victim inhale the warm moist air of a steam kettle or vaporizer. A vaporizer can be improvised in an emergency by pouring boiling water into a bowl and forming a "tent" over the steaming bowl with a large towel or sheet, or by placing a large paper bag over the bowl and cutting an opening at the closed end of the bag so the face can be exposed to the steam. The hot water can contain a bit of camphor or menthol, if available, to make the warm moist air more soothing to the throat, but this is not necessary.

Continue the use of the vaporizer for several days, as needed. The victim should not use the vocal cords any more than absolutely necessary. If the infection does not subside within the first few days, a doctor should be consulted.

Leeches

EMERGENCY TREATMENT: Do not try to pull leeches off the skin. They will usually drop away from the skin if a heated object such as a lighted cigarette is held close to them. Leeches also are likely to let go if iodine is applied to their bodies. The wound caused by a leech should be washed carefully with soap and water and an antiseptic applied.

Lightning shock

EMERGENCY TREATMENT: If the victim is not breathing, apply artificial respiration. If a second person is available to help, have him summon a doctor while artificial respiration is administered. Continue artificial respiration until breathing resumes or the doctor arrives.

When the victim is breathing regularly, treat him for shock. Keep him lying down with his feet higher than his head, his clothing loosened around the neck, and his body covered with a blanket or coat for warmth. If the victim shows signs of vomiting, turn his head to one side so he will not swallow the vomitus.

If the victim is breathing regularly and does not show signs of shock, he may be given a few sips of a stimulating beverage such as coffee, tea, or brandy.

Motion sickness

EMERGENCY TREATMENT: Have the victim lie down in a position that is most comfortable to him. The head should be fixed so that any view of motion is avoided. Reading or other use of the eyes should be prohibited. Food or fluids should be restricted to very small amounts. If traveling by car, stop at a rest area; in an airplane or ship, place the victim in an area where motion is least noticeable.

Drugs, such as Dramamine, are helpful for control of the symptoms of motion sickness; they are most effective when started about 90 minutes before travel begins and repeated at regular intervals thereafter.

Muscle cramps

EMERGENCY TREATMENT: Gently massage the affected muscle, sometimes stretching it to help relieve the painful contraction. Then relax the muscle by using a hot water bottle or an electric heating pad, or by soaking the affected area in a warm bath.

A repetition of cramps may require medical attention.

Nosebleeds

EMERGENCY TREATMENT: Have the victim sit erect but with the head tilted slightly forward to prevent blood from running down the throat. Apply pressure by pinching the nostrils; if bleeding is from just one nostril, use pressure on that side. A small wedge of absorbent cotton or gauze can be inserted into the bleeding nostril. Make sure that the cotton or gauze extends out of the nostril to aid in its removal when the bleeding has stopped. Encourage the victim to breathe through the mouth while the nose is bleeding. After five minutes, release pressure on the nose to see if the bleeding has stopped. If the bleeding continues, repeat pressure on the nostril for an additional five minutes. Cold compresses applied to the nose can help stop the bleeding.

If bleeding continues after the second five-minute period of pressure treatment, get the victim to a doctor's office or a hospital emergency room.

Poison ivy/poison oak/poison sumac

EMERGENCY TREATMENT: The poison of these three plants is the same and the treatment is identical. Bathe the skin area exposed to poison ivy, poison oak, or poison sumac with soap and water or with alcohol within 15 minutes after contact. If exposure is not discovered until a rash appears, apply cool wet dressings. Dressings can be made of old bed sheets or soft linens soaked in a solution of one teaspoon of salt per pint of water. Dressings should be applied four times a day for periods of 15 to 60 minutes each time; during these periods, dressings can be removed and reapplied every few minutes. The itching that often accompanies the rash can be relieved by taking antihistamine tablets.

Creams or lotions may be prescribed by a doctor or supplied by a pharmacist. Do not use such folk remedies as ammonia or turpentine; do not use skin lotions not approved by a doctor or druggist. Haphazard application of medications on poison ivy blisters and rashes can result in complications including skin irritation, infection, or pigmented lesions of the skin.

Rabies

See ANIMAL BITES.

Sciatica/lower back pain

Although lower back pain is frequently triggered by fatigue, anxiety, or by strained muscles or tendons, it may be a symptom of a slipped or ruptured disk between the vertebrae, or of a similar disorder requiring extensive medical attention.

EMERGENCY TREATMENT: Reduce the pressure on the lower back by having the victim lie down on a hard flat surface; if a bed is used there should be a board or sheet of plywood between the springs and mattress. Pillows should be placed under the knees instead of under the head, to help keep the back flat. Give aspirin to relieve the pain, and apply heat to the back. Call a doctor if the symptoms do not subside overnight.

Scorpion stings

EMERGENCY TREATMENT: Apply ice to the region of the sting, except in the case of an arm or leg, in which event the limb may be immersed in ice water. Continue the ice or ice-water treatment for at least one hour. Try to keep the area of the sting at a position lower than the heart. No tourniquet is required. Should the

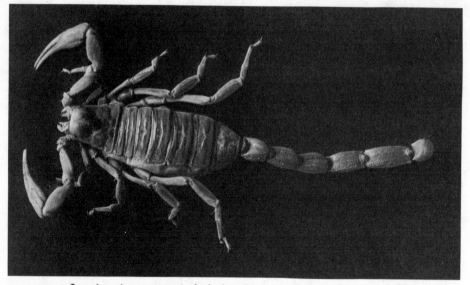

Scorpion stings are particularly dangerous for children under six, who may experience convulsions that require prompt medical treatment.

breathing of a scorpion sting victim becomes depressed, administer artificial respiration. If symptoms fail to subside within a couple of hours, notify a physician, or transfer the victim to a doctor's office or hospital.

For children under six, call a physician in the event of any scorpion sting. Children stung by scorpions may become convulsive, and this condition can result in fatal exhaustion unless it receives prompt medical treatment.

Snakebites

Of the many varieties of snakes found in the United States, only four kinds are poisonous: copperheads, rattlesnakes, moccasins, and coral snakes. The first three belong to the category of pit vipers and are known as *hemotoxic* because their poison enters the bloodstream. The coral snake, which is comparatively rare, is related to the cobra and is the most dangerous of all because its venom is *neurotoxic*. This means that the poison transmitted by its bite goes directly to the nervous system and the brain.

HOW TO DIFFERENTIATE BETWEEN SNAKEBITES: Snakes of the pit viper family have a fang on each side of the head. These fangs leave characteristic puncture wounds on the skin in addition to two rows of tiny bites or scratches left by the teeth. A bite from a nonpoisonous snake leaves six rows—four upper and two lower—of very small bite marks or scratches and no puncture wounds.

The marks left by the bite of a coral snake do not leave any puncture wounds either, but this snake bites with a chewing motion, hanging on to the victim rather than attacking quickly. The coral snake is very easy to recognize because of its distinctive markings: wide horizontal bands of red and black separated by narrow bands of yellow.

SYMPTOMS: A bite from any of the pit vipers produces immediate and severe pain and darkening of the skin, followed by weakness, blurred vision, quickened pulse, nausea, and vomiting. The bite of a coral snake produces somewhat the same symptoms, although there is less local pain and considerable drowsiness leading to unconsciousness.

If a doctor or a hospital is a short distance away, the patient should receive professional help *immediately*. He should be transported lying down, either on an improvised stretcher or carried by his companions—with the wounded part lower than his heart. He should be advised to move as little as possible.

EMERGENCY TREATMENT: If several hours must elapse before a doctor or a hospital can be reached, the following procedures should be applied promptly:

1. Keep the victim lying down and as still as possible.

2. Tie a constricting band *above* the wound between it and the heart and tight enough to slow but not stop blood circulation. A handkerchief, necktie, sock, or piece of torn shirt will serve.

3. If a snakebite kit is available, use the knife it contains; otherwise, sterilize a knife or razor blade in a flame. Carefully make small cuts in the skin where the swelling has developed. Make the cuts along the length of the limb, not across or at right angles to it. The incisions should be shallow because of the danger of severing nerves, blood vessels, or muscles.

4. Use the suction cups in the snakebite kit, if available, to draw out as much of the venom as possible. If suction cups are not available, the venom can be removed by sucking it out with the mouth. Although snake venom is not a stomach poison,

it should not be swallowed but should be rinsed from the mouth.

5. This procedure should be continued for from 30 to 60 minutes or until the swelling subsides and the other symptoms decrease.

6. You may apply cold compresses to the bite area while waiting for professional assistance.

7. Treat the victim for shock.

8. Give artificial respiration if necessary.

Splinters

EMERGENCY TREATMENT: Clean the area about the splinter with soap and water or an antiseptic. Next, sterilize a needle by holding it over an open flame. After it cools, insert the needle above the splinter so it will tear a line in the skin, making the splinter lie loose in the wound. Then, gently lift the splinter out, using a pair of tweezers or the point of the needle. If tweezers are used, they should be sterilized first.

Wash the wound area again with soap and water, or apply an antiseptic. It is best to cover the wound with an adhesive bandage. If redness or irritation develops around the splinter wound, consult a doctor.

Sprains

A sprain occurs when a joint is wrenched or twisted in such a way that the ligaments holding it in position are ruptured, possibly damaging the surrounding blood vessels, tendons, nerves, and muscles. This type of injury is more serious than a strain and is usually accompanied by pain, sometimes severe, soreness, swelling, and discoloration of the affected area. Most sprains occur as a result of falls, athletic accidents, or improper handling of heavy weights.

EMERGENCY TREATMENT: This consists of prompt rest, the application of cold compresses to relieve swelling and any internal bleeding in the joint, and elevation of the affected area. Aspirin is recommended to reduce discomfort. If the swelling and soreness increase after such treatment, a physician should be consulted to make sure that the injury is not a fracture or a bone dislocation.

Sting ray

EMERGENCY TREATMENT: If an arm or leg is the target of a sting ray, wash the area thoroughly with salt water. Quickly remove any pieces of the stinger imbedded in the skin or flesh; poison can still be discharged into the victim from the sting-ray sheath. After initial cleansing of an arm or leg sting, soak the wound with hot water for up to an hour. Apply antiseptic or a sterile dressing after the soak.

Consult a physician after a sting-ray attack. The doctor will make a

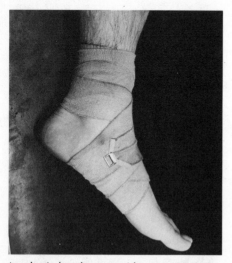

An elastic bandage provides temporary support for healing tendons or ligaments following a strain or sprain.

thorough examination of the wound to determine whether stitches or antibiotics are required. Fever, vomiting, or muscular twitching also may result from an apparently simple leg or arm wound by a sting ray.

If the sting occurs in the chest or abdomen, the victim should be rushed to a hospital as soon as possible because such a wound can produce convulsions or loss of consciousness.

Strains

When a muscle is stretched because of misuse or overuse, the interior bundles of tissue may tear, or the tendon which connects it to the bone may be stretched. This condition is known as strain. It occurs most commonly to the muscles of the lower back when heavy weights are improperly lifted, or in the area of the calf or ankle as the result of a sudden, violent twist or undue pressure.

EMERGENCY TREATMENT: Bed rest, the application of heat, and gentle massage are recommended for back strain. If the strain is in the leg, elevate the limb to help reduce pain and swelling, and apply cold compresses or an ice bag to the area. Aspirin may be taken to reduce discomfort.

In severe cases of strained back muscles, a physician may have to be consulted for strapping. For a strained ankle, a flexible elastic bandage can be helpful in providing the necessary support until the injured muscle heals.

Stroke

Stroke, or apoplexy, is caused by a disruption of normal blood flow to the brain, either by rupture of a blood vessel within the brain or by blockage of an artery supplying the brain. The condition is enhanced by hardening of the arteries and high blood pressure, and is most likely to occur in older persons. A stroke usually occurs with little or no warning and the onset may be marked by a variety of manifestations ranging from headache, slurred speech, or blurred vision, to sudden collapse and unconsciousness.

EMERGENCY TREATMENT: Try to place the victim in a semi-reclining position, or, if he is lying down, be sure there is a pillow under his head. Avoid conditions that might increase the flow of blood toward the head. Summon a doctor immediately. Loosen any clothing that may be tight. If the patient wears dentures, remove them.

Before professional medical assistance is available, the victim may vomit or go into shock or convulsions. If he vomits, try to prevent a backflow of vomitus into the breathing passages. If shock occurs, do not place the victim in the shock position but do keep him warm and comfortable. If convulsions develop, place a handkerchief or similar soft object between the jaws to prevent tongue biting.

Sty on eyelid

Sties usually develop around hair follicles because of a bacterial infection. Like cold sores, they are most likely to develop in association with poor health and lowered resistance to infection.

EMERGENCY TREATMENT: Apply warm, moist packs or compresses to the sty for periods of 15 to 20 minutes at intervals of three or four hours. Moist heat generally is more penetrating than dry heat.

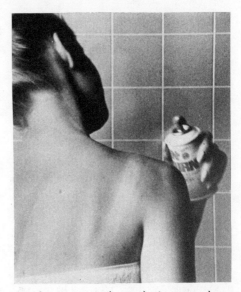

Avoid using topical anesthetics on sunburnt skin. They may cause allergic reactions. Use a soothing lotion such as baby oil.

The sty should eventually rupture and the pus should then be washed carefully away from the eye area. If the sty does not rupture or is very painful, consult a doctor. Do not squeeze or otherwise handle the sty except to apply the warm moist compresses.

Sunburn

EMERGENCY TREATMENT: Apply cold wet compresses to help relieve the pain. Compresses can be soaked in whole milk, salt water, or a solution of corn starch mixed with water. The victim also may get some relief by soaking in a bathtub filled with plain water. Soothing lotions, such as baby oil or a bland cold cream, can be applied after carefully drying the skin. Don't rub the burn area while drying. Avoid the use of "shake" lotions, like calamine, which may aggravate the burn by a drying action. The victim should, of course, avoid further exposure to sunlight.

If pain is excessive, or extensive blistering is present, consult a physician. Avoid application of over-the-counter topical anesthetics that may cause allergic skin reactions.

A severe or extensive sunburn is comparable to a second-degree thermal burn and may be accompanied by symptoms of shock; if such symptoms are present the victim should be treated for shock. See also BURNS, THERMAL.

Sunstroke

See HEATSTROKE.

Tick bites

EMERGENCY TREATMENT: Do not try to scrape or rub the insect off the skin with your fingers; scraping, rubbing, or pulling may break off only part of the insect body, leaving the head firmly attached to the skin. Rubbing also can smear disease organisms from the tick into the bite. To make the tick drop away from the skin, cover it with a heavy oil, such as salad, mineral, or lubricating oil. Oil usually will block the insect's breathing pores, suffocating it. If oil is not readily available, carefully place a heated object against the tick's body; a lighted cigarette or a match that has been ignited and snuffed out can serve as a hot object.

Carefully inspect the bite area to be sure that all parts of the tick have been removed. Use a pair of tweezers to remove any tick parts found. Then carefully wash the bite and surrounding area with soap and water and apply an antiseptic. Also,

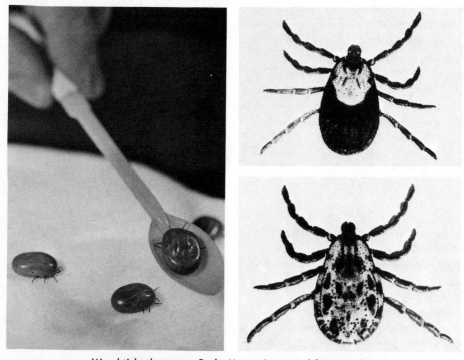

Wood ticks that cause Rocky Mountain spotted fever, in the engorged state *(left)*, and in the unengorged state *(right)*. The female is at the top right, the male at the bottom right.

wash your hands and any equipment that may have come in contact with the tick. Consult a physician if symptoms of tick fever or tularemia, such as unexplained muscular weakness, occur following a bite.

Toothaches

EMERGENCY TREATMENT: Give an adult one or two aspirin tablets; a young child should be given no more than one-half of an adult tablet. The aspirin should be swallowed with plenty of water. Do not let it dissolve in the mouth or be held near the aching tooth. Aspirin becomes effective as a pain-killer only after it has gone through the digestive tract and into the bloodstream; if aspirin is held in the mouth, it may irritate the gums.

Oil of cloves can be applied to the aching tooth. Dip a small wad of cotton into the oil of cloves, then gently pack the oil-soaked cotton into the tooth cavity with a pair of tweezers. Do not let the tweezers touch the tooth.

If the jaw is swollen, apply an ice bag for periods of 15 minutes at a time, at intermittent intervals. Never apply heat to a swollen jaw when treating a toothache. Arrange to see your dentist as soon as possible.

Tooth, broken

EMERGENCY TREATMENT: Apply a few drops of oil of cloves to the injured tooth to help relieve pain. If oil of cloves is not available, give an adult one to two regular aspirin tablets. One-half of a regular tablet can be given to a young child.

Make an emergency filling from a wad of cotton containing a few drops of oil of cloves. An emergency filling also can be made from powdered chalk; it is important to protect the cavity from infection while providing pain relief.

If the tooth has been knocked out of the socket, retrieve the tooth, because it can be restored in some cases. Do not wash the tooth; ordinary washing can damage dental tissues. A dentist will take care of cleaning it properly. Wrap the tooth in a damp clean handkerchief or tissue or place the tooth in a container of slightly salty warm water for the trip to the dentist.

Unconsciousness

Unconsciousness is the condition which has the appearance of sleep, but is usually the result of injury, shock, or serious physical disturbance. A brief loss of consciousness followed by spontaneous recovery is called *fainting*. A prolonged episode of unconsciousness is a *coma*.

EMERGENCY TREATMENT: Call a doctor at once. If none is available, get the victim to the nearest hospital. If the loss of consciousness is accompanied by loss of breathing, begin mouth-to-mouth respiration. If the victim is suffering cardiac arrest, administer cardiac massage. Don't try to revive the victim with any kind of stimulant unless told to do so by a doctor.

Vertigo

See DIZZINESS.

CHAPTER 34

Safety

SAFETY IN THE HOME

Approximately 30,000 people will die in home accidents this year, and many more will sustain serious, lasting injury. The most likely accident victims are those under the age of 5 or over 65, but accidents can happen to anyone. The most tragic aspect of most home accidents is that they could have been prevented. Making a home safe to live in is not difficult or time-consuming, especially considering the peace of mind it provides.

In Your Own Backyard

Home safety begins with inspection of the site the home is on. Prospective home buyers and builders should inspect a house with safety features in mind, but if a home with unsafe grounds is already owned, bear in mind that most features can be improved and made safe. Attractive landscaping of grounds is certainly important, but a homeowner should make certain that there is good drainage for both rain and

snow, and that hedges, trees, and shrubs are not placed so that they obscure the view of the street from the driveway.

Homes set on hillsides are certainly picturesque, but are balconies, terraces, or steep grades protected by a railing? Drives and walkways should be well lighted and paved with a nonskid surface. Any broken pavement should be repaired as soon as possible. During the winter months drives and walks should be kept clear of snow and ice.

A wide roof overhang should protect porch and house entrances from rain and snow. If snow or ice does collect in these places, it should be swept or shoveled clear immediately. Any large trees around the house should be healthy and well maintained. Tree limbs need to be checked periodically, especially those that overhang the house, and all dead ones should be removed. Awning and casement windows should not project over walks and other traffic areas where they can cause bumps and bruises. Sidewalks or paths with sharp drops in grade or single steps are also potential hazards. Chimneys should always be kept in good repair, at the bottom as well as the top.

Checking the Garage

Garage doors should open easily from both inside and out. At least one window to provide ventilation should be present. Even if the window is open, a car should never be started or kept running if garage doors are closed, no matter how cold it gets in winter. Carbon monoxide fumes are extremely dangerous and can be fatal.

Installing a light switch near the door will prevent any possible falls or bumps when groping in the dark. If the garage holds two or more cars, lanes painted down the garage floor or along the wall opposite the door will help prevent one car from taking up too much space.

Children should be taught that bikes and other possessions must not be left in the driveway. But no matter how well trained the children are, whenever pulling out of a garage, the driver should always carefully check the rear-view mirror, looking for both people and obstructions. All cars that are parked even for a short time should be set in "Park" or have their handbrakes pulled.

Turning On the Heat

The home itself should be checked for basic structural soundness, fire and emergency exits, the use of fire-resistant materials, including paint, and an adequate amount of nonglare light. Fuel-consuming heating units should be

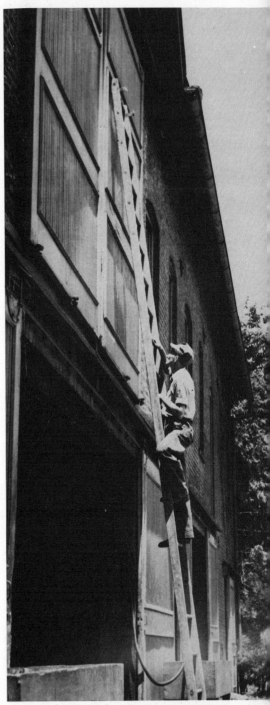

This man is using a ladder dangerously. The angle is too vertical, and as he nears the top his weight is likely to send it toppling over backwards.

vented to the outside, directly or through a chimney, and appropriate dampers and draft hoods should be installed. All heating equipment should be in good condition, and water heating units should have a temperature or pressure valve that can be easily tested by a home owner. Sprinkler heads placed over heating units are an extra precaution.

Most homes and apartments have main gas and water switches or valves, and all adult family members should know where these are located and how to turn them off in case of emergency. The valves should be distinctly tagged for quick identification. If a leaky gas pipe or valve is suspected, the gas company should be called immediately.

Adults in the home should also be familiar with the procedure for lighting the pilot light on a furnace and water heater. If the home has a fireplace, correct procedure for lighting should be taught and observed here, too. Kerosene, a dangerously flammable liquid, should never be used to start a home fire, and the fire should be screened at all times. Safety authorities warn that fires in a home fireplace are unsafe unless the hearth projects at least 16 inches into the room.

Avoiding Live Wires

The homeowner's increasing dependence on modern electrical appliances makes a well-designed electrical wiring system a must. The wiring and its installation can be considered safe if they comply with the standards of the National Electrical Code or the National Electrical Safety Code, and with state and local ordinances. The best outlets to use are those that will accept grounding-type three-pronged plugs. The plugs should require turning to expose the openings or be fitted with plastic insert covers to prevent curious youngsters from getting hurt.

There should be enough branch circuits in the wiring system so that plugs are not overloaded and extension cords do not have to be used except as a temporary expediency. Permanent cords must be placed carefully. They should not be run through holes in walls, ceilings, or floors, nor should they be wrapped around a pipe or other possibly warm objects, fastened to a building surface, placed where they constitute a tripping hazard, or put in areas where they will get excessive wear, such as under a rug. Permanent and extension cords should be inspected frequently, and thrown away if worn places or any sign of a defect appears.

PRECAUTIONS AGAINST ELECTRIC SHOCK: All home appliances should carry the label of the Underwriters' Laboratory (UL) which guarantees that they have been tested for shock hazard. The cords and plugs of all appliances should be examined regularly for fraying, wire exposure, or loose parts, and repaired promptly if necessary. If there are young children in the family, all unused but active electrical wall outlets should be completely covered with layers of masking tape.

FUSES: Both the fuse box and the circuit breaker are good, safe methods of controlling a wiring system if proper precautions are followed. When changing a fuse, the suspected appliance or other source should be unplugged and the main switch pulled to be sure the current is off. While standing on a dry surface—such as a board, tile floor, or rubber mat—to reduce the chance of shock, a new fuse of the proper size should be installed. Makeshift devices, including copper pennies, are dangerous substitutes. They destroy the purpose of a fuse, which is to cut off power and thus prevent overheated wires. After the fuse has been installed, the main switch should be turned on. If the fuse blows again, a qualified electrician should be called in, since this is an indication of major trouble.

CIRCUIT BREAKERS: If a circuit breaker pops to the "open" or "off" position, the cause should be located and corrected. The breaker can then be reset. If it opens again, there is a fault in the circuit, and an electrician should be called in for repairs.

No matter which system is used, if lights dim repeatedly, the wiring should be checked by an electrician to avert the possibility of fire.

Creating Traffic Lanes

Living space within the home should be carefully considered in regard to traffic patterns. Rooms should be arranged in relation to one another so a smooth pattern, as short and direct as possible, is created. Doors should open against walls so they do not swing into a line of traffic. Once a traffic lane has been established, any objects likely to tip or be stumbled over should be removed. Furniture should not be moved from an accustomed place, particularly into a traffic lane, without first warning the family of the impending move. Unnecessary changes in floor level and any sharp corners or projections that could cause falls should be avoided.

When not in use, objects such as children's toys, sewing boxes, and the like, should be kept off the floors. Spilled liquids and foods should be wiped up promptly, and small articles such as rubber bands, paper clips, and pencils should be picked up as soon as possible, since they can cause someone to trip. It is much easier to keep floors clear if a room has adequate storage space. It is often worthwhile to build a closet or storage hutch which will allow things to be stored away safely.

Floors

Bare floors should be kept in good repair, free from uneven or rough areas, loosened tiles, or wide cracks that could catch a heel. If floors are to be waxed, the job must be done properly. It is important to choose the right wax. Paste or liquid polishing waxes are good for wooden floors, but self-polishing water-base waxes should be used on asphalt tiles. Before waxing, floors should be rinsed well, since any cleansing agent left on the floor can soften the wax, making it slippery. The wax should be applied in a thin coat and buffed thoroughly, following manufacturer's directions. Applying new wax on top of old wax too frequently is not a good idea, since this can create a slippery surface that may cause falls.

When cleaning waxed floors, a dry dust mop should be used; an oiled or chemically treated one can soften the wax.

If carpeting is used to cover floors, it should be securely anchored. Area rugs, particularly small ones, are not safe unless made with nonskid backing or used with a rubber pad. Floor coverings which have tears, holes, frays, or loose or curled edges can cause falls and should be replaced.

Stairs

The stairs in a home can be hazardous, but measures can be taken to make them safer. Whether they are indoors or outdoors, short flights of stairs with a landing are preferred over a long, single flight. All steps should be the same height and width. The height of each step should not exceed eight inches, and the tread should be a minimum of nine inches deep.

At least one railing on a flight of stairs is a good safety precaution. Bannister spindles should be close enough together to prevent a small child from placing his head between them. Attic and basement stairways in particular, and other stairways, where practicable, should be provided with doors at top and bottom, doors that swing open away from the stairs—not over them. If a door leads to a landing, it is best that the landing be at least 30 inches in width. To protect the family while they sleep, the stairway door should be kept closed; a closed door, particularly if painted with a fire retardant paint, can help prevent the spread of fire.

A runner or carpeting to cover stairway steps and landings must fit snugly and be securely anchored. Any materials with holes or worn spots should be replaced, since they can easily catch a heel and cause a fall. Steps should be kept clear of all articles or objects. If there are small children in the home, gates at the top and bottom of the stairs are essential.

It is often helpful, particularly on outdoor stairs, to have a white strip painted on the edge of each step, or

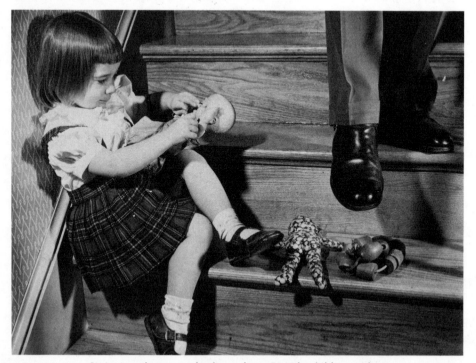

Stairs in a home can be hazardous. Provide children with a place to enjoy their toys that is away from normal family traffic.

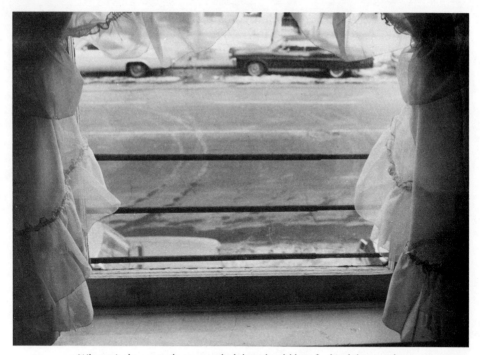

When window guards are needed they should be of a kind that can be removed easily and that are not in violation of local fire regulations.

to have the top and bottom step of a flight of stairs painted white to make the stairs more visible. During winter months, outdoor stairs should be kept free of ice.

Good lighting on the stairs is important, and switches should be located at both the top and bottom of a flight of stairs. Light fixtures should be placed so they illuminate all steps. Bare bulbs create glare, which could result in a fall, so bulbs that are covered or shaded in some way will prove the safest. If there are any windows in stairwells, they should be located where they can be easily and safely cleaned.

Glass

Windows, particularly those on or above a second story, should have bars or heavy screens if there are youngsters in the home. If there are glass doors leading to a patio or balcony, they should be made out of one of the three types of safety glass available on the market; tempered glass, wire-embedded glass, or laminated glass.

Even safety glass can break, however, and certain safety precautions should be observed in homes that have glass doors. Children should be taught that they should never play around a glass door, since many accidents happen when children fall or are accidentally pushed against the door.

To prevent people from walking through a glass door they've failed to see, doors can be marked to make them more visible. Decorative decals can be applied, bars can be mounted on the surface at doorhandle level, or the door can be sanded, etched, painted, or gilded.

If a sliding or swinging glass door is adjacent to a fixed glass panel, the panel should be identified in some way to prevent anyone's mistaking it for the door. A table, large potted plant, or a planter, for example, would serve this purpose.

The Childproof Home

When planning children's bedrooms, playrooms, and dens, a special effort should be made to make these rooms safe for children. Traffic lanes should be made as wide as possible, since the likelihood of tripping and bumping into objects is greater than for adults. Furniture should be as unbreakable as possible, with no rough edges or sharp corners that can catch at clothes. Glass and other breakable objects and knickknacks should be kept out of reach if they are used in these rooms at all.

Toys Should Be Fun

As early as possible, children should be trained to look after their toys, since toys left lying around are a tripping hazard for both children and unwary adults. Children will be easier to train if they are given a designated storage space for their toys. Easily accessible low shelves are good, since the child can then see his toys on display, and not have to dig to the bottom of some box for a favored possession.

It cannot be assumed that every toy currently available is a safe toy. In many cases toys are extremely dangerous, and careful thought must be given to each one bought or given a child. Very young children should have toys that are washable, too large to fit in the mouth, ear, or nose, and light enough not to cause the child injury if he drops them on himself. The toys should not be made of glass or other brittle or sharp material. The eyes on a stuffed animal or doll should be embroidered, or, as a second choice, sewn on. They must never be attached with pins.

All toys should be sturdy enough to withstand investigation by curious children. Wheels on toys should be attached with screws, and pull cords should be fastened with staples (not tacks) or tied through a hole in the toy. Edges should be rolled or turned in and corners rounded; a sharp corner can cause serious injury. Toys with loose parts, worn edges that have become sharp, and defective wiring in electric toys, can be dangerous, so parents should check for these potential hazards frequently. If toys are repainted, a leadfree paint must be used.

The construction of toys such as horns, whistles, and bubble blowers, which are meant to be put in the mouth, is very important. In badly constructed toys, a loose part can be sucked into the throat. Children old enough to play with paints, crayons, and pencils should be taught that these objects must never be put in the mouth. Each year about 350 children die from an obstruction, suffocation, or puncture, and many of these accidents result from swallowing or trying to swallow toys and similar objects.

Toy tools given to children should be sturdy and well made. The heads of hammers and mallets should be securely fastened to the handle so they will not come loose and fly off. Cutting tools such as saws should be sharp. (A dull edge is more likely to cause injury, since the child must push harder to get the job done.)

Children too young to use tools should not be given construction toys that require hammering.

Electric toys operating on house current should carry the Underwriters' Laboratories marker on the cord and toy to ensure safe construction. If possible, electric toys should operate on a transformer which reduces house current to 6 to 12 volts. Children must be taught early that electric toys must never be used while hands or clothing are wet. Though often more expensive to operate than electric toys, battery-operated toys are safe to use, since they eliminate shock and cord hazards.

A child's maturity, rather than mere chronological age, should be the main factor to consider before giving him such equipment as a bicycle, skis, skates, a tool kit, chemistry set, archery set, sharp knives, or an air rifle. The child should be mature enough to understand the danger involved in a particular plaything. Before being allowed to use such an item, he should be carefully taught its safe use and care.

The Basement

The basement of a home is often used as utility room or workroom, and for storage and recreational purposes. If so, it should have a ceiling of fire-resistant material.

The Utility Room

The utility room usually holds a washing machine and dryer. Ironing and sometimes sewing may be done there as well. Before an electric washer and dryer are installed, they must be properly grounded. A *ground* is a connection which con-

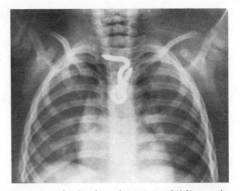

An X ray of a hook and eye in a child's esophagus. Objects small enough to be swallowed should be kept away from children.

ducts electricity between an electric circuit and earth, and can protect people from electrocution. The grounding should be installed or inspected by a qualified electrician.

LAUNDRY: The laundry area should be adequately lighted. Electric laundry equipment should not be used in wet areas, or by someone standing on a damp surface. Gas dryers, if so designed, should be vented outside. Before using washers and dryers, the operator should know how to operate emergency releases. Safety switches that automatically shut off a washer or dryer when the lid is raised or door is opened should be checked. Keep appliance cords dry. Before running the washing machine, the load of clothes should be checked to make sure it is evenly balanced. After each use of the dryer, the lint filter should be cleaned.

IRONING: When ironing, one should use a well-balanced, sturdy ironing board with noncumbustible board and asbestos cover. A steam iron should not be plugged into an outlet until after it is filled, and should be placed on its heel when it is not in use. Irons should never be left on the

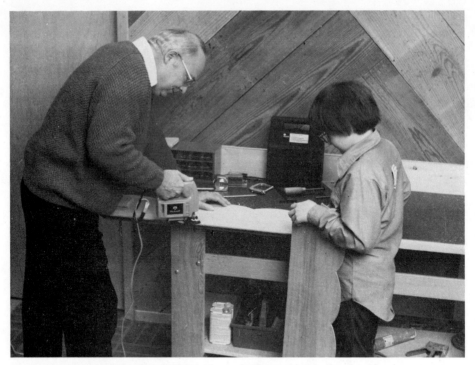

Children like to work with tools, and, if properly taught, they develop the good habits that enable them to use tools safely and with confidence.

ironing board unattended, and should be disconnected from the outlet when not in use.

SEWING: When sewing, pins and needles should always be put in pin cushions, never held in the mouth. Sharp objects should not be put in the lap, even momentarily. Scissors and other sharp objects should be sorted in holders or in a secure place out of the reach of children.

When first learning to operate a sewing machine, slow speed should be used. The cord should be placed so it does not rub against the motor belt when the sewing machine is in use. The machine should be unplugged when not in use. Fingers should be kept away from the path of the needle. If the sewing table has a leaf, excessive weight or pressure should not be put on it.

The Workroom: Caring for Tools

The workroom can constitute a hazard if care is not taken. Children should be warned that they are not to enter the room without adult supervision, and all tools should be kept locked up or otherwise out of the reach of children. No tool should be used without a proper understanding of how it works and what it can best be used for. Accidents can result quite easily if a tool is used for a job it was not intended for.

All tools must be kept in good condition, and stored in a safe place when not in use. A tool cabinet or tool rack hung on the wall is one of the best storage places for most tools. However, items such as chisels or other edged tools should not be kept in wall racks, since it is quite easy to bang against them when reaching for another tool. Sharp-edged tools should be kept flat in a drawer or tray, with the edges covered.

Tool handles should be checked periodically to make sure they are firmly attached to the tool itself. Any wooden handles should be firm and smooth to minimize the possibility of slivers and splinters. Blades and edges on tools should be kept sharp. More pressure must be exerted on dull tools, which may cause injury, and they may slip, stick, or slide more easily than a sharper one. Bent tools should be straightened or discarded. Tools should be periodically rubbed with an oiled cloth to prevent rust.

HAMMERS: The misuse of hammers, the most familiar home tool, has caused many smashed fingers and thumbs. The handle should be held firmly and close to the end, and the object struck should be hit squarely. Striking at an angle can cause chips to fly. When hammering anything that looks as though it will chip, goggles should be worn.

To drive a nail safely, the nail should be held lightly between thumb and forefinger near the point of the nail. The nail should be given one or two light blows to hold it in place. The fingers should then be withdrawn before hammering firmly. If the nail must be held in place throughout the hammering, a gripping tool should be used.

Hammers should be kept in good condition. The head should be checked often to make sure it is firmly attached to the handle and will not fly off when a blow is struck.

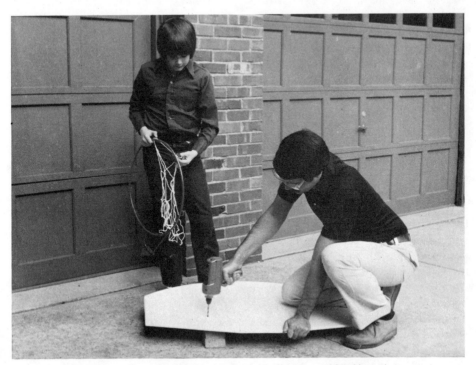

This boy will enjoy using his new basketball hoop and backboard. In addition, he is learning a valuable lesson in how to use tools properly.

The head and handle should be kept free of grease and oil, which can cause slipping.

SCREWDRIVERS: All screwdrivers should have smooth, firm, unsplintered handles and blades that have not become broken, chipped, or rounded. Screwdriver blades can be ground, reworked, and retempered if they get in poor condition. If they cannot be fixed, discard them.

It is both handy and safe to own screwdrivers in a variety of sizes and shapes. Only a screwdriver that fits the screw should be used. The work to be done should never be held in one hand while the screwdriver is in the other, since it can easily slip and cut the hand holding the work. Only screwdrivers with insulated handles should be used for electrical work. Most important of all, screwdrivers should never be used as a substitute for hammers, chisels, or any other type of tool.

PLIERS AND WIRE CUTTERS: Pliers and wire cutters should be kept clean, and the joint pin should be oiled occasionally. Pliers should not be used often on hardened surfaces, since this can dull the teeth, causing the pliers to slip. Neither pliers nor wire cutters should be used to cut spring wire, since they are usually not heavy enough for this job.

If wire under tension or in coils is to be cut, both ends of the wire should be secure or covered to prevent a loose end from flying up into the face of the cutter. It goes without saying that a live wire must never be cut.

HATCHETS, AXES, AND ADZES: Hatchets, axes, and adzes are quite safe when used properly. The piece to be hit should not be held while swinging, and feet and legs must be kept out of the way. Before swinging, any obstructions that might be in the way should be cleared, and no one should be standing close enough to be hit by flying chips. Blades should be kept sharp, and handles should be of good material that will not crack or splinter. When not in use, it is best to embed the cutting edges of these tools in a block of wood or store them in a leather case. Many accidents with these tools have occurred when the cutting edge was unintentionally handled.

SAWS: Hacksaws and handsaws should be kept as sharp as possible, oiled to prevent rusting and, when stored, hung by the handles or otherwise placed to protect the teeth. Whenever possible, a sawhorse or bench should be used as a work support.

CHISELS: Chisels come in two types. Cold chisels, the safest of which are made from high-carbon steel, are used for cutting metal. Wood chisels, with strong substantial handles, are the familiar workshop variety. Goggles should be worn when using cold chisels to protect oneself from flying fragments. A screen placed around work in progress is necessary to protect any bystanders from flying chips. If the head of a chisel, punch, or similar tool flattens out at point of impact, it can be restored by grinding.

BARS: Ripping or pinch bars, also called crowbars, should be kept in good condition, with the point kept sharp. They are best stored on racks. Crowbars should be used only when the hands are dry and the footing secure.

PLANES: Planes should be used only when the user is perfectly balanced, since the plane may jump and cause the unbalanced user to lunge forward. Planing done toward the body is dangerous. The front part of the plane should be pressed downward at the beginning of the stroke, the rear part of the plane when completing strokes. The plane should be raised slightly on the backward stroke to prevent the blade from dulling.

VISES: If a vise is used it should be solidly mounted on a two-inch plank directly over workbench legs. The solid jaw should extend at least half an inch beyond the plank edge. The vise should be heavy enough to handle the work to be done. After using a vise, the object in it should be gripped firmly before loosening, so that it will not fly out or fall when the vise is released.

POWER TOOLS: If any power tools are kept in the workshop, they should be disconnected or the switches kept in the lock position when not in use. Grounding may be necessary. Follow the manufacturer's directions.

PREVENTING WORKSHOP FIRES: Good ventilation in the workshop is a must, and all work areas should be well lighted so that the work in progress can be clearly seen. If paints, paint thinners, or solvents are kept in the workroom, they should be stored in metal cans. Any oily rags kept around for convenience should be stored in airtight metal cans. In addition to a fireproof ceiling, a dry-powder carbon dioxide or all-purpose fire extinguisher should also be kept handy.

Storage Areas

If the basement—or any other areas of the home, including the attic—is used as a storage area, cer-

tain safety precautions should be observed. First, the storage area should not be used as a place where items not immediately needed for use are simply dumped indiscriminately. Unless all articles, particulary combustible materials, are stored neatly and with care, the storage area could quickly become a fire trap.

COMBUSTIBLES: Potentially combustible materials kept at home should be stored in metal containers. Heavy objects to be stored should be placed on lower shelves or on the floor. Light and small articles can be kept on upper shelves—but keep a sturdy stepladder or stool nearby at all times to prevent the temptation of climbing over boxes or barrels to reach an article stored away on an upper shelf. Cabinet or cupboard doors and any drawers should be closed immediately after use. Other articles can best be stored in cabinets or shelves along a wall or walls. Unless these shelves are free-standing, they must be fastened securely to the walls.

POISONS: Poisonous materials or dangerous compounds, including lyes, bleaches, and insecticides, should be clearly labeled and kept in their original containers when stored away. Accidental poisonings are often caused by storing poisonous materials in containers that originally held food. All poisonous materials, including materials that are not thought of as poisonous but that can be dangerous if inhaled or used indiscriminately, such as aspirin, aerosol sprays, and so on, should be locked up or stored out of the reach of children. Any canned, packaged, or preserved foods that are kept in the storage area should be placed well away from poisonous materials. Any-

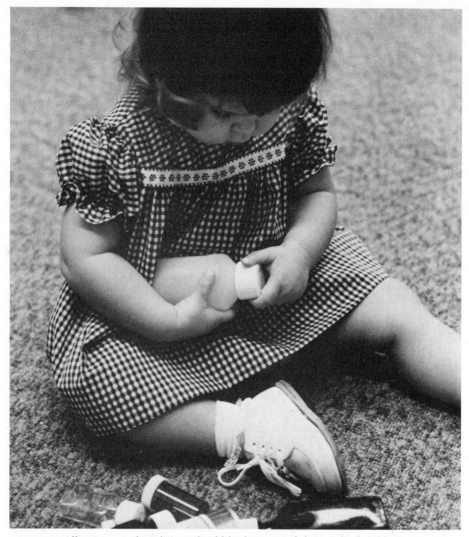

All poisons and medicines should be kept out of the reach of children, whose curiosity may lead them to taste or swallow a dangerous substance.

thing that comes in an aerosol container should be kept away from heat, which can cause it to burst.

The Kitchen

Safety in the kitchen begins with the plan of the kitchen itself. Large pieces of kitchen equipment and counter space for working are most often arranged in a "U", "L", corridor, one wall, or island shape, depending on kitchen size and personal preference. All of these arrangements are safe if the appliances and counter space naturally divide into three distinct work areas:

• The sink area, which should also contain the dishwasher if there is one. For right-handed persons, the dishwasher should be to the right of the sink (to the left for left-handed persons). Since foods that are washed and dried before storing are cleaned in this area, it should be convenient to the refrigerator, which will lessen the chance of dropping items to be refrigerated.

• The storage and mixing area, containing the refrigerator, should have enough counter space to ensure good working conditions, and have sufficient electrical outlets for any small appliances used in this area.

• The stove area, where food is cooked and served, should be nearest to family eating areas. The range should not be placed under a window, where low-hanging curtains can easily catch fire.

All three kitchen centers should flow naturally into one another to eliminate unnecessary steps. The normal traffic pattern should be considered, so that congested areas where family members might constantly bump into one another are not created. Each kitchen center should contain good lighting (including over the stove and in the oven, if possible), enough electrical outlets to eliminate the need for any trailing cords which can create a tripping hazard, and enough storage space for the supplies, utensils, and small appliances needed for each area's work.

If possible, cabinets should be made with sliding doors instead of those which open out, to avoid bumps and bruises. If items must be stored in hard-to-reach cabinets, a stepladder should be kept handy; using chairs or climbing on counters is hazardous. No matter how scant storage space is, sharp knives and utensils should never be stored in the same drawer as table silver. The best place for sharp working knives

and steak knives is in a case or wall rack.

Allowance should also be made for adequate ventilation, which not only rids the kitchen of cooking odors, but also decreases the possibility of accumulation of gas in a gas range. If there is no window in the kitchen, an exhaust fan will prove helpful in getting rid of fumes, odors, and excessive heat.

Appliances

Before buying any new appliances and equipment, check their safety features. Electrical products should have circuit breakers and overload features. Controls and knobs should remain cool to the touch and easy to reach while the product is in operation. Signal lights should indicate when equipment is on. All appliances and equipment, large and small, should be installed, grounded if necessary, cleaned, and used according to the manufacturer's directions.

On large appliances, doors should be flush and handles located so that clothing does not catch easily. Laundry and dishwashing equipment should have safety switches which automatically shut off action when the door or lid is opened. Any pull-out shelves and racks should have a lock position that prevents them from being completely pulled out unintentionally. Refrigerator and freezer doors should have a latch designed to open easily from the inside, particularly if there are young children in the house. Any removable part should come out readily and be easy to clean.

Smaller appliances should be well insulated at the base to protect table and counter tops, and should stand firmly. Those that come apart for cleaning, and, if possible, are totally immersible in water, are easier to keep clear of food particles and germs. Cords on appliances to be used on wet surfaces should be waterproof. Handles should be comfortable to use, and strong enough to support the appliance's weight. Electrical equipment that starts automatically when plugged in is dangerous. Look for appliances that come with an off-and-on switch.

All appliances should be checked for noise level. Modern studies have proved that everyday noise can cause fatigue and temper outbursts, thus creating an atmosphere of potential danger. The pneumatic jack-hammer has a decibel rating of 94 (a *decibel* is a unit for measuring the intensity of sound) and, surprisingly, a standard dishwasher, disposal unit, and exhaust fan going at the same time add up to 91 decibels. Therefore, the more quietly an appliance runs, the better and more pleasant it will be for the home. If noisy equipment must be used, it should be run while the kitchen is empty. Using insulated or acoustical floors and ceilings and placing appliances on casters or rubber pads will also help to keep the noise level down.

Appliance cords should be stored by rolling them up loosely and keeping them in a cool dry place. They should never be used on a wet surface, hung on a nail or sharp object, or run under a door or rug. Any cords that are cracked, crumbled, or worn should be replaced. Appliances should always be switched off when being plugged in or disconnected, and should be disconnected by pulling on the plug, not the cord. If a tingle or slight shock is received while handling an appliance, it should be checked for loose wires or poor insulation.

Portable appliances should be used on firm, level surfaces, with enough space allowed around heating appliances in use so that they do not burn or ignite nearby items. If lights dim when appliances are turned on, chances are the circuit is overloaded, and fuse sizes should be checked. All appliances should be allowed to cool before storing.

Safe Work Habits

Even though the kitchen itself has been made as safe as possible, a number of accidents can be caused by careless work habits. When cooking, all pot handles should be turned toward the counter or range top (though a handle should not be placed directly over another burner). This prevents any accidental brushing against the handle or having it catch on clothes, thus upsetting the pot's contents, and also avoids tempting a toddler or slightly older youngster who might hear water boiling and grab the pot handle in an effort to investigate the sound. Using back burners that are not easily reached by a child is preferable to using front burners.

Always using a pot holder is another good safety rule. Using dish towels, apron corners, and other improvisations can result in burns. A spare pot holder should always be convenient to the stove. When checking on pots whose contents are being cooked by steam, the lid should always be lifted in a direction that allows the steam to escape away from the face.

Good work habits should also be observed while preparing and serv-

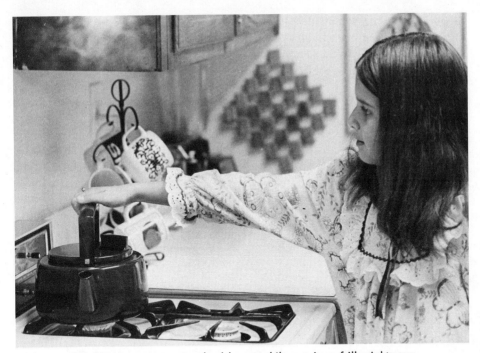

Reaching across a stove to a back burner while wearing a frilly nightgown can lead to a serious accident. Close-fitting clothes are more sensible.

ing food. Small objects should never be held in one hand while cutting with the other. A cutting board should always be used, and the knife should always be pointed down and away from the body. It is important to use the proper-sized knife for each choice. Large butcher knives, for example, should not be used for paring. Knives should always be kept sharp, since greater pressure must be exerted in using dull ones, thus increasing the chance of accident. Finger guards on large knives help prevent slippage. When serving food, hot bowls and decorative pots brought directly to the table should be carried with pot holders. Cracked or chipped plates, cups, and glassware should be discarded.

What is worn in the kitchen can be as important a safety habit to develop as learning the right way to hold a knife. Flimsy nightgowns and robes with long flowing sleeves can brush against a flame or catch on a sharp object or pot handle, causing spillage or cuts. Long hostess gowns, glamorous lounging pajamas, and floppy slippers can cause trips and falls. Practical, close-fitting clothes should be worn at all times. If the arrival of guests calls for an unsafe outfit, the menu should be planned so that after the host and hostess are dressed, nothing more arduous than tossing a salad or heating up a previously cooked main dish is called for.

Falls in the kitchen, particularly in homes with older people or very young children, can be avoided by keeping it well lighted, without glare or shadowy areas. If scatter rugs must be used, they should be the kind that have nonskid backs. If any water, grease, or food spills on the floor, be sure it is wiped up immediately. Floor waxes should be applied in thin, even coats, and should be buffed to a hard, dry finish. Old wax should be stripped fairly frequently.

Food Spoilage

Most food poisoning is caused by a bacterium called *staphylococcus aureus,* or *staph.* It flourishes between temperatures of 40 and 140 degrees, particularly in cream-filled foods, dishes made with mayonnaise and other creamy dressings, cheese, cooked meats, casseroles, and moist prepared foods. None of these foods should be unrefrigerated for more than three hours, and on hot summer days, even less.

If sandwich fillings or other cooked foods are to be mixed with salad dressing or mayonnaise for a picnic, there will be less chance of food spoilage if the two are carried separately to the picnic spot and actually mixed just before eating. When preparing stuffings for chicken, turkey, or other poultry, do not stuff the bird until it is ready to go into the oven. Leftover stuffing should be stored in a separate dish, not left in the cavity of the bird.

Foods that are meant to be served hot should be served that way, and not allowed to stand indefinitely at room temperature. Until serving or cooking, foods should be kept properly chilled, and the refrigerator should be checked occasionally to make sure it keeps foods at temperatures below 40 degrees. Anyone with an intestinal upset or infection should not be allowed to help with food preparation, and everyone's hands should be cleaned thoroughly before touching any food.

The Bathroom

The bathroom is potentially one of the most dangerous rooms in the home. Each year, approximately 200,000 people sustain some kind of accidental injury in the bathroom. Most of these accidents can be avoided if proper safety precautions are followed.

Electrical Shocks

Because water and electricity are often brought together in the bathroom, accidental electrocution is always a hazardous possibility. Electrical switches, fixtures, and appliances should never be turned on while standing in the bathtub or shower or on a damp floor, or if the body is still wet. As a precaution, electric switches and outlets should be located out of reach of the tub and shower, to avoid accidents due to forgetfulness.

Care should be exercised before buying items such as electric razors and electric toothbrushes, and other appliances used chiefly in the bathroom. If such appliances have been labeled by the Underwriters' Laboratory or other qualified testing agency, it can be assumed that their motors or vibrators have been properly sealed against all possible contact with water. If extension cords are used, they should be of the rubber-insulated variety. Because there is often excessive humidity in the bathroom, check cords frequently for signs of deterioration.

Many bathrooms still have a light over the washbowl that is controlled by a pull chain. Whenever possible, the chain should be replaced by a wall switch. If that cannot be done, the metal chain should be replaced by a cord, or equipped with an insulating link near the socket. Otherwise one might be severely shocked by simultaneously touching the metal chain of the light and a metal water faucet or some other metal object.

Electric heaters should be used in the bathroom with great care, and should be used only if labeled by a nationally recognized testing agency. Heaters should be kept in good condition, and a worn cord should be replaced with one of the same type and quality as the original. The manufacturer's directions should be checked, since some heaters require rubber-covered cords and others asbestos-covered ones.

Avoiding Slips and Falls

Falls cause a large percentage of bathroom injuries. The chance of a fall can be greatly reduced by making certain that the bathroom floor has a nonslip finish and that the tub or shower has a nonskid surface. Either a suction-type mat or safety strips may be used in the tub. If the bathroom is being remodeled, tubs with permanent slip-resistant bottoms are now available.

A good grab bar that offers the bather firm support while getting in and out of the tub is a big help in preventing falls, particularly for older people. The L-shaped bar offers the most support. Shower curtain rods should be anchored firmly into the walls with long screws (which should reach the studding, not just the lath or plaster), since a bather may grab a shower curtain or rod for support if he feels himself slipping. If shower doors and tub enclosures are used instead of curtains, they should be made of safety glass or shatterproof plastic. Soap should be kept in a soap container, preferably the built-in type. When bathing and showering, soap should be placed in the dish when not in use, not in the tub or on a ledge, where it can easily slide down into the tub and become a hazard.

Many slips and falls in the bathroom are caused by wet floors. Bath mats should always be used when showering and bathing to catch stray water. If the bathroom is also used as a place to hang clothes while they are drying, they should be hung so that they drip into the tub and not on the floor. Any spills and drips should be mopped up immediately.

Leaving a night light on in the bathroom is a good idea. It not only helps prevent slips and bumps, but can also help prevent the taking of medicine or pills from the wrong bottle in the dark. Keeping the medicine cabinet door closed whenever it is not in use will also help avert painful bumps. If there are clothes hooks on doors or walls, they should be placed above eye level, to prevent face or eye injury.

Water Control

Bathroom sinks, tubs, and showers should all contain mixer valves, to prevent scalding from hot water. A thermostatic or pressure regulating control valve is also useful. Bath and shower water should always be tested before stepping in. It is particularly easy for young children and elderly persons to get scalded by water that is too hot.

All faucet and valve handles should be made of an unbreakable material, such as metal. Old-fashioned porcelain handles can break easily and cause severe cuts. The

Home Safety Quiz

• Are you always alert for tripping hazards (mops, brooms, scatter rugs, wires)?

• Do you light your way ahead of you into rooms, and up and down stairs?

• Do you carry only small loads up and down stairs, so that you can see where you are going?

• Do all stairs have handrails, and do you use them?

• Are broken stairways and handrails, loose floor boards, and wobbly railings promptly repaired?

• Is there a safe hand hold or grab bar for bathtub and shower?

• Are nonslip rubbers mats or adhesive strips placed in bathtub or shower?

• Are all rugs anchored, do scatter rugs have skidproof backing, and is worn carpet or linoleum repaired?

• Are stairs, halls, exits, and traffic lanes free from clutter?

• Is furniture placed so that it doesn't block normal walking areas?

• Are practical shoes worn for household activities, instead of floppy bedroom slippers?

• Are electrical cords in good condition?

• Do you avoid plugging more than two appliances or lamps in each double outlet?

• Are open hearth fires always screened?

• Are pan handles turned toward the back of the stove?

• Are short or close fitting sleeves worn when cooking, or are wide sleeves fastened back with pins or rubber bands?

• Are matches lit before the gas oven is turned on?

• Are electrical appliances disconnected when not in use?

• Is bath or shower temperature checked with a hand before showering or bathing?

• Do you observe the rule "No Smoking in Bed"?

• When cooking, are pot holders used instead of aprons or dish towels?

• Are all medicines clearly labeled?

• When taking medicine, do you first read the label?

• Is just one night's supply of pills taken from the medicine chest and placed by the bedside?

• Do you strictly follow doctor's instructions when taking medicine?

• Do you have a separate place for cleaning agents and food supplies?

• Do you have a family escape plan in case of fire?

• Do you know how to phone the fire department?

• Do you avoid using storage areas as a dumping ground?

• Do you know how to locate and quickly turn off gas and water valves?

• Can you light the pilot light on furnace and water heater?

• Can you change a fuse?

• Do you know how to turn off the main electrical switch?

• Are appliances grounded?

• Are knives kept in a rack or otherwise safely separated from silverware?

• Is a sturdy stepladder or stool used to reach high places?

• Are oily rags and other potential flammables kept in airtight metal cans?

• Are glass doors and shower enclosures made of safety glass?

• When sewing, are pins and needles kept in a pin cushion, not in your mouth?

• Are the ironing board and its cover of noncombustible material?

• Is lighting adequate over all work centers?

• Does electrical equipment comply with the standards of Underwriters' Laboratories?

• Do you use wooden tongs instead of a metal fork to remove toast stuck within an electric toaster?

• Are frayed floor coverings replaced and bare floors kept in good repair?

• Are spills always wiped up immediately?

• Are medicines and dangerous household products locked up out of reach of children?

potential danger of used razor blades can be minimized by disposing of them in a closed container, with a slot just large enough for a blade. The container should be kept out of reach of small children.

Storing Medicines

Bathrooms are often storerooms for potentially poisonous items such as medicines, cleaners, and disinfectants. All poisons and substances which would be harmful if taken internally should be clearly marked. Taping the bottle cap or sticking pins into the cork will also help to mark these bottles. As an extra safety measure, it's a good idea to store medicines and other compounds that should be taken internally in a different place from those items meant for external use.

All family members should make it a rule never to take medicine in the dark. Labels should always be double checked to make sure the right medication is being taken. After it has served its purpose, all prescription medicine should be discarded to prevent its being taken accidentally by someone else. Medicines and other potential poisons to be discarded should be emptied down the drain, and the containers should be rinsed. Aerosol cans should be disposed of according to the manufacturer's directions, and should never be put down an incinerator.

Flammable products such as hair sprays, nail polish, and many other cosmetic preparations that usually come in aerosol cans, should be stored away from a source of heat. They should never be placed next to a radiator or hot water heater, especially a gas heater with an open flame.

Childproofing the Bathroom

Because children are so curious, the bathroom can be extremely hazardous to them. Even seemingly inaccessible medicine cabinets can be reached by children, as by climbing from the toilet to the washbowl, and thereby to the medicine cabinet. Therefore, all drugs, medicines (both prescription and patent), laxatives, astringents, mouthwashes, antiseptics, sleeping tablets, and so on, should be kept in medicine cabinets or storage units that lock, or that have separate compartments that can be locked. Older children should be taught that they must never take anything out of the medicine cabinet without permission.

If one's bathroom is steam heated and has radiators or floor-to-ceiling steam pipes (called *risers*), these should be covered. A child who has just been bathed can get a nasty second-degree burn by backing into a hot steam pipe or radiator. The lower part of risers should be covered with asbestos insulation—and, incidentally, it's a good idea to cover all risers in this way if children are about. Radiators should also be screened or covered to protect curious or careless children.

Very young children and babies should never be left alone in the bathroom, and particularly not in the bathtub. Children can drown in very small amounts of water. As a safety measure, some parents remove all locks from the bathroom door. If an inside lock is kept, it should be one which can also be opened easily from the outside. This will provide quick access to the bathroom if a child should lock himself in, and can also help others reach anyone who might have had an accident while locked in the bathroom. If a lock that unlocks from the outside cannot be used, and some sort of inside lock is desired, a simple hook and eye lock is probably best, but be sure to position it very high, well beyond the reach of small children.

The Bedroom

All bedrooms should have a lamp within reach of the bed, and all family members should faithfully observe the rule of no smoking in bed. If medication within reach of the bed is needed for any reason, only the exact amount needed for one dose should be kept handy, to prevent the accidental taking of an overdose. All medications, and all items that might be kept in the open in an adult's bedroom, such as nail clippers, nail polish and remover, hairpins and clips, and similar items, should be kept out of the reach of children. Heating pads should be unplugged when not in use, and should be used only according to the manufacturer's directions.

In Case of Fire

Fire kills about 7,500 people each year, and ranks second as a cause of death among home accidents. A few simple precautions will reduce the chance of home fires and can save lives, not to mention property. The most basic rule is to formulate a family escape plan which outlines an alternative way out if the normal route through a front or back door is blocked by flame.

When formulating a family escape plan, the importance of getting out of

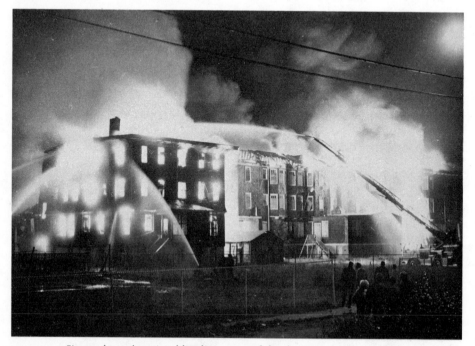

Fire ranks as the second leading cause of death among home accidents.
Every family should have an agreed-upon plan for escape in case of fire.

the house quickly must be stressed. Children are especially apt to panic in a fire and try to hide under a bed or in a closet. Adults sometimes forget that lives are at stake, and may return to a burning home for a valued possession. The following escape rules should be gone over with the whole family.

• Everyone should sleep with the bedroom door closed at night, since a closed door can delay the spread of fire and keep out deadly gases and smoke. If this is impractical—as it is, for example, with young children in the house—close off as much of the house as possible.

• A floor plan of the home with well-marked escape and alternate routes should be made and posted in a prominent place. Since night-time fires are the most serious, particular attention should be given to bedroom escapes. All windows designated as escape routes should be checked to make sure they are not painted shut or blocked by air-conditioners. Children should be told how to break glass with a chair or heavy object, and how to clear away any remaining pieces of glass in the frame with a shoe or similar object. If ropes or folding ladders are needed, they should be purchased.

• Provision should be made for very young children, elderly people, and pets, who will need help in escaping.

• A method of alarm, such as pounding on the walls, yelling, or using a whistle should be decided upon in case fire blocks hallways and prevents family members from reaching one another's bedrooms.

• Family members should be instructed to leave the house immediately in case of fire, and not

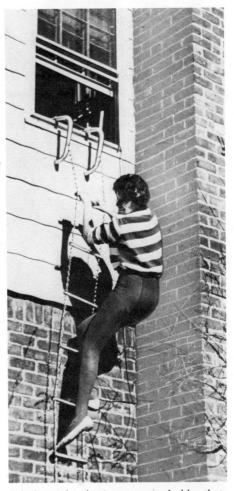

A lightweight aluminum escape ladder that fastens securely to a windowsill is important to have in the house in case of fire.

waste time getting dressed or packing prized possessions.

• Instruction should be given on the proper way of testing doors if fire is suspected. If panels or knobs are warm, the door should be kept closed and the alternate escape route used. A cool door can be opened cautiously, bracing the foot and hip against it, to prevent its blowing open. The door is probably safe if no hot air or smoke comes through the opening.

• If anyone is forced to remain in a room, he or she should stay near a slightly opened window and place towels or cloths in the door cracks. Smoke-filled rooms should be crossed by crawling, with the head held about 18 inches from the floor.

• A family meeting place outside the house where everyone will assemble as soon as he or she escapes should be decided upon.

• Plan to call the fire department as soon as possible after everyone is safely outside the house.

• Fire drills should be held to practice the escape route.

Extinguishing Fires

The most important thing to remember if someone's hair or body is on fire is to grab the thickest piece of material nearest to hand and cover the flame with it. Smothering fire with a coat, rug, or blanket is usually quicker and more effective than wasting time getting enough liquid to do the job.

Only if absolutely no other method is available for extinguishing flames should an attempt be made to beat out a flame with bare hands. Severe injury can result both to the victim and the rescuer in such cases.

FIRE EXTINGUISHERS: A fire extinguisher that is simple to operate is an essential part of household equipment. Two of the safest and most effective means of putting out small fires are water and sand. A hose connected to a special faucet for this purpose can be stored under the sink ready for emergency use. Several fire buckets filled with sand can be stored in a utility closet, pantry, or on the back porch.

Don't use water to put out flames caused by burning fat, oil, or sol-vents. One of the quickest ways to extinguish a fire in a pan of burning oil is to drop a lid on it immediately. Another method is to sprinkle the fire with the contents of a box of bicarbonate of soda that should be kept on the kitchen shelf for such emergencies.

Chemical fire extinguishers in aerosol cans should be kept in the kitchen, basement, and garage, since they are easy to use and effective against flaming oil, grease, gasoline, and chemical solvents. Avoid the use of extinguishers that contain carbon tetrachloride, and make sure that children understand that no extinguisher is meant to be played with.

FIRE SAFETY: Every household should be carefully checked for fire hazards.

Even when a fire begins, the proper and prompt use of an extinguisher can usually put it out. However, if the flames aren't brought under control immediately, the most important thing to do is get everyone out of the house and then notify the fire department.

Avoiding Fire

Fire can break out from a variety of causes. Most common causes are carelessness with smoking and matches; faulty electrical wiring or misuse of electrical equipment; defective or misused heating and cooking equipment; and carelessness involving flammable liquids, combustible home furnishings, or construction materials.

SMOKING: Fires caused by careless smoking habits and improper use of matches, the major cause of home fires, can be prevented by never smoking in bed; by keeping matches and lighters out of the reach of small

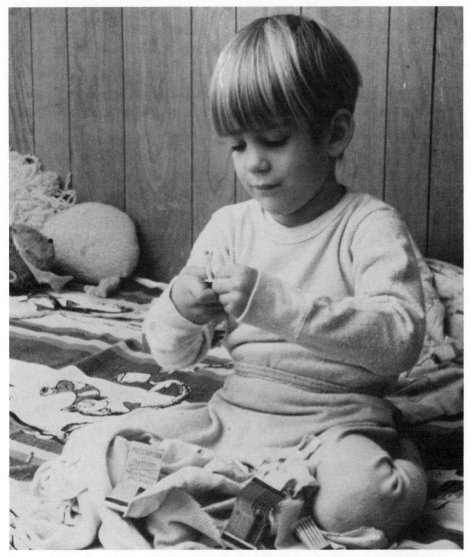

Many fires have been caused by unattended children who have experimented with matches. Keep matches in a safe place where children cannot get them.

children; by providing ashtrays that hold cigarettes and cigars securely; by disposing of ashes safely before retiring; and by selecting furniture and bedding that do not easily ignite and burn.

ELECTRICAL EQUIPMENT: To prevent fires caused by defective wiring and appliances and the misuse of electricity, wiring in the home should be checked, and rewiring undertaken if the system is inadequate. Worn and damaged cords should be replaced, defective appliances repaired or replaced, overloaded circuits remedied. Too many appliances should not be attached to one circuit; extension cords, unless a temporary arrangement, should be replaced with permanent wiring;

makeshift fuses should be replaced with adequate ones.

HEATING EQUIPMENT: Fires caused by defective or overheated heating equipment can be prevented by having all heating equipment, chimneys, and flues checked annually; by providing a door to the basement (or whatever area in which heating equipment is located), and keeping it closed; by protecting floors, walls, ceilings, and partitions near furnace, stoves, or heating pipes with noncombustible materials or with air

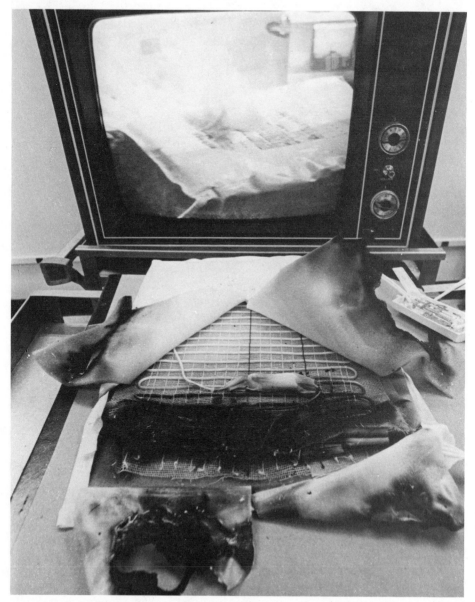

In the foreground is the back panel that has been removed from a defective television set. Note the extensive charring of the insulating material.

space; and by exercising special caution when using portable heating equipment.

USE OF FLAMMABLES: Flammable liquids such as kerosene and gasoline, used for cleaning purposes or to start fires, are always a fire hazard. A good safety precaution is to keep only small quantities of flammable liquids in the home, store them in safety cans, and label them. Never do home dry cleaning with gasoline or naphtha; never kindle a fire with gasoline or kerosene.

HOME FURNISHINGS AND CONSTRUCTION MATERIALS: To prevent fires caused by unsafe home furnishings and construction materials, curtains, drapes, upholstery and rugs made of comparatively noncombustible fibers should be selected. If rebuilding or remodeling, materials in walls, ceilings, floors, and partitions should be treated to make them fire-retardant; hollow walls should be filled with fire-resistive insulation; solid doors or doors painted with fire-retardant paint should be used on all bedrooms and at the tops and bottoms of stairways.

FIRE DETECTION: The longer a fire burns undetected, the more damage it can do. Therefore, a reliable fire detection or smoke detection system is of prime importance. In any system of heat or smoke detection, the component parts should be listed and labeled by Underwriters' Laboratories, Inc. (UL), or Factory Mutual Laboratories (FM), to ensure maximum protection.

Preventing Firearm Accidents

Most gunshot accidents occur at home as a result of carelessness. Families who own firearms *of no*

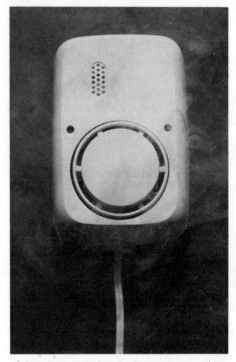

A fire detection device that emits an alarm when smoke is present may be a good investment for home owners.

matter what type should therefore observe the following rules, especially if there are children in the house:

1. A loaded gun should never be kept indoors.

2. Even before a hunting trip, a gun should never be loaded in the house or in a car.

3. Guns should be stored in a locked cabinet and ammunition stored elsewhere so that both are inaccessible to children.

4. Adults should *never* show off or play with a gun in the presence of children, nor should irresponsible remarks be made in their presence about shooting.

5. A child who is afraid of a gun should not be encouraged to handle one.

SAFETY IN THE CITY

The rapid pace and impermanence that characterize life in today's cities have a direct relationship to safety. Nevertheless, an awareness of the dangers and potential hazards will enable you to make your home, whether it be in an apartment building or in a house, both more secure and more private.

A Good Lock

Begin at the beginning. Whenever you move into a new dwelling, replace all existing locks on doors and windows. A certified locksmith can advise you on the best locks for your particular doors and install them correctly. Dead or double bolts are a must; spring latches are easily opened by burglars.

A peephole in the front door gives you a look at whoever is standing outside. A sturdy chain is another efficient safety device, enabling you to receive small packages and sign delivery slips without opening the door completely. Use either or preferably both of these safety devices and never automatically open your door in response to the doorbell.

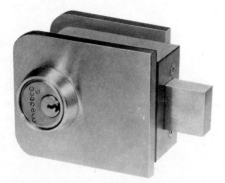

A deadlock (*above*), bolted by turning a key or a knob, is safer than a spring lock, which latches automatically as the door is closed.

Most newer apartments have intercom systems so that residents can avoid admitting any caller into the building itself until they know his identity. Be sure to use it; never admit anyone until he has responded through the intercom—even if you are expecting someone. Since houses do not have this device, a good, stout chain is a wise investment.

ADMITTING STRANGERS: Never admit any stranger into your apartment or house without proper credentials or identification, even if you have requested a visit from a washing-machine repairman, for example, or an upholsterer. If in doubt, telephone the company involved to confirm whether a representative has been sent to your home. Apartment dwellers should telephone the superintendent to check on workmen whose faces are unfamiliar.

LOST KEYS: The most effective lock system in the world, however, will do no good if you are careless with your keys. Don't put your name and address on your key ring. If you lose an unidentified set of keys there is less chance that a burglar will be able to trace them. But even without identification, lost keys are a potential danger; have your lock tumblers changed at once if keys are missing.

Avoid keeping house keys and car keys on the same ring, thus preventing a parking attendant from duplicating them while your car is parked in a lot or garage.

All windows on the ground floor and those that open onto fire escapes or other accessible areas should be protected with window locks or grilles. No grating should bar quick access to a fire escape, however. Check with your local fire department to find out what kind of gratings, if any, may be used.

SAFEGUARDING VALUABLES: Try not to draw attention to yourself by ostentatious display. If you own valuable paintings, antiques, or silver, don't advertise the fact. Keep any expensive small possessions such as jewelry, deeds, and stocks, in a safety deposit box.

Make a note of the serial numbers of all electrical appliances, typewriters, cameras, bicycles, etc., in your household, and keep this list in a safe place. It is especially important to have a record of all credit card numbers so that in case of loss or theft you can report the loss promptly. In the event of a burglary, the police have a better chance of returning your property if you can provide them with concrete identification.

When hiring cleaning women, baby sitters, or handymen, ask for references and check carefully to confirm the workers' honesty as well as their efficiency.

Vacations

Vacations and travel leave the vacant apartment or house especially vulnerable to burglary. Try to leave your house looking as lived-in as possible. Cancel newspaper and other deliveries before leaving and arrange to have a friend pick up mail and any circulars that may be left near the door. Don't broadcast details of a forthcoming vacation. Upon leaving, give your house a normal appearance by adjusting window blinds or shades at various levels; a house with all its windows covered is an announcement that no one is home.

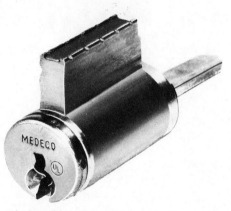

A lock tumbler. If your keys are lost, have your lock tumblers changed at once.

One good investment is an automatic timer that turns lights on and off at intervals each day in your absence.

Do inform a reliable friend about your trip so that he can keep an eye on your house. Vacationers have been known to return home only to find their house stripped of everything they own. Unless you tell someone otherwise, neighbors who notice the furniture being moved might assume that the burglars were legitimate moving men working under your orders.

Apartment dwellers should notify the superintendent of their forthcoming trip and make arrangements for him or an available friend to keep a set of keys in case something should go wrong while they are away. Water pipes might burst, fuses might blow, a gas line might spring a leak. Do make sure that your door will not be broken down for a minor problem because you forgot to make this simple arrangement before your departure.

Car Theft

If you own a car and live in the city, take precautions against automobile theft. On an average day in New York

City, 123 automobiles are reported stolen. It is a good idea to observe the following rules whenever possible:
- Don't park on dark streets or in deserted areas.
- Make it harder for someone to break in by always locking all doors and the trunk, upon leaving the car.
- Packages and clothing should not be left in plain view.

Many cars today are equipped with burglar alarm systems, but even these are no deterrent to a determined thief. The safest place to leave your car is in a reputable garage or parking lot. Always keep registration and insurance papers in the house or on your person, not in the glove compartment. If your car should be stolen, having them will simplify matters for you.

Safety Tips on Coping with Crime

Precautions for Women

Women who live in urban areas should take precautions regarding their personal safety. Become familiar with a neighborhood before walking through it at night. Avoid short cuts through deserted alleys and parks. Try not to place yourself in an isolated position. As a rule it is best not to enter an elevator if the only other occupant appears suspicious or odd in any way.

Should you suspect you are being followed, try to attract attention. Go into a store or restaurant. If there are no stores open and you are really frightened, ask a male passer-by who looks trustworthy to accompany you for as long as it takes to discourage the person or persons following you. If there are no passers-by, step out into the street and try to flag down a passing car. Familiarize yourself with the location of police call boxes along your accustomed route.

Street Crime

Whether you are a man or a woman, if you should be held up, the safest policy is to hand over your property and do as you are told. You have no way of knowing whether your assailant is armed, nor how ready he is to use violence. He may even have an accomplice nearby. What you *can* do is to observe your assailant as carefully as the circumstances allow. Note in particular any distinctive features of his appearance that might give the police clues for identification.

Purse snatching is, unfortunately, a fairly common city street crime. Women should keep a firm grip on their pocketbooks to foil the ordinary take-and-run purse snatcher—often a young boy or a group of boys. But they should never put up a struggle if the purse snatcher tries to use force. There is no sense in risking injury or disfigurement. Especially if you must be out alone at night, you might try to do without a pocketbook and carry your money in a pocket wallet or in a carryall that doesn't look as valuable as a purse.

Burglary

It is probable that a thief in your home wants to meet you even less than you want to meet him. Never enter your apartment or house if it looks as though someone has forced an entry. Call the police. But should you enter and then discover a stranger in your house, don't panic. Sudden movements or hysterical gestures could provoke him into attacking you.

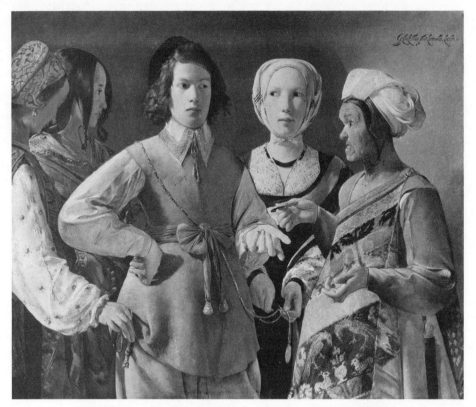

Pickpockets are hardly a creation of modern big cities—as this 17th-century painting by Georges de la Tour proves. Called *The Fortune Teller,* it shows the victim suspiciously accepting his change from an old crone while her accomplices pick his pockets and clip his gold chain.

Instructing Children

City children should be taught simple rules that help to insure their safety. Show them the best routes to take to and from school, the playground, and other frequented haunts. Don't let them carry any more money than is necessary. As a rule, children should be escorted when out in the streets after dark.

Teach your children, without terrifying them, to refuse rides or invitations from strangers, and to report any older person who loiters about near them. Know your children's schedules and be alert to any variation that might indicate trouble.

Pickpockets

Crowds are an inescapable part of the urban scene, and as a city dweller, you are constantly exposed to both the excitement and the dangers inherent in large groups. As people press about you on the streets, in stores, in buses, and in subways, be aware that pickpockets thrive in crowds, and don't let yourself become one of their victims.

Men should carry their wallets or money in an inside jacket pocket or a front trousers pocket. Women should bury their wallets deep in their handbags and be sure that the bag has a reliable clasp. Be suspicious of

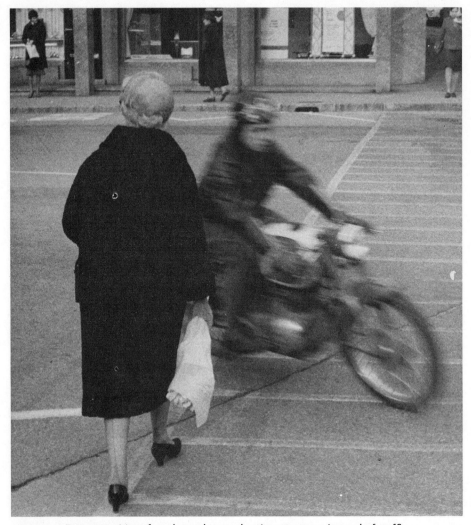

European cities often depend on pedestrian crossways instead of traffic
signals. Travelers abroad need to be especially alert to avoid accidents.

persons who brush up heavily against you, placing a hand on your shoulder to steady themselves. Pickpockets often work in groups of two; one bumps into you, and while you are distracted, the other picks your pocket.

Accidents

Impatient pedestrians are often tempted to jaywalk or rush pell-mell across the street even though the light is beginning to change. It is estimated that 7 out of 10 urban pedestrian deaths occurred while the victims were crossing or entering the street. Two-fifths of all these accidents happened between intersections. Allow yourself sufficient traveling time to avoid the carelessness that results from rushing.

Driving in city traffic can be nerve-wracking, but if you leave sufficient time for the trip you can at

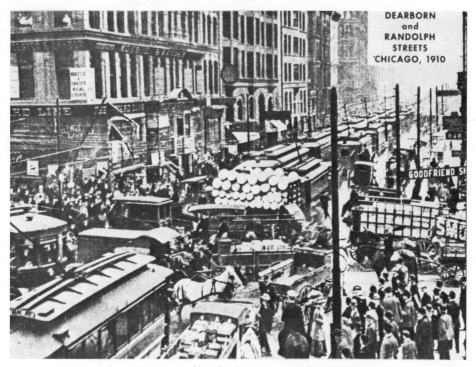

DEARBORN
and
RANDOLPH
STREETS
CHICAGO, 1910

If you think city traffic is bad now, you may be comforted
to know that it used to be even worse. Photo below is a
recent view of the same intersection pictured above.

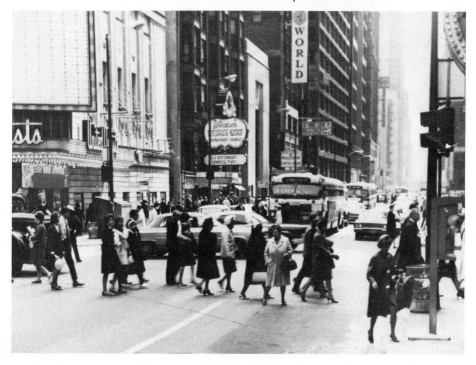

least grin and bear it. Try to keep your temper. Don't slam on the brakes, tailgate, or come to a stop on the crosswalks. Be on the alert for pedestrians, bicycles, and delivery carts that may suddenly seem to appear out of nowhere. The good driver is always prepared for the unexpected.

Elevators

Haste can work against you in other areas, too. It is haste that impels you to leap frantically into an elevator as the doors begin to close. Automatic elevators are equipped with devices that trigger the door to open as soon as an object intercepts an electric beam. But machines can malfunction, and the few seconds you may save by leaping into elevators will bring little satisfaction the day a coat or a hand gets caught in the door.

If you are in an elevator that loses power and stops between floors, or one in which the doors refuse to open, remain calm. Use the intercom system to summon help. If there is no intercom, look for the emergency button and ring it at regular intervals. If the button does not work, call out. Never attempt to leap to safety or crawl out of the top. Most elevators are adequately ventilated even if they seem stuffy, so don't let the fear of suffocation overcome you. You will be perfectly safe until an elevator repairman or the building superintendent comes to your assistance.

Never use the elevator in case of fire. Find the fire steps and walk down. No story is more tragic than that of people trapped in an elevator and asphyxiated by smoke after the power has failed.

Construction Accidents

Be especially careful while passing construction sites. A sponge dropped by a tenth-floor window-washer might not be dangerous, but a bucket is a different story. Ropes and cables lying on the sidewalk, planks with rusty nails, broken sidewalks—all are commonplace at construction sites, and all are hazardous. High winds can dislodge stray bricks and construction equipment from the upper stories of buildings being demolished. Watch where you are going and make detours when necessary.

Coping With "Characters"

Cities are famous for characters. On some days it may seem to you that there are really nothing *but* characters living in your city and that all of the ordinary everyday types have moved away. Loneliness contributes to the rather erratic behavior of some city dwellers. Bizarre behavior can also be the result of mental illness, or the misuse of drugs or alcohol.

If you are accosted by a person who does not appear mentally stable, try to extract yourself from the situation with as little fuss as possible. Many people who are mentally ill have the delusion that they are being persecuted and therefore may regard everyone around them with suspicion, fear, or open hostility. If you react with anger or abusive language, you will simply reinforce their delusions of persecution and are likely to increase their hostility. It is far better simply to walk away briskly, or move on while responding in a civil manner to the person's question or comment.

City residents are often accused of ignoring people in trouble. Do take a good look at any person who acts ill. The "drunk" slumped forward in his seat may be in a diabetic coma or may be suffering a heart attack. Make an effort to evaluate the situation properly and use good judgment.

SAFETY ON THE FARM

To a city dweller, the farm may seem a bucolic and tranquil place, but in fact agriculture ranks third among major industries in the number of accidental deaths each year. Because the farm worker is often long miles and precious minutes away from prompt medical aid, he should be aware of the hazards associated with his work, and take the necessary precautions to avoid them.

A thorough knowledge of first aid should be top priority. Local Red Cross chapters, 4-H Clubs, and other farm groups usually offer classes in emergency treatment for accidents. Make first aid kits standard equipment in all outbuildings and on farm

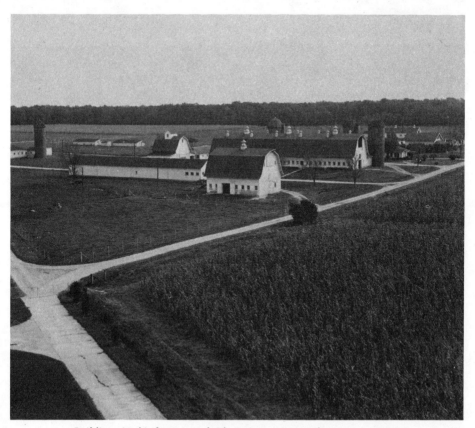

Buildings in this farm were laid out in a staggered pattern, not too close together. A fire in one building will not easily spread to others.

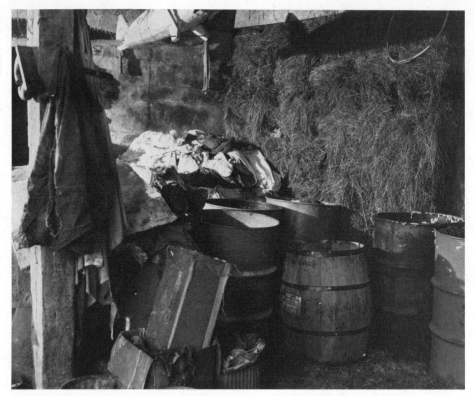

Accumulated rubbish is a common cause of fire on farms. Rubbish should be kept in metal-covered containers and removed regularly.

machines. Make yourself familiar with the more likely first-aid procedures. See *Medical Emergencies,* p. 1065.

Fire Prevention

Of all the dangers a farm dweller must look out for, perhaps the most disastrous is that of fire. Because of the quantity of combustible materials used on farms and the distance from professional fire-fighting equipment, effective fire prevention should be of vital concern to every rural dweller.

HAZARDS: The simplest way to avoid fire is to eliminate fire hazards. Some farm buildings are little more than fire traps, constructed of dry, easily combustible wood. Keep weeds and brush cleared away from buildings, and don't allow piles of old lumber and refuse to accumulate. Have all of your buildings equipped with well-grounded lightning rods. Check the wiring regularly and replace any that is worn.

With many farm vehicles to be fueled and crops to be sprayed, the farmer often has to keep a store of flammable liquids. They should be stored in a well-ventilated place away from any direct heat source. The door should be locked to keep children out. When bringing a vehicle into the area for refueling, be sure that the motor is shut off before beginning to pump. Take pains to avoid careless spills. Gasoline slicks and nearly empty containers are a potential hazard. It goes without saying that smoking should not be permitted in such areas. It's a good idea to post signs in no-smoking areas, and to provide buckets of sand or an ample supply of tin cans to encourage employees to cooperate.

FIRE-FIGHTING EQUIPMENT: All buildings and farm machinery should be equipped with fire extinguishers. Be sure that you have the proper kind of extinguisher for each area: a container filled with water will not help in a grease fire. The best type of fire extinguisher for tractors and similar equipment is the all-purpose dry chemical extinguisher. It is effective against all three major causes of fire—ordinary combustibles, flammable liquids, and electrical fires.

Your workers should be familiar with fire-fighting equipment and know what they are expected to do if fire breaks out. Family members should know escape routes in case of a house fire. Ladders or ropes should always be accessible to second-story dwellers.

Using Equipment Safely

Farm machinery is a major cause of accidental death. Tractors alone claim over a thousand deaths annually. Mangled fingers and hands are an all too common result of mishandling farm machinery, whether it be combine, corn picker, hay baler, chain saw, or mower. Make it a cardinal rule to turn off the motor before attempting to adjust or repair any piece of machinery.

Tractors

All tractors should be properly equipped with safety belts and overturn bars. An estimated 93 out of every 100 tractor fatalities could have been prevented had such equipment been employed. The overturn bar keeps the driver from being crushed while the seat belt holds him securely in place, protecting him from serious injury if the tractor should overturn.

Be on the alert for obstacles that could overturn your tractor. Don't

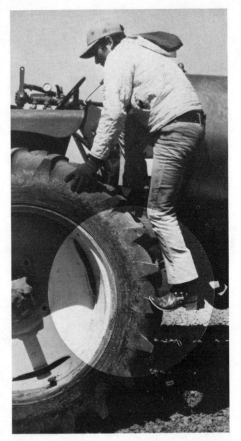

Always use the steps for mounting a tractor. Never climb up the lugs of a tire, which invites a fall, especially if the tire is wet.

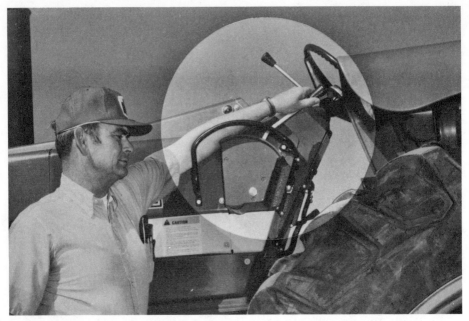

Never operate the hydrostatic drive from an off-the-seat position. Too much pressure on the lever and the machine may lurch and run over the operator.

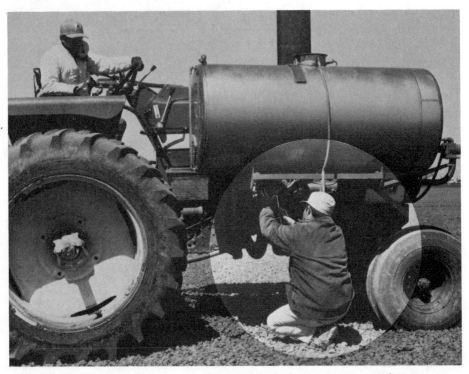

Don't get under a tractor to work on it while the engine is running. When changing a tire, block other wheels to keep the machine from moving.

speed through high grass or go racing home at dusk. Learn to use the right gear for each type of job and the proper speed for work safety. The PTO (Power-Take-Off) shield is put on for your protection. Always check to see that it is in place before starting your machine.

When using your tractor to pull loads on the public roads, make sure it is marked with a slow moving vehicle (SMV) sign across both front and back. In fact, use this sign for any slow vehicle you drive on public roads.

Wagons

When pulling a wagon, a safety hitch pin and safety chain should be used to keep the load from swerving into the path of an oncoming vehicle or rolling into a ditch. Never permit passengers to ride on your wagon on paved surfaces. Incidentally, when you are carrying passengers on the farm, signal them before starting up so that they have time to brace themselves, and once underway, don't speed up suddenly or slam on the brakes. Falls account for 60 percent of all wagon injuries.

Every farm machine comes with a manual that describes how to use it efficiently and how to care for it. Study the manual before attempting to work with your machine. Have someone who is familiar with the machine demonstrate its use, or, if possible, oversee your efforts to be sure that you are using it properly.

It's a wise precaution to teach all young children to stay away from

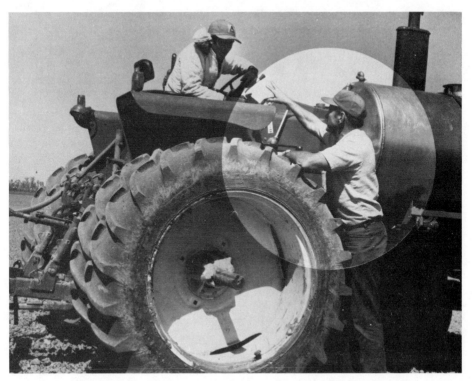

Never stand next to a tractor wheel to talk to a driver whose machine is running. If it lurched suddenly, you might be seriously hurt.

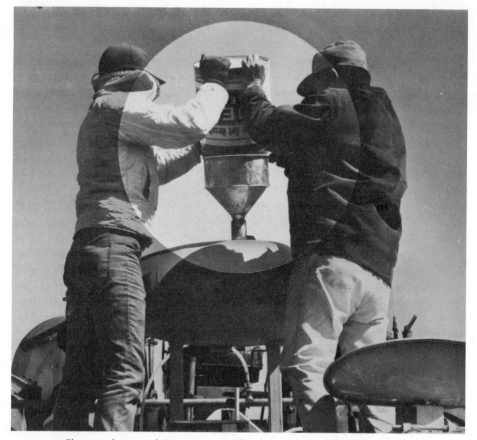

These workers are dumping a pesticide into a tank. Both should be wearing safety goggles, and the man at right should wear protective gloves.

farm equipment. Impress them with the fact that machines can be dangerous and are not to be used as playthings.

Rural Traffic Safety

Every year in the United States well over 1,000 people are killed at rural railroad-grade crossings, as contrasted with less than 500 in urban areas. Most of these deaths could have been prevented had the driver heeded the warning signs. Follow the rules for road safety, no matter how isolated your areas. Only one collision can end a life.

If your children travel to school by bus, check to see that the driver is qualified to drive a bus and that he is aware of all safety regulations regarding school buses. He should be especially careful when crossing railroad tracks. Make sure, too, that the buses themselves are kept in good repair.

Safe Use of Chemicals

Farmers employ a host of chemicals to spray crops, fertilize the soil, and check rodents. Safety precautions must be taken in the mixing and use of these products. Follow directions carefully, and protect the hands, eyes, and other exposed areas. Check spraying equipment before filling to insure that it is working properly. If the day is windy, postpone the spraying; the wind could blow the chemical into another field or even into your face.

As soon as you have finished using chemicals, wash your hands and face; change clothes before entering the house. Store the chemicals in their original containers so that they remain clearly labeled. If you put them in empty milk bottles or fruit juice cans, you might forget what they are at a later time, or a child may find the containers and harm himself. When disposing of empty containers, rinse them and break them up; bury them if possible. When burning paper containers, stand away from the smoke and make sure it is not carried into the vicinity of children or animals. Avoid inhaling pesticides or spraying them around food or water supplies or livestock.

Livestock

An animal that has always been friendly and gentle may be a different creature with newborn young. Farm workers and children should respect such protective instincts of animals and handle them as little as possible. Any breeding livestock, such as a dairy bull, should be handled only by highly experienced personnel, and should always be approached with caution.

Pens, fences, and loading areas must be kept sanitary and in good repair. Broken or splintered boards and protruding nails can cause nasty wounds to both humans and animals.

Animals Bites

Rabies

Rabies is a very real danger in rural areas. Such animals as skunks, foxes, and bats can become infected as well as cats and dogs. A staggering gait and glazed eyes are often symptoms of the disease. Do remember, however, that hot summer weather can cause many animals to drool and act drugged, and healthy dogs frequently foam at the mouth when they run in hot weather. The best rule of thumb is to have domestic animals inoculated against rabies and to avoid any animals behaving suspiciously.

If bitten or scratched by an animal that may be rabid, try to identify it so that it may be examined by a veterinarian. A series of rabies shots is required for anyone who has been bitten by a rabid animal. The sooner the shots are begun, the more effective they are. It is, therefore, of the greatest importance—quite possibly a matter of life or death—to seek medical advice *immediately* after being bitten by an animal suspected of being rabid. For further information about exposure to rabies, see *Animal bites*, p. 1089.

Snakebites

Farm residents should wear high, heavy boots when working in weeded areas or thick brush and should keep a snakebite kit close by in case of emergency. For recommended treatment of snakebites, see p. 1116. Since snakes are helpful in ridding the farm of vermin, it is worth your while to be able to distinguish between harmless and poisonous varieties instead of killing all snakes indiscriminately.

SAFETY ON THE HIGHWAY

Though it may not be categorized as such, the automobile is a deadly weapon. In its 75-year history in the United States, the automobile has taken nearly two million lives and crippled and injured millions of others. In a single July 4th weekend a few years ago, 609 people were killed and 28,000 were injured.

Causes of Accidents

Three out of every four people killed in automobile accidents are killed within five miles of their home, with over half of all wrecks taking place at speeds of less than 40 miles an hour. Perhaps people relax too much in familiar surroundings. Careless driving is no less dangerous on your home street than on the highway.

Driving and Drinking

The most critical aspect of automobile accidents today, however, is that of the drunken driver. Roughly one-half of all automobile fatalities in the United States are caused by drivers under the influence of alcohol. Drinking accounts for more than two-thirds of accidents involving a single car running off the road.

An individual whose blood contains 0.10 percent or more alcohol is legally intoxicated—driving under the influence of alcohol. Some authorities are convinced, however, that a blood-alcohol level of as little as 0.04 percent can be a contributing factor in accidents.

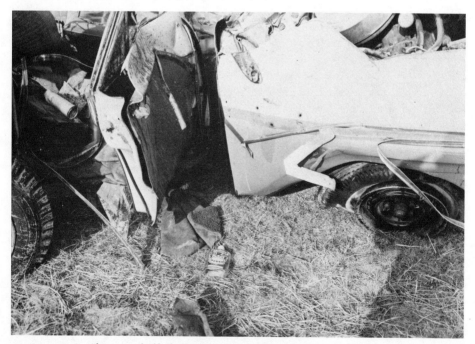

About one-half of all automobile fatalities in the United States are caused by drivers who are under the influence of alcohol.

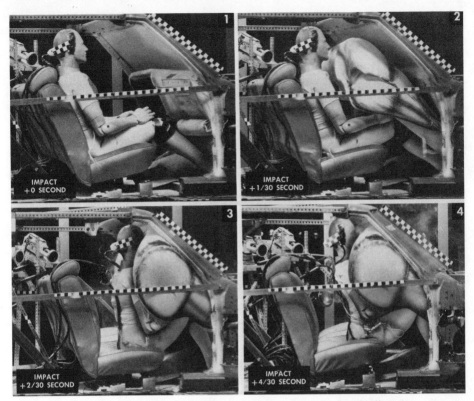

This series of photographs shows what happens in a simulated collision when the occupant is not wearing a seat belt. These tests were conducted to try out the air bag safety device—a bag that inflates instantaneously upon impact, thus protecting the occupant from serious injury.

In a typical driving crisis, three-fourths of a second pass before the driver reacts to the situation. Since alcohol, even in small amounts, depresses brain processes, precious instants are lost before the driver can respond.

The moral to the story is plain: do not drive when you have been drinking, and discourage other drinkers from taking the wheel. Drinking affects judgment; a drinker is certainly no judge of whether he is capable of driving. The feeling that one is different from other drinkers and in complete control is an illusion of a particularly dangerous kind. See also Ch. 31, p. 1022.

Driving and Drugs

Quantities of cold pills, pep pills, diet pills, and tranquilizers are consumed by millions of Americans every day. Any of these products can affect your driving performance. Antihistamines cause drowsiness. Amphetamines—often taken by long-distance truckers to keep them awake—can leave the user in a highly excited or nervous state. And when they suddenly wear off, the user is completely exhausted. See also Ch. 32, p. 1045.

Drugs taken to relieve circulatory problems or headaches also retard normal responses. It is best to con-

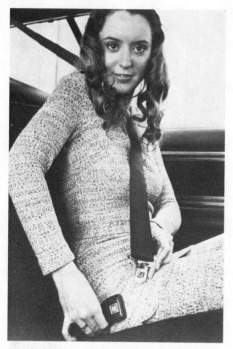

Seat belts do indeed save lives. Fatal injuries can occur even at low speeds, and seat belts can and do prevent them.

sult with your doctor when taking any type of medication, and follow his advice in regard to driving safety.

Avoiding Accident and Injury

Equipment failure is a major cause of accidents. Give your car a regular checkup just as you do your body. Brakes, of course, should be checked during regular servicing appointments and at the first sign of any irregularity. Tires, too, should be checked periodically and rotated when necessary. Always carry a good spare tire and the necessary equipment for changing a flat.

Seat Belts

Wear seat belts! Having seat belts in your car—and they are now considered standard safety equipment —does no good if they are not worn by the driver and each passenger. Research tests with actual cars crashed at varying speeds prove that seat belts do indeed save lives. In the event of a sudden stop, as in a collision, seat belts can keep you from flying out of the car or being crushed against the dashboard. Since a fatal injury can occur at 12 miles an hour as well as at 60, it is wise to use the seat belt every time you get into the car—even if it's just to go a few blocks to the supermarket. The shoulder belt provides even more protection and should also be worn.

An estimated 10,000 lives a year could be saved if only people would make a habit of fastening their seat belts. Moreover, the courts have actually denied personal injury judgments to people involved in wrecks who were not wearing their safety belts.

Emergencies

The careful driver, although relaxed, is always alert to the possibility of the unexpected. Although it may never happen to you, an emergency calls for an instantaneous response. It is wise, under these circumstances, to know beforehand what to do in certain hazardous situations.

BLOWOUTS: In the event of a blowout, take your foot off the gas and try to keep a firm grip on the wheel. Slow down gradually and come to a stop, getting your car off the road if you can. Sudden braking may make the car swerve into oncoming traffic.

SKIDS: Should your car go into a skid, turn the wheels in the direction of the skid, if possible, until you feel the tires grip the road again. Whatever you do, don't turn the wheel sharply in the opposite direction; that can turn the car over.

The best way to come out of a skid is never to get in one. Heed signs that warn of dangerous driving conditions. Use snow tires in winter weather. Drive at a speed that takes into consideration road conditions and visibility. If you observe these basic precautions, you will keep your car on the road with you in control.

SAFETY ON A BICYCLE OR SKATEBOARD

Bicycling, long a popular pastime and means of transportation for children and teenagers, has in recent years experienced a phenomenal growth in popularity among adults. Many factors have contributed to this bicycle boom: high gasoline prices, awareness of the environmental damage caused by automobiles, appreciation of the inexpensive and healthful exercise cycling provides.

Against the health and environmental benefits of cycling, however, must be set a rising rate of bicycle accidents, a number of them involving fatalities. While most victims of bike accidents are children between the ages of 5 and 14, the accident rate for adult riders has been rising steadily in recent years. A knowledge and application of the basic rules for safe cycling could have prevented many of these accidents.

Maintaining a Safe Bicycle

Bicycle safety begins with a machine that is in good working order, fitted to the individual rider, and outfitted with the proper safety devices. Before you buy a bike for yourself or another member of the family, you should take into account the purposes for which the bike will be used

(recreation, transportation to school or work, long-distance travel), the amount of traffic in the neighborhood, and the proficiency of the rider.

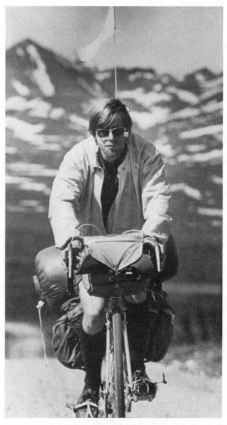

A bicycle designed for long-distance travel must have features other than those in a bike used for short trips or recreation.

The Right Bike for You

Most adults will find a lightweight bike suitable for their needs. A three-speed model should prove serviceable for recreation, errands, and short-distance commuting. Cyclists who are interested in long-distance touring or competitive racing, or who plan to do a great deal of riding in hilly terrain, may want to invest in one of the more expensive ten-speed models, with gears that can be adjusted to fit varying road conditions and gradients. (Avoid bikes with the gear shift located directly in front of the saddle; they can cause serious injury in the event of a sudden stop or spill.)

BUYING A CHILD'S BIKE: For a child who is just learning to ride, a middle-weight bike is easier to control; as he develops skill and confidence, he can graduate to the faster and more maneuverable lightweight model. Since many young children do not have a strong enough grip to operate a hand brake properly, a first bike should be equipped with coaster brakes instead of, or in addition to, a hand brake.

"Banana seats" have a backrest or riser which makes stunt riding easier by allowing the rider to shift his weight backward and lift the front wheel off the ground. Such riding is extremely dangerous; parents would do well to discourage their children from attempting such stunts. Bikes with risers also make it difficult for a rider to dismount quickly in an emergency; although these bikes may be more attractive to children, parents should weigh these safety factors before buying them.

Buying a bike that's too large for a child, in the expectation that he'll "grow into it," is both foolish and dangerous. It's better to replace an outgrown bike after a year or two than to risk an accident on a bike too big for a child to handle safely.

HOW TO MAKE SURE YOUR BIKE FITS YOU: When buying a bike, take time to make sure that it fits your physical proportions (or can be easily adjusted to fit). This extra care will pay you important dividends in riding comfort and safety.

The following simple tests will help you gauge the proper fit of your bike. They apply to all types of adults' and children's bicycles except track racing models.

1. Stand astride the bike in front of the saddle with both feet flat on the ground. Your body should clear the top of the frame by at least a half inch.

2. Sitting on the saddle, place one foot on the pedal in the lowest position. You should be able to extend your leg fully without stretching or shifting your position.

3. Bending your upper body forward, grip the handlebars. Your arms should be almost straight, with elbows relaxed.

If the saddle or handlebars are not comfortable for you, they can easily be adjusted. A child's bike will probably need frequent adjustment as he grows, anyway. Remember, when adjusting saddle height, to leave at least 2½ inches of the seat post in the frame.

Preventive Bike Maintenance

In order to keep your bike in top riding condition, you should have it inspected and overhauled by a competent mechanic twice a year. Pedals and handlebar grips should be replaced when they show signs of wear.

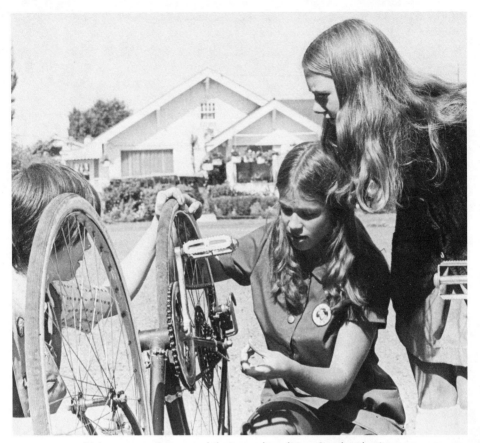

It's important to keep your bike in good condition. See that the tires
are properly inflated and repair leaks as soon as they develop.

Even if you're not very mechani-cally minded, you can keep your bike in good condition by perform-ing a few simple maintenance tasks each month.

Lubricate front and rear wheel hubs with a few drops of lightweight oil or grease. Lubricate brake and shift cables, and pivotal points of hand brakes, with a few drops of lightweight oil. Use medium-weight oil to lubricate pedals at each end; use only a few drops. Remove the chain, soak it in solvent, then in lightweight oil, drain, and reinstall. (Remember to use the solvent in a well-ventilated room or, if possible,

outdoors.) Finally, clean the saddle with warm water and soap.

Wipe off the metal parts of the bike with a damp cloth whenever they become soiled. Polishing these parts with auto wax every few weeks will keep them shiny and prevent rust.

KINDS OF TIRES: Children's bikes, and the less expensive adult models, are equipped with clincher tires. They are sturdy and relatively easy to repair, since the inner tube can easily be detached from the tire.

Tubular tires are lighter and more vulnerable to blowouts and punc-tures. They are used on the more ex-pensive touring and racing bikes, since they permit greater speeds. Because of its light weight and flexibility, a tubular tire can be folded and carried in the basket or under the saddle as a spare.

Some cyclists who use their bikes both for city riding and for cross-country touring have interchangeable sets of wheels, one with clincher tires and one with tubular tires.

CARE OF TIRES: Bicycle tires should be kept inflated to the correct pressure (usually printed on the sidewall). A hand pump is best, since the air pumps at most service stations are designed for automobile tires and can blow out bicycle tires with a sudden surge of pressure.

Many variables affect the condition of your tires. If you're riding with a heavier than normal load, the tires should be inflated to a slightly higher pressure than usual. It may be necessary to let a little air out of the tires periodically in very hot weather, since heated air expands. Tubular tires will need to be inflated more often than the clincher type, since their porous walls allow air to escape gradually.

Inexpensive puncture-repair kits are available at hardware and sporting-goods stores. It's a good idea to carry one of these kits whenever you go on a long bike ride far from repair shops.

Safety Equipment

There are many devices designed to make a bike more easily visible and audible to motorists. Some of these, such as a headlamp visible from 500 feet at night, a rear reflector visible from 300 feet, and a horn or bell, are mandatory in many states. Check with your state highway department for safety equipment regulations in your state.

Strips of reflecting tape can be applied to the metal parts of your bike to increase night visibility. A bright-colored pennant on a long pole can be attached to the rear of a bike to alert drivers at a distance in traffic.

Safety Programs

Many communities sponsor annual or semiannual bike safety days,

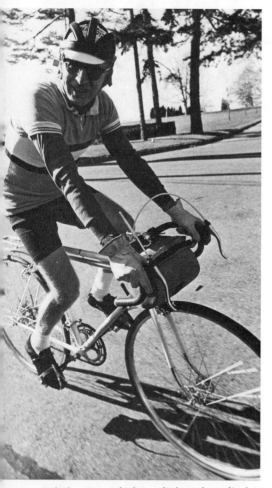

Tubular tires, which are lighter than clincher tires, are used for racing bikes or for long-distance travel.

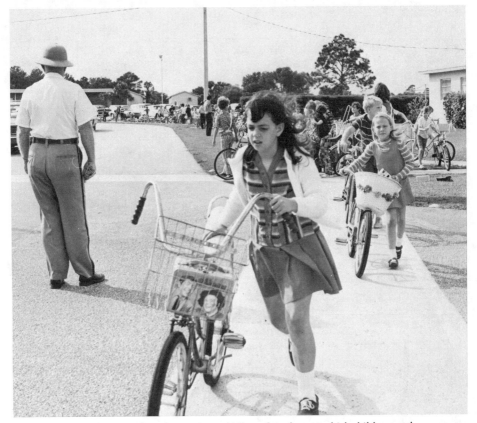

Many communities sponsor annual bike safety days at which children and adults can have their bikes inspected for proper fit and maintenance.

at which children and adults can have their bikes inspected for proper fit and maintenance, and test their riding skills and knowledge of safety rules. These programs are often combined with a campaign to register bikes with the local police department as a deterrent to bicycle theft.

Dressing Safely for Cycling

Cycling is an easygoing, informal kind of recreation that requires no special clothing. However, the following pointers should increase your comfort and safety while cycling.

Wear clothing that is loose enough to be comfortable, but not so loose as to be a safety hazard. Long trailing scarves and billowy skirts that could catch on pedals or in spokes, or be snagged by stationary objects such as trees and cars, should be avoided.

Shorts are comfortable in hot weather, but give little protection against abrasions in the event of a spill. It's better to wear long pants when riding on hard surfaces. Trousers that are very long or wide at the bottom should be rolled up or fastened securely around the ankles with bicycle clips.

In cold weather, several layers of sweaters topped by a lightweight

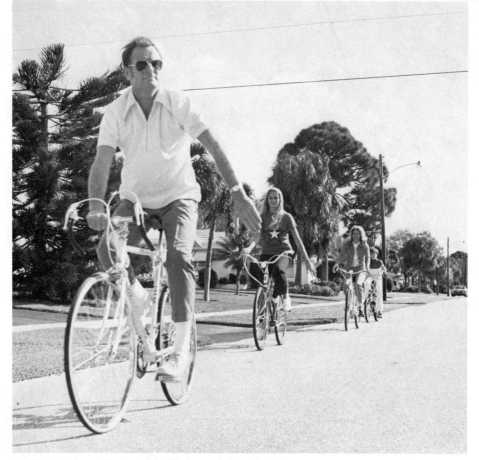

Wear comfortably loose clothing for biking, but not so loose
as to get snagged in the spokes or caught in the pedals.

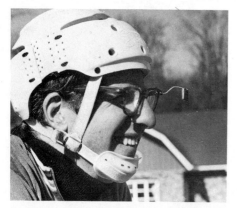

Anyone doing a lot of cycling in city traffic
should consider getting a protective helmet
with a rear-view mirror.

parka are safer and more comfortable
than a long, heavy coat. Shoes should
have low heels or none. Rubber and
crepe soles grip the pedals best.
Gloves should be flexible enough to
permit clear hand signals and easy
operation of the hand brake. Leather
palms provide a firm grip on the
handlebars. Hats and scarves should
not interfere with the rider's side vision. For night riding, jackets with
reflector strips or patches are available in clothing and sporting-goods
stores. Reflectorized tapes can also
be sewn onto clothing.

Rules of the Road

Too many cyclists think of themselves, when riding a bike, simply as speedier pedestrians, with a pedestrian's flexibility—free to travel two and three abreast, move on and off sidewalks at will, and dart across intersections against the light. Actually, a bicycle is a vehicle (legally defined as such in all states), although it is not motorized. A bicycle rider should observe the same rules of the road as those followed by motorists, plus a few others designed to guard against the special hazards of cycling.

Obey all traffic regulations—stop signs, one-way streets, traffic lights, etc. Keep right, riding with traffic, not against it. Ride single file and in a straight line. Use proper hand signals for turning or stopping; signal a half block in advance. Slow down at all intersections. Look both ways and proceed with caution. At very busy intersections, with cars turning in several directions, get off and walk your bike across.

Always give pedestrians the right of way. Keep off sidewalks, unless road traffic is very heavy and pedestrian traffic very light. (Parents of small children should exercise discretion in letting them ride on the sidewalk in areas where there is road traffic.)

Watch for cars pulling into traffic and for car doors opening on the street side. Don't carry passengers,

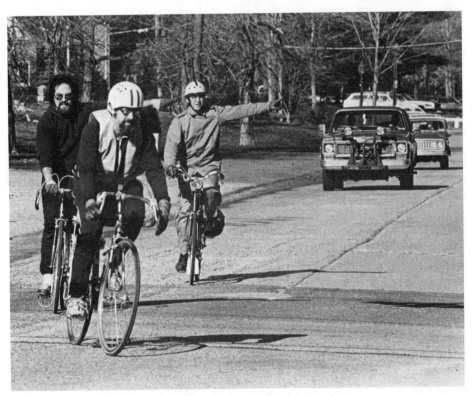

Bicyclists should observe the same rules of the road as motorists, including signaling when they are about to make a turn.

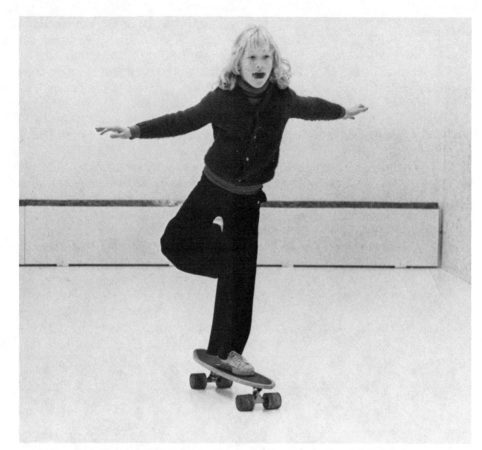

Skateboarding is fun, but it can also be dangerous. Over 27,000 skateboarding injuries were treated in hospitals in the U.S. in one recent year.

or packages that interfere with vision or control. Never "hitch a ride" on a bus or any other vehicle.

BE ALERT TO THE UNEXPECTED: Safe cycling requires constant alertness to road and traffic conditions. Even on roads with light traffic, the cyclist should always be watching the road several feet ahead for possible hazards. These include potholes, sewer gratings, loose sand and gravel, broken glass, and oil slicks. A cyclist should also listen carefully to the sounds of street traffic so that he can react quickly to such situations as a car pulling into traffic behind him or stopping suddenly ahead.

Guarding Your Bike Against Theft

Along with the growing popularity of bicycles in recent years has come, unfortunately, a corresponding sharp increase in the number of bicycle thefts. Expensive ten-speed and racing models are especially attractive to thieves.

A few precautions will help reduce the possibility of your bike being stolen, or aid in recovering it if it is.

CHAIN IT: Never leave your bike unattended, even for a few minutes, without locking it to a sturdy stationary object. Use a heavy-duty, case-hardened chain and lock with a shackle at least ³/₈ inch in diameter. Run the chain through both wheels and the frame before locking.

Leave your bike locked in a conspicuous, well-lighted place where any tampering with it will be noticed by passers-by. Never leave it outdoors overnight. If your bike is equipped with quick-release hubs, remove the front wheel and take it with you, if possible.

KEEP RECORDS: Record your bike's serial number (found on the head tube under the manufacturer's name). If your community has a bicycle registration program, register the number with the local police. Have your bike marked with your Social Security number or other identifying number. Take a color photograph of your bike to aid the police in identifying it.

Skateboard Safety

Skateboarding, which had a brief flurry of popularity in the 1960s, entered a new phase in the mid-70s. The new boards featured polyurethane wheels mounted on axles which permitted the rider to change direction simply by shifting his weight. As millions of youngsters— and some grown-ups, too—have found, skateboarding is fun. The balance, coordination, and dexterity that skateboarding requires are skills to be encouraged. But if not properly used, a skateboard, like a bicycle, can be dangerous.

The hazards of skateboarding are illustrated by the fact that over 27,000 skateboarding injuries were treated in hospital emergency rooms across the U.S. in one recent year. One of the most common injuries in

this sport is fracture of the tip of the elbow, which doctors have come to call "skateboarder's elbow."

Children and teen-agers who zoom along or do stunts on crowded sidewalks endanger not only themselves, but pedestrians as well. Beginners should practice on level ground before trying to negotiate a slope, and they should find a place away from pedestrians.

Safe Skateboarding Equipment

Parents can help protect their children against serious skateboarding injuries by making sure that a child's board is sturdy, well maintained, and suited to his age and skill. Beginning skateboarders may feel more secure on a fairly wide board, which makes balancing easier.

WHEELS: Wheels should be made of rough-surfaced polyurethane. They should be properly aligned and spin freely. If wheels become stiff, squirt a little powdered graphite into the ball bearings. Never use oil; it will only collect dirt and make matters worse, and if any gets on polyurethane wheels it will disintegrate them.

TRUCKS: The "trucks" which attach the wheels to the board should be cast iron, and should be bolted all the way through the board. They should be loose enough to permit the board to turn easily. They can and should be adjusted according to the weight and skill of the rider.

Avoid cheap plastic skateboards, which can break. The safest boards are made of fiberglass, aluminum, or Lucite.

There's probably no way to prevent a youngster from attempting stunts once he feels confident, but if possible, have him wear a helmet and knee and elbow pads. These can minimize otherwise serious accidents.

Safe Places for Skateboarding

Skateboarding should be permitted only on streets with light traffic, and on sidewalks little used by pedestrians. Better still is a neighborhood area set aside exclusively for skateboarding—a section of a town park or playground, or a school parking lot after hours and on weekends. Parents should contact local government officials and park departments about establishing such a skateboard zone.

SAFETY IN A BOAT

Boating is one of the most popular recreation sports in the United States today. It provides an escape from the everyday, a chance to skim about in the sunshine and fresh air in attractive surroundings. One can go to lovely remote places for picnics or swimming or use the boat for water sports such as skiing. Once the cost of a boat was prohibitive, but now millions of families can afford one; and, even if no body of water is nearby, it is an easy matter to transport the boat to a suitable area.

Basic Information

Perhaps feeling that there is safety in numbers, many boat owners do not bother to inform themselves about either the mechanical functions of their boats or the various safety rules that apply to boating. Yet there are certain basic facts about safety that every boat owner should know in order to protect himself and his family from converting a carefree outing into a grim disaster.

Buying a Boat

Before buying a boat you should answer these questions: What is the boat to be used for? How many people are going to be using it? Where will the boat be used? What are the facilities for repairing and servicing it? Is your family car big enough to haul it? What are the maintenance costs likely to be?

The first thing the new owner should do is familiarize himself with the workings of his craft. The boat salesman should be able to explain some of the boat's practical points. In the case of a motorboat or sailboat with auxiliary motor, he should tell you how much fuel it holds and help you calculate how far one can go with it at what speeds. He can also give an idea of how the boat is expected to perform. For example, a 14-foot outboard motorboat cannot be expected to take four large people for a ride at the same time briskly tow water skiers.

But such advice is merely the beginning. Classes given by a local boating club, a Coast Guard Auxiliary group, or a similar organization are a must for any inexperienced boat owner. There you can receive expert instruction on right of way, boating signals, the meaning of various types of buoys, management of

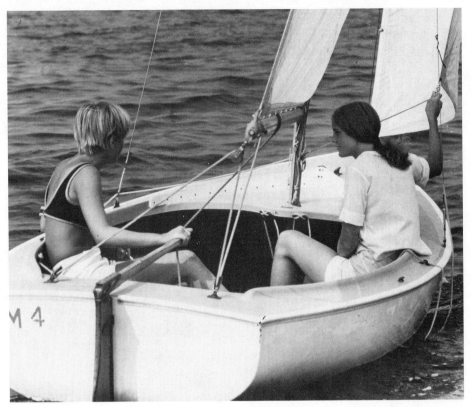

With the availability of inexpensive sailing and motor craft, boating has become an increasingly popular pastime in all parts of the country.

the boat in rough water, and many other details which will make you a confident skipper instead of a Sunday driver.

Safety Equipment

All boats should carry the following safety equipment: lifesaving devices (one per person, in the proper size for each passenger), compass, first-aid kit, flashlight, distress signal, fire extinguisher, oars, small tools, some sort of bailing device, and anchor and cable. This may seem like a lengthy list, but each of these items is essential. Most will fit neatly into a small waterproof box. Oars and larger equipment can be stored along the sides of the boat.

Swimming Safety

Since the greatest danger when boating is that of drowning, the best thing you can do for your family is insure that they are all good swimmers. Various organizations such as the American Red Cross and the YMCA offer classes in swimming and lifesaving techniques for nominal sums. Knowing that everyone in your family can swim eliminates much of the worry in boating.

Even though all of your passengers are swimmers, you should be on the alert for possible dangers. If you are swimming in an unfamiliar area, be careful about diving deep beneath the surface. Submerged

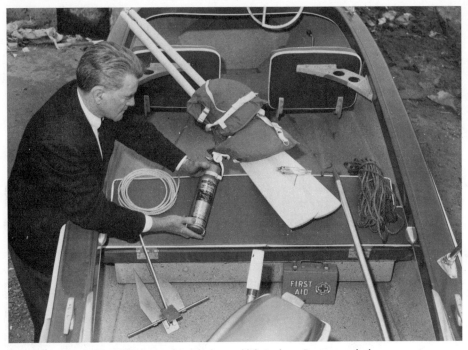

Every boat must have lights and life jackets. Recommended
are a fire extinguisher, oars, a whistle to signal for help,
a boathook, extra line, an anchor, and a first-aid kit.

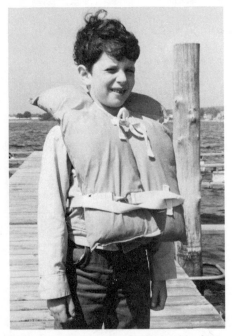

Young guests on water craft should always
wear life jackets even if they can swim.

branches, wires, or weeds can catch a swimmer's arms or legs and hold him beneath the surface. If boating in bays and sea areas, keep an eye out for undertows and dangerous tides.

The buddy system, though it may bring back memories of childhood summer camps, is still the best way to insure that each swimmer is looking out for and being watched by another. In large parties of swimmers, one person can disappear and his absence not be noted for some time. With the buddy system, this risk is minimized.

CRAMPS: Contrary to popular opinion, swimming after a meal is no guarantee that you will get swimmer's cramp. Nevertheless, any violent exertion immediately after a meal is apt to cause digestive difficulty. No one should swim when tired or chilled, when muscle cramps *are* likely to occur.

SUNBURN: Reflection makes the sun's rays more intense on the water than they are on land. Be careful about sunburn, wear a hat, and use a protective cream or oil on the most exposed skin areas.

Drowning

Anyone attempting to rescue a distressed swimmer who is far away from shore should have the proper training and credentials for doing so. Too many double deaths have oc-

curred because of good intentions and inadequate skill.

RESCUE: A child or adult who appears to be drowning near shore, or near a boat from which he has fallen, can be rescued even by someone who can't swim. The rescuer can lie prone and extend his hand or foot, or he can extend the longest available pole or branch or an oar to pull the bather to safety.

If the swimmer is too far from shore to be reached in this way, a ring buoy attached to a long rope can be tossed in his direction. If a rowboat is available, row to the victim as

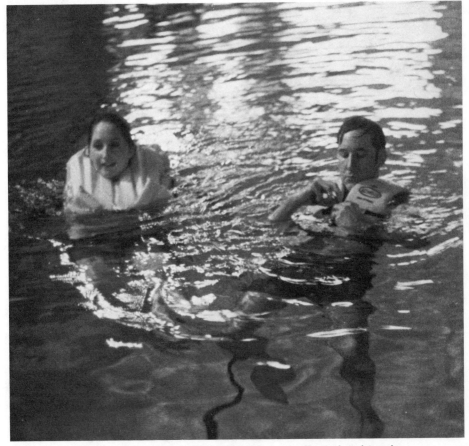

This picture demonstrates how life jackets work effectively to keep the head well above the water. Every boat should be equipped with them.

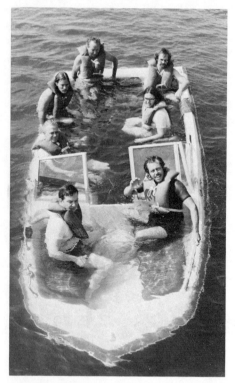

A new level flotation standard now required of outboard boats means that they must float level when swamped, as seen here.

quickly as possible and extend an oar that will bring him around to the stern so that he can hang on while being brought to shore.

EMERGENCY TREATMENT: If normal breathing has been impaired, administer mouth-to-mouth respiration, described on p. 1066, at once.

PREVENTION: Drowning is one of the major causes of accidental death. As in many major accidents, the chief contributing factor is poor judgment.

Boating Sports

WATER SKIING: When practicing sports such as water skiing, the skier should wear a life jacket. It may not flatter the figure, but it will keep him floating should he fall and strike his head or be injured. Avoid exercising strenuously for too long a period; fatigue makes you much more susceptible to accident.

Don't ever use your boat for showing off. One young man, bent on im-

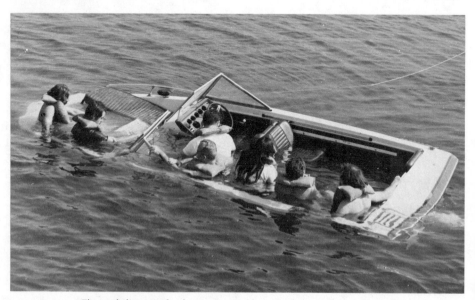

The stability test for boats is met when the boat will not capsize with all passengers on one side, even when the boat is swamped.

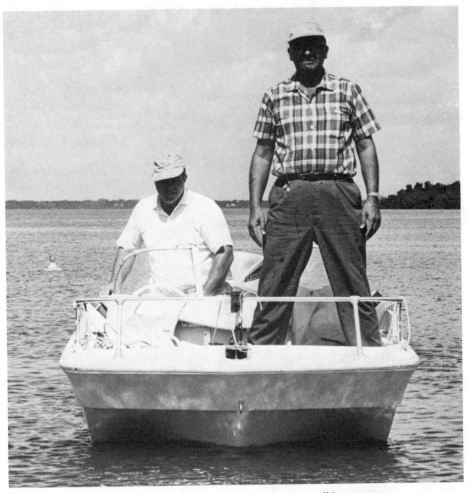

Don't stand up in a small boat. Standing up in a small boat may capsize it, and a shift in speed or direction could send this man overboard.

pressing onlookers on a nearby dock, was performing various turns at a high speed while sitting casually on the edge of his craft when he slipped and fell overboard. The boat, left running at full speed, headed straight into the dock and smashed to pieces. In a sense, this man was lucky. Normally an unattended boat running with open throttle will circle. Many people who have fallen overboard have been run down and killed by the propeller of their own boat.

FISHING: Fishing, the most popular boating activity, may look tame in comparison with water skiing, but it is fishing that accounts for over 55 percent of all boating accidents. In the excitement of the catch, fishermen sometimes simply forget where they are, and may leap to their feet, lose their balance as the boat lists sharply, and fall into the water or swamp the boat.

When fishing, watch where you are going. While searching for a likely fishing hole, you might run the

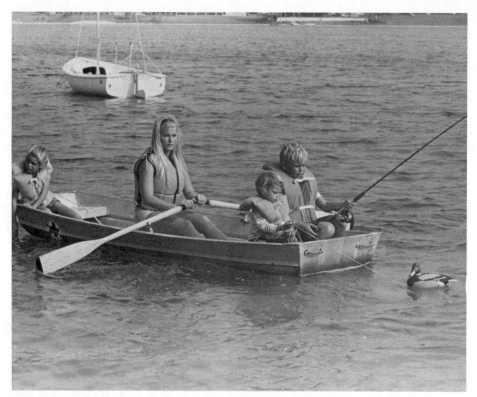

Landing a fish can be exciting, but it should not make anyone forget that
he is on a boat and that basic boating safety rules must be observed.

boat into the bank or onto a partially submerged log or sandbank. Lines can become tangled in underwater obstacles or overhanging trees. Keep your temper; don't jerk your line about and run the risk of hooking a companion or yourself.

Fishing is a sport that fluctuates between moments of tranquillity and moments of intense excitement. Never permit yourself to become so distracted you forget you are in a boat, not on land, and that the basic rules of boating safety must prevail at all times.

Emergencies

FIRE: Two serious hazards that may occur when boating are fires and passengers falling overboard. If a fire breaks out on your boat and there is danger of an explosion, get away from the boat. If there is no immediate danger of explosion and the fire can be checked, head the boat into the wind so the flames will flow away from the cockpit, and use your fire extinguisher. If possible, throw the burning material overboard.

MAN OVERBOARD: If a passenger falls overboard, the driver's first thought should be to keep the propeller away from him. Throw him a life jacket. Even if the man overboard can swim, he may be stunned or dizzy from his fall. If you are the only person in the boat, be especially careful while helping him aboard or you may fall out too, and there won't be anyone around to help.

MOST LIKELY ACCIDENTS BY AGE

According to statistics gathered by the National Safety Council, accidents are the leading cause of death among all persons aged 1 to 37. They are the fourth leading cause of death among persons of all ages.

Unsettling as these figures are, they scarcely account for the even greater number of nonfatal accidents that result in major disabilities, not to mention the mishaps that necessitate hospital and medical care as well as absence from work or school. It is calculated that in a recent year the cost of accidents to the nation in terms of wage loss, medical fees, insurance settlements, and property damage amounted to more than 22 billion dollars.

Infancy to 4 years

Although it used to be thought that suffocation was a leading cause of death in infancy, it is now believed that such fatalities are generally the result of a sudden overwhelming infection that has nothing to do with being smothered by blankets. In the group of young children from one to four, most accidental deaths are caused by motor vehicles. Taking this into account, it is important that families with very young children see to it that they are never left to play alone on city streets, and that adequate fencing—as well as firm instruction—prevents them from playing on roads and highways.

For children in this age group, the second leading cause of accidental death is fire, as a result of being trapped in a burning building, often because they have been left alone "for just a few minutes." Drowning ranks third, and usually occurs not at beaches or in pools, but at some place close to home, such as a nearby brook, pond, or well.

Poisoning is another major cause of accidental death in very young children, as is suffocation from the blockage of respiration by a foreign object or by food swallowed "the wrong way."

From 5 to 9 years

As children get a little older, they may learn to become more careful, but they are also likely to be bolder

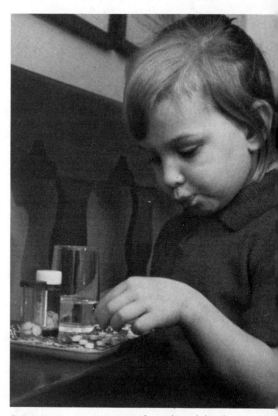

Poisoning is a major cause of accidental death in young children. Flavored medicines, which are taken for candy, are especially dangerous.

and more experimental. From five to nine, the chief cause of accidental death is still the motor vehicle, followed by drownings. The third factor in fatalities is fire. Fewer children die of poisoning during these years since they are less inclined to put everything they see into their mouths.

From 10 to 14 Years

As children approach adolescence, the motor vehicle is still the main cause of fatal accidents, not only in pedestrian fatalities but also in smashups involving young passengers. Drownings are the next cause, and firearms the third. Deaths caused by gunshot usually occur because of parental carelessness in matters of storing weapons or supervising their use.

Nonfatal Accidents to Children

The most common injuries sustained by children at home are usually the result of cuts and falls. In accidents involving falls, the part of the body most often affected is the head, and in decreasing frequency, the hand and fingers, the shoulder and arm, and the legs.

Fire, suffocation, and poisoning are ever-present dangers to children at home, and they should never be left unattended. The presence of a baby sitter, whether it is a neighbor who agrees to be on hand for half an hour or a teen-ager who will be paid for a whole evening, is absolutely essential when parents are away. Baby sitters should be briefed on how to handle various emergencies and how to reach help if necessary.

Teen-Agers

Motor vehicles, drownings, and firearms are the chief causes of fatal accidents in adolescence. Both major and minor injuries are also likely to occur during participation in athletic activities. These are also the years when experimenting with drugs and alcohol can have disastrous consequences.

Young Adults

According to the National Safety Council, the largest number of fatalities involving motor vehicles occurs in the age group from 15 to 24—in a recent year almost 16,000 deaths. The figures for similar fatalities during the same year for other age groups are approximately 13,000 for people from 25 to 44, and approximately 11,000 for those from 45 to 64. It is also significant that there are three times as many accidental deaths from all causes in the age group from 15 to 24 as in the group from 5 to 14: over 21,000 in the older group as compared to over 7,000 in the younger one.

From 25 to 44 Years

In this age group, motor vehicles account for 12 times as many fatalities as those caused by drowning, falls, or fire. This is a period when men are likely to have a high rate of major or minor accidents on the job, and when women have serious or lesser mishaps at home while cleaning or cooking. Also, excessive use of alcohol begins to be an important factor not only in deaths from motor vehicle accidents, but also in serious injuries resulting from falls.

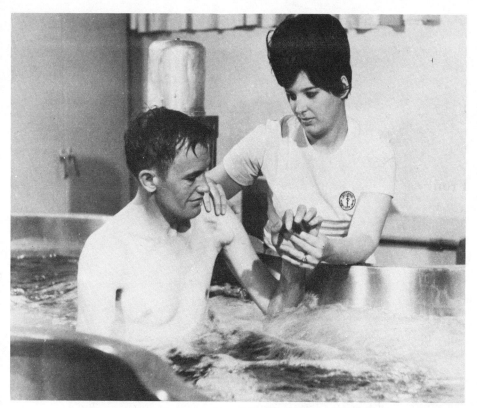

A physical therapist works with a victim of an industrial accident in a Hubbard tank to restore the use of his shoulder and arm muscles.

From 45 to 74 Years

Although motor vehicles account for the largest number of accidental deaths in the group from 45 to 64, their number is lower than for the preceding age group, and the number of deaths because of falls is higher. Fires and drowning are the next most significant causes of fatalities. In the decade from age 64 to 74, these figures remain about the same.

75 Years and Over

The major cause of accidental death for the old is falling. It is with this age group that motor vehicles are no longer the major hazard, as can be seen from the following figures: at 75 years and older, the number of deaths reported in a recent year because of falls was about 11,500, and because of motor vehicles, about 3,200. It should be obvious that in families that include an aging member, accident-proofing the home against falls must be considered the same kind of special problem and have as high a priority as making the home safe would have in the case of a very young child.

An awareness of the chief causes of fatal or serious accidents should make everyone more vigilant about safety—in the home, on the road, or on vacation.

CHAPTER 35

Physical Fitness

One of the most important health studies of our time was started by the National Institutes of Health back in 1949. The population of an entire community was put under continuous scrutiny by a team of doctors who recorded the daily habits of thousands of men and women. For more than a quarter of a century, the citizens of Framingham, Massachusetts, have been observed at work, at play, and in the home. They have been measured and weighed repeatedly, their food analyzed, their cigarettes counted, blood pressure checked, and so on, without interfering with the normal life styles of the individuals.

The Framingham Study

Results of the Framingham Study of a generation of a typical American community reveal certain links between a way of life and the most common cause of death, which is cardiovascular disease. The links were found to be too many calories, mainly in the form of saturated fats and sugar, too many cigarettes, and too little exercise. Dr. William B. Kannel, Medical Director of the Framingham Study and a member of the Harvard Medical School faculty, reported that the most sedentary, or least active, men had about three times the heart attack risk as the most physically active. The rate of risk of cardiovascular disease seemed to be generally proportional to the degree of obesity, resulting from too many calories. The use of cigarettes was found to be associated with all manifestations of cardiovascular disease. One other link, which is still being explored, is high blood pressure.

The Framingham Study of the adult lives of some 5,000 subjects confirms what most doctors have suspected for many years—that

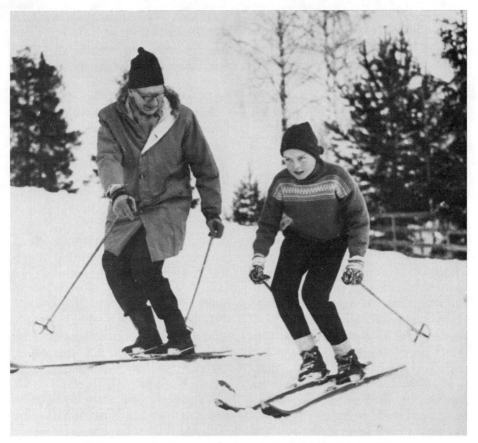

Outdoor exercise is especially important during the winter. This father and son have found an enjoyable winter recreation in skiing.

physical activity helps counteract the effects of overweight, diets rich in fats and sugar, blood pressure, and similar factors. Dr. Kannel's report added another explanation: physical exercise probably helps extend the life and health of even those people with cardiovascular disease by developing collateral circulation. In other words, a person who might otherwise develop heart trouble because of a diminished blood supply in his coronary arteries can forestall that threat to his life by physical exercise which promotes the increased flow of blood through alternate blood vessels.

There is a valuable lesson in the Framingham Study for every reader of this book: daily exercise, which requires no greater investment than a more efficient use of free time, can extend your life and retard certain organic diseases of the heart and blood vessels—diseases that account for more than half of the "natural" deaths in America each year.

Winter Exercise

If you are a typical American adult, the chances are that you are a "fair weather athlete." Although some men and women enjoy a hike through the freshly fallen snow to an outdoor ice skating rink, or an occasional visit to a ski run, too many individuals use the period between Indian summer and the return of spring as a time to take things easy, and indoors. That television producers save their best shows for the fall and winter months suggests that their careful surveys find most families indoors at that time. Sales of phonograph records and tape cassettes reach a peak as winter advances. And despite the letdown in physical activity, the long periods of relaxed entertainment seem to stimulate tremendous appetites for high-carbohydrate goodies like potato chips, pretzels, candy, beer, and soft drinks. This seasonal irony is compounded by the fact that autumn usually is marked by an increasingly heavy schedule of cocktail parties, business or club lunches, dinner parties, and holiday feasts that may stretch through several days.

The Value of Physical Fitness

The ancient Greek physician Hippocrates may have established the first rule of physical fitness some 2,400 years ago. He outlined what he called the Law of Use which governs the living organism: "That which is used develops; that which is not used wastes away." Modern medical practice still follows that Hippocratic concept in preventive medicine as well as in the rehabilitation of surgical patients. Dr. Harry J. Johnson, Chairman of the Medical Board of the Life Extension Institute, expresses the Hippocratic Law of Use this way: "Life itself is movement. Even the developing embryo moves

and stretches within the uterus by the fifth week of life—long before the mother becomes aware of it. And what does the mother say when she feels the first detectable stirring? She says she 'feels life.' "

After the birth of the baby, doctors have found that the mother recovers more quickly from the effects of childbirth if she gets out of bed and into action as soon as possible instead of lying in bed for a week or more to recuperate. The baby, during its hours of wakefulness, is in almost continuous motion—crawling, grasping, walking, running, jumping; the joy of activity continues in most normal children until adulthood.

There are exceptional people who almost literally keep moving throughout adult life. For example, Senator William Proxmire of Wisconsin is a strong advocate of jogging and regularly runs from his place of residence to his office on Capitol Hill. President Truman kept newsmen panting at his heels during his brisk morning walks. Individuals in all walks of life who spend a good deal of time in an office recognize the importance of daily exercise.

When Dr. Leonard Larson was president of the American Medical Association, he explained the importance of exercise in developing greater strength, stamina, endurance, and recuperative powers of the human body. "During exercise," said Dr. Larson, "the muscles need more oxygen and food. The blood circulates faster to meet the needs of the muscles and to carry off wastes. Body cells increase so that muscles gain strength and flexibility. There also is improved neuromuscular coordination."

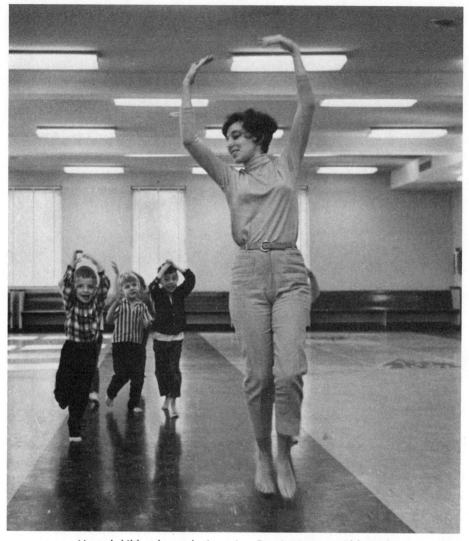

Normal children love to be in motion. Dancing is a natural form of exercise and a fine way to maintain muscle tone and good posture.

Everyday Emergencies

A frequently overlooked fringe benefit of physical fitness is an improved ability to survive everyday emergency situations that create a sudden demand for physical strength and endurance, which in turn require greater than normal performance by the heart and blood vessels, lungs, nerves, and muscles.

This was illustrated during a meeting of physicians to discuss the health hazards of flying. The medical director of one of the major airlines was asked if he had any records of passengers on his airline dying of a heart attack. "Yes," the medical director replied matter-of-factly. "Last year, seven of our passengers died of heart attacks. But not while they were flying. In each case, the pas-

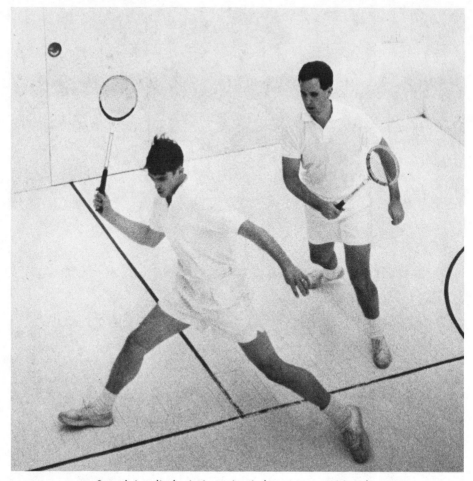

Squash is a lively, invigorating indoor sport requiring the stamina, alertness, and agility that develop physical fitness.

senger was running down a corridor to catch a flight when he collapsed and died." Each of the victims, it must be assumed, was "out of condition," perhaps a bit paunchy and flabby from lack of exercise, and unable to meet the ultimate test to fitness: the sudden demand on the body's organs to meet a brief modern emergency of running with suitcase in hand to reach the airline counter before the gates closed.

Running for a plane, running for a bus, running for a commuter train, pushing a stalled car, carrying an air conditioner up a flight of stairs— these are civilization's equivalents of the primitive human's battles with wild animals or hand-to-hand combat with tribal rivals. But the primitive man probably had a better chance for survival in an emergency because he maintained muscle, heart, and lung strength and endurance through the daily demands of his prehistoric life style.

Vigorous Recreational Activities

The alpine lakes of the mountains of Idaho were once stocked with trout that were carried there in milk cans strapped to the backs of husky college boys. Some years out of college and softened by sedentary jobs, the same individuals, burdened only by sack lunches and fishing rods, had to stop several times for their "second wind" when they returned recently to the same lakes. There are still duck hunters who travel each autumn to a hilltop on the California-Oregon border; it is a favorite hunting ground for waterfowl that skim over the hill which separates two

lakes on the Pacific Flyway. To reach the hilltop, the hunters have to scale a thousand feet of slippery lava rocks, and many drop out along the trail because of dizzy spells, painful leg cramps, and other discouraging symptoms. The peak bears the nickname of "Cardiac Ridge."

The point here is that true physical fitness involves more than a few easy or specialized exercises. A man can be a championship weight lifter with the physique of Mr. America, but he may not be able to compete in

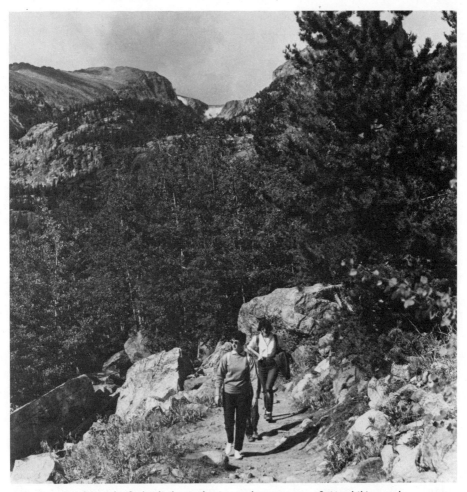

For those who find calisthenics boring and sports too confining, hiking and camping combine exercise with the ever-changing variety of nature.

running, swimming, or other sports activities unless he has developed and maintained strength and endurance in the heart, lungs, and muscles used for functions other than weight lifting. Conversely, an individual who considers himself in good physical condition because he has been jogging for the past two years might be unable to lift a portable TV set. The goal for anyone seeking an exercise program should be all-around physical fitness, with good heart and lung conditioning in addition to muscular strength.

Weight Control and Exercise

While no single set of exercises will guarantee physical fitness, neither will exercise alone control an overweight problem—although the Framingham Study has suggested a complementary relationship between exercise and weight control. The catch is that it takes a lot of exercise to get rid of a pound of fat. It would require, for example, about 90 minutes of swimming to burn up the calories you gain by eating a 450-calorie piece of chocolate layer cake; for most people, it would be easier to control weight by skipping the cake.

One pound of body fat is equivalent to about 3,600 calories of food. That amount of fat is about equal to a food intake of ten calories a day over a period of a year. In other words, you can add or lose a pound of fat by altering your diet by approximately ten calories a day. A three-inch cookie averages about 120 calories, slightly more than the amount of calories in ten medium potato chips. Translated into weight-control terms: if you eat one cookie a day beyond your body's normal food

requirements—or ten potato chips more—you should gain about 12 pounds in a year. Or if you regularly munch on such goodies, you should be able to reduce your weight by approximately 12 pounds a year simply by eliminating one cookie per day, or its equivalent.

Calorie Consumption During Normal Activities

An average human body needs about 1,500 calories a day just to survive; it burns about one calorie per minute in maintaining such simple body functions as breathing, keeping the body temperature at a normal level, and so on. A person who spends most of his time sleeping or watching TV doesn't need much more than a calorie per minute of food energy. A person who operates an electric typewriter for an hour requires only about 20 calories more for that period of work than a sleeping person. Driving a car for one hour might increase the body's need for calories by about 100 more than the amount needed for sleeping; one tablespoon of mayonnaise or a half-dozen saltine crackers will provide enough calories for one hour of driving.

By matching the calories in snack foods with the calorie needs of the human body for such low levels of inactivity as driving a car, watching TV, or operating an office machine, it is easy to see how pounds of body fat can accumulate within a short period of time.

Even walking, which is considered a mildly active way of utilizing calories, burns only three calories per minute above the basic needs of the body. So you would need to walk two hours to burn an extra 360

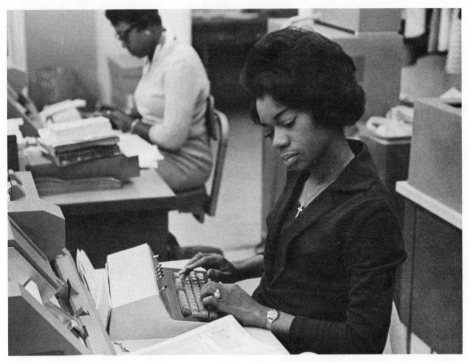

Sedentary workers such as key punch operators burn up relatively few calories and should avoid snacks of calorie-rich foods.

calories—the equivalent of a slice of cherry pie. The next time a friend assures you that you can burn up the calories in a piece of fruit pie by walking back to the office after lunch, make the friend promise to walk with you because it will require six miles of walking.

Lack of Exercise and Weight Gain

Nevertheless, it is better to walk for two hours after eating a piece of pie than to remain inactive after adding hundreds of excess calories to your body's fuel supply—if you can't resist the temptation to add the calories—because there *is* a relationship between weight control and exercise. Some people apparently gain weight even though they eat no more than their friends and relatives who remain slim. Careful studies made of obese people who ate only small or average amounts of food—in some cases as few as 1,800 calories a day—showed that they were simply less active than their slim friends and relatives who consumed the same amount of calories.

In one instance involving students, motion pictures were taken of the obese youngsters working out with their classmates in physical education classes. The investigators discovered by watching the movies that the overweight students were in effect faking the exercise routines; that is, they did not play enthusiastically, but merely went through the motions.

What about the need for fat deposits in the body as a source of energy? The answer is that while fat is indeed a rich source of energy for the body, the human body chemistry is geared to convert protein to energy, if needed. But the body is not equipped to build protein molecules from fat. As for sugar in the diet, the body gets all it needs from carbohydrates in fruits, vegetables, and other food sources.

Planning Your Own Physical Fitness Program

Any weight control program in connection with physical fitness improvement should be tailored to your individual needs and directed by a physician. Only your doctor knows for sure about your individual nutrition needs, and no two individuals are precisely alike. The same rule applies to physical conditioning: you could have a hidden bodily deficiency that would not cause problems in a sedentary life style. But a sudden strenuous program of jogging, calisthenics, or other athletic activity could be enough to push you over the brink. After an examination, the doctor can recommend a program that will permit certain types of exercise but restrict or eliminate others. There are so many methods of exercise available today that an effective program can be built around any individual physical problems.

Exercises Keyed to Age

Age ordinarily is one factor in determining which exercises are most suitable for an individual, although

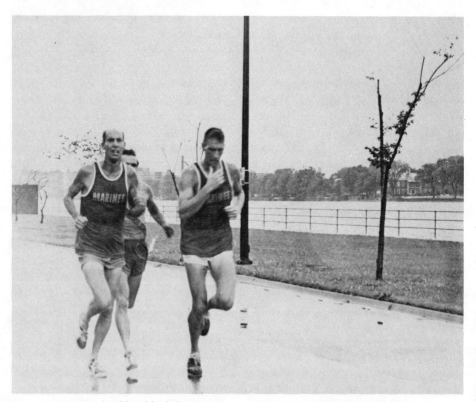

No one should suddenly begin a strenuous activity such as running without having a complete physical examination, preferably including a stress test.

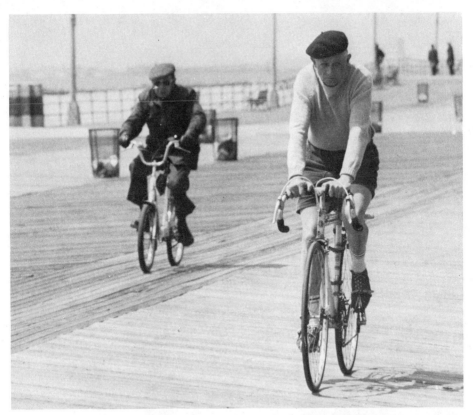

Bicycling is an excellent way to maintain physical fitness after age 50, as it exercises the whole body and provides the benefits of fresh air.

everybody knows people who seem young at 60 and others who appear to be old at 30. The general rule for determining whether it is safe to begin an exercise program is this: if you are still in your 20s and have passed a standard physical examination within the past year, it should be safe to begin a progressive program of conditioning without further examination. But if you are over 30 years of age, you should have passed a complete physical examination that included an electrocardiogram within the past 90 days.

If you are over the age of 50, you can still begin a physical fitness program, but it should be a medically supervised program. For the over 50 group, the doctor may advise that certain activities, such as jogging and competitive sports, be restricted or eliminated. Jogging can be damaging to the spine in persons beyond the age of 40 and can aggravate signs of arthritis. But walking, golf, swimming, bicycling, and exercising on a stationary cycle are alternate types of exercising for the past-middle-age set.

Fitness and Mental Health

In addition to the physical benefits gained by exercise, Dr. Ernest Simonson of the University of Minnesota Medical School found in a study of 10,000 persons that physical activity can be a definite aid to men-

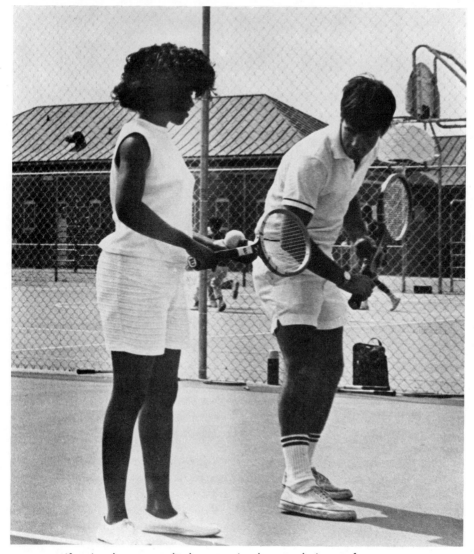

If you've always wanted to learn tennis, why not make it part of your regular physical fitness program? A vacation is a good time to begin lessons.

tal health. Typical comments by his subjects reflect that they "feel more alive" when they exercise. Dr. Simonson reported after analyzing the improved mental health of his subjects: "It is common logic that if one feels better, his attitude toward others will be more congenial. When one is in a cordial, happy frame of mind, he will likely make wiser decision, and his world in general will look better."

The late Dr. William Menninger, one of the world's foremost experts on mental health, explained that

Good mental health is directly related to the capacity and willingness of an individual to play. Regardless of his objections, resistances, or past practice, an individual will make a wise investment for himself if he will budget some of his time each day for his play —and take it seriously.

Dr. Menninger added that play provides an outlet for instinctive aggressive drives that enable a person to "blow off steam." Physical activity, he said, is a necessary supplement to daily work.

At the Beginning

Two things to remember in planning your own physical conditioning program are:

• Tailor the exercises and sports to your own needs and interests. If you have wanted to ride a bicycle, or learn water skiing, or take regular fishing trips, this is your opportunity to begin.

• Follow a progressive program in which you start at the bottom and improve gradually over a period of weeks or months. Don't expect overnight miracles, and be willing to cut back on the pace of your workouts if you find the going tough; you may be pushing yourself too fast. Your goal is to improve your own physical condition to the highest level feasible for your age and other possible limiting factors. Don't expect to set any new world records; just try to do the best you can—for your own health.

WARM-UP EXERCISES: The easiest place to begin your exercise program is in your own home, with the kind of warm-up exercises that you performed each day in high school. The main difference is that you will be on your own, unless you can find a friend or family member to participate in the workouts. You can do your own counting.

The purpose of the warm-up exercise is to increase the blood flow to the muscles and gradually limber up the body. And a warm-up period of at least 20 minutes should be used before any strenuous exercise. Otherwise, you may experience strains and sprains, or worse. It is quite possible to rupture a tendon or injure a joint by starting with certain strenuous exercises without a preliminary warm-up period. Also, remember to taper off a workout period with mild muscular activity, such as walking, until breathing and body temperature have returned to normal levels.

The warm-up exercises include body benders, situps, pushups, bend and stretch, ankle stretch, knee lifts, straddle hops, walking, running-in-place, and rope-skipping workouts, among a wide assortment of calisthenics. You can select from the assortment of warm-up exercises illustrated on pp. 1204–1207 those that are best suited to your own situation. If you live in a house or apartment where you are likely to disturb your neighbors by running in place or skipping rope, you can find other exercises that stimulate the general body circulation. But if you have facilities, such as a basement or garage, or a ground-floor bedroom where there is room for straddle hops or rope skipping, the exercises that provide the better range of action should be followed. Most of the exercises can be done in a small area; airline personnel investigating a strange thumping in a jet aircraft at 30,000 feet altitude one morning discovered a passenger running in place in the rest room.

Although no special equipment is necessary, don't hesitate to invest in a few items of gym equipment— dumbbells, weights, a stationary cycle, or whatever you think you need to help you in your own fitness program. For the cost of one or two days in a hospital, you can buy enough exercising equipment to keep yourself out of the hospital for several years.

MUSCLE SORENESS: You can expect some muscular soreness for the first two or three weeks of the toughening stage of physical conditioning, particularly if you have shunned exercise for several years. Later on as you progressively increase the work load on your body you may experience some stiffness or soreness. Usually this is only a warning sign that you are moving up the fitness scale too quickly. On the other hand, if the muscle soreness is relatively mild and goes away overnight, you can assume that you are not overdoing the exercise routine.

If your muscles and joints appear to suffer from the exercise load, simply slow down to an easier pace and work back up the scale again at a more gradual rate. By working at your own pace, with only the goal of improving your muscular strength and endurance, you can build a lot of flexibility into your fitness program. You don't have to compete with others; if you need an extra day or week to advance from one stage to the next, take the extra time. It's your own conditioning routine, and the suggested benchmarks or guidelines for the accompanying exercises can be adapted to your own needs.

The Indoor Exercise Program

Based on the U.S. Army's 6–12 conditioning project, the Indoor Exercise Program on pp. 1208–1219 includes six sets of exercise routines. Each set requires 12 minutes a day

to complete. Each of the sets, from I to VI, is in turn divided into three levels of activity. They are labeled A, B, C. The entire program, therefore, is designed to provide a progressive scale of physical conditioning for 12 minutes a day over a period of 18 weeks. You should begin at the C-level of set I and follow that routine for the first week. At the start of the second week, you progress to the B-level exercise routine of set I, and to the A-level routine at the beginning of the third week. Then, assuming that you follow the schedule according to its original design, you advance to the C-level routine of set II of the 6–12 exercises at the start of the fourth week, and so on.

The progression guides accompanying each table of 6–12 exercises represent suggested goals for healthy males. Women generally are not expected to match the suggested pace, although some may be able to do so. To follow the progression guide of Table I, read the first vertical column of numbers under the word *Exercises*. Under Exercise 1, in the age group of 17–29, are the numbers 15, 13, 11. These numbers show the repetitions of Exercise 1 to be completed within two minutes, the number indicated at the bottom of the column. The beginner in that age group should attempt to complete 11 side straddle exercises within two minutes, or at least he should work toward that primary goal. He also should try to complete 14 of the modified pushups in 1 minute, 12 situps in 1 minute, and so on. If he can accomplish the C level goals in the first week, he progresses to the B level goal of 13 side straddle exercises within two minutes, 16 modified pushups, 13 situps, and so on.

You will note that the total of the minutes suggested for the various exercises is 12 regardless of the age group or exercise level chosen. The greatest amount of time is allocated to running in place, and the number of steps ranges from a beginning level of 30, or six per minute, for men over 60 to a maximum of 250, or 50 per minute, for a young man in good condition.

Adapting the Program to Meet Your Needs

There is considerable flexibility in adapting this program to suit your own physical abilities, whether you are a man or woman. Each individual is as different in his physical strength and endurance as his fingerprints or other traits. The important thing about these sets of exercises is that most normal adults can perform most or all of them at one of the beginning levels, and with the beginning level as a benchmark the individual can gradually follow the progression guidelines to a higher level of fitness.

Some individuals may already be in such good condition that they can work up to the A-level of Table VI at the ninth week instead of the 18th week without any of the muscle stiffness or soreness that would indicate too fast a rate of advancement. Others may feel more comfortable if they spend two or three weeks at the C or B-level of Table I before moving to another level. There are no fixed rules to this program; the progression guides are merely suggestions that can be altered to fit your personal needs.

But don't go through the exercises half-heartedly. One purpose of exercising is to maintain a modest over-load on the muscles and the heart and lungs, which builds up a good reserve of strength and endurance. So you have to push a bit every day to make the plan work; if some of the exercises are less demanding of your muscles and circulatory system than your daily work responsibilities, you may be wasting your time. A man who moves pianos for a living would do little to improve his strength by lifting six-pound dumbbells for exercise.

On the other hand, there are people over the age of 45 who should be cautious about advancing beyond set IV of the Indoor Exercise Program. If they experience discomfort at the C-level of set V, they should drop back to the A-level of Table IV. This program is designed to fit all sorts of individual needs and abilities; some individuals probably should not advance beyond the Table III set of exercises. If there is any question about the level at which you should taper off your personal progressive program, discuss the matter with your doctor.

Maximum Performance Plateau

The rate of improvement in your physical condition will seem to be quite rapid at first, then increase slowly as you reach a plateau about halfway through the 18-week program. You can tell when you have reached your peak performance because you will begin to experience the huffing and puffing effects of an oxygen debt when you try to push yourself beyond that particular level—even though you have learned to overcome the need to pause for a "second wind" that you may have experienced earlier in the program.

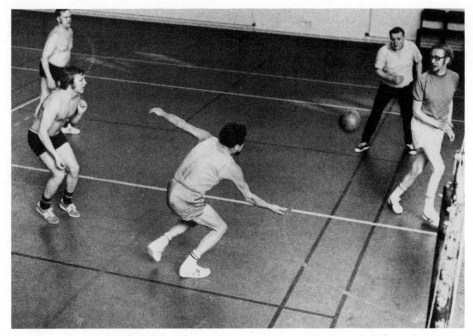

Volleyball, if played with intensity, requires agility, speed, and split-second timing. It is an excellent physical conditioner.

There is a practical limit to the performance of anybody—even Olympic champions —when the heart and lungs simply cannot supply oxygen fast enough to sustain the activity of the muscles. The muscle cells can "borrow" oxygen that is dissolved in the blood and other tissues in order to function temporarily, but eventually that debt of oxygen has to be repaid. This is why you may occasionally see track stars collapse in a series of agonizing gasps after they reach the finish line: they have run their oxygen debt to the point of bankruptcy.

In your own conditioning program based on the 6–12 exercise schedule, you may reach a point where, for example, you can do all of the exercises at the A level of Table V without experiencing an oxygen debt, but you can't make it through the Table VI routines without huffing and puffing. Then you will know that you are at your personal plateau of maximum performance. But you don't quit exercising at that point; you simply continue working out at the highest level that is comfortable for you. If you drop out of the program after reaching the level of your maximum performance your physical condition will deteriorate within two or three weeks.

There are still goals ahead and skills to be developed after you reach your maximum performance plateau—development of strength and endurance for participation in certain sports or improvement of the function of special muscle groups used in athletic activity. Rope skipping, a traditional conditioning exercise, always a favorite of professional boxers in training, is an example of an athletic activity that requires a high level of coordination, muscular function, and heart-lung perfor-mance to do well. Anyone who has tried high-speed rope skipping for more than three minutes without missing a jump knows it is more than a playground game; in fact, such a test has been used by the army in training soldiers for combat duty.

Weight Lifting

Another special method of develop-ing strength and endurance is weight lifting practice. See pp. 1220–1224. Weight lifting may be one of the oldest known sports that utilizes equipment; youths who wanted to participate in the ancient Greek Olympics in about 800 B.C. were required to lift a heavy iron weight to prove their strength be-fore they were accepted into the ritual. Weight lifting as a formal com-petitive sport was popular in Europe for many generations, but it did not attract much attention in North America until the 1930s when the United States organized its first weight lifting team for Olympic com-petition.

Exercising With Barbells

Although competitive weight lift-ing generally is considered a mas-culine activity, there is no reason why women could not work out with barbells if they wanted to do so. Body weight is not necessarily a fac-tor; U.S. championship weight lift-ing has a minimum body weight class of 114.5 pounds while A.A.U. competition is held in a 123-pound body weight class. However, most women probably are not interested in developing the muscle groups that would benefit from lifting barbells. The type of weight lifting that is more compatible with female physi-cal fitness goals, exercising with dumbbells, is described later in this chapter.

There are two approaches to weight lifting as a part of physical conditioning. One approach is to use barbell weights in competitive lift-ing in which the participant lifts a tremendous amount of weight off the floor and holds it aloft for a brief period of time. The other approach is to use weights to develop the strength and tone of major muscle groups in the arms, legs, back, trunk, and shoulder girdle. The effect is to improve the blood flow to the mus-cles through more efficient pumping volume of the heart and distribution by the capillaries.

Muscle Overload

The principle of muscle overload-ing is particularly applicable in weight lifting because of the added demands made on the muscles by lifting progressively heavier weights. A person normally has no more muscular strength than he seems to need for daily work and play routines. There is, therefore, lit-tle or no reserve for emergencies un-less you create an artificial need by overloading the muscles with heavy weights three or four times a week. The body responds to the extra de-mand by providing the extra muscle fibers.

Each time you stimulate the body to reach a certain plateau of muscle overloading, you begin working to-ward the next higher level by adding more weight to your barbell. You may begin, for example, with 40 or 50 pounds of weight and add five pounds when you are able. But do not overload the muscles to the point of a strain or a joint dislocation. Also,

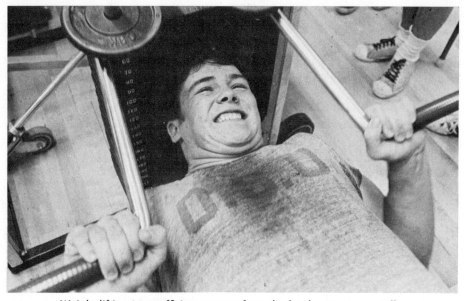

Weight lifting is an efficient means of muscle development, especially of the back and shoulders. Achievement depends on steady practice.

as you follow the basic barbell exercises described in this chapter, begin at the minimum number of repetitions. After you have learned to do six squats with 50 pounds of weight, continue at that rate for four or five days, then try seven squats with the same amount of weight. Do not advance to 55 pounds until you can handle 10 or 12 at the starting weight level.

WARM-UP EXERCISES: As mentioned above, you should go through a period of warm-up exercises before you begin a weight-lifting routine. Another factor to remember is that most weight-lifting exercises require postural control—which means you must hold the back straight during the lifting phase. Always squat to grasp the barbell from the floor; the bend-and-stretch technique could result in a serious back injury.

OTHER TIPS FOR WEIGHT LIFTING: Begin with the feet spread about 12 inches apart and the toes under the bar; otherwise the bar will tend to swing toward the feet when the lift movement begins. For most barbell exercises, grasp the bar overhand with the thumbs hooked under the bar; keep the arms spread apart by at least the width of the shoulders. For performing curls, reverse the hold with an underhand grip and the thumbs hooked above the bar. Breathe through the mouth and inhale as you lift; exhale on the return movement. Keep the weight evenly distributed between the hands.

Exercising With Other Weights

Another type of weight lifting is performed with dumbbells. There are at least ten different exercises that can be executed with these small, inexpensive weights to develop muscles from the waist to the shoulders and arms. Like the barbell exercises and the 6–12 program, they should be followed in a progressive order. Start with the minimum number of repetitions and advance gradually by adding one or two repetitions per week.

Dumbbells are somewhat deceptive in that they appear easy to handle when first viewed on the counter of a sporting goods store. And a pair is no heavier than a bag of groceries. But when the exercise routines with dumbbells are followed according to directions, you will discover muscles you didn't know you had.

Still other weight-lifting exercises designed to develop specific muscles are the war club swings and the twist grip. See the illustrations on p. 1224. The war club weighs about 20 pounds with a handle 14 inches long attached to the weight. It is swung in circles with one or two hands or swung as a hatchet or a baseball bat. It is intended to improve the function of muscle groups in the trunk, back, and shoulders, but provides fringe benefits for the arms and waist also.

The twist-grip exerciser, which is used to develop muscles of the arms and hands, can be made at home from such simple objects as a foot-long piece of pipe, a length of rope, an empty container, and about 20 pounds of cement. The rope is attached to the pipe at one end and the other end is attached to the weighted container. By holding the pipe at arm's length and turning the pipe in the hands, the weight is raised and lowered, using alternately an underhand and overhand grip on the pipe.

Isometrics

Still another method of developing specific muscle groups is known as isometrics. Although isometrics was once popularized as an easy way to exercise, most physical fitness experts agree that there is no such thing as an easy exercise. This opinion applies especially to isometrics; if isometric exercises are performed according to the rules, they can be as difficult as any other kind of exercise. In fact, most isometric exercises should not be performed by an individual who has not been examined by a physician first. The effects of straining some muscle groups while holding the breath can prove dangerous for a person whose heart is not in good condition.

The term isometrics is used to describe a technique in which the muscle is contracted without moving the body part involved, and the muscle is held in contraction for about ten seconds before it is relaxed. Isometrics also are called static exercises, as contrasted with dynamic exercises or isotonic muscle activity in which the muscles not only contract but flex and extend extremities. Some exercise routines may include both isometrics and isotonics; in weight lifting, isometric muscle contractions are used to grasp the weight at the floor and to hold the weight in an overhead position but an isotonic contraction is involved in moving the weight through a curl or press between the isometric phases.

It should be understood that a specific isometric exercise generally is designed to develop only one specific group of muscles. To get the comparable benefits of a warm-up series of exercises and a 6–12 program you would have to perform a very large number of different isometric exercises to involve all of the body's muscles that need daily exercising. Also, they do not provide the aerobic effect of the more active exercise routines. *Aerobics* refers to the kind of physical activity that requires maximum or nearly maximum effort for at least four minutes in order to get the heart and lungs, as well as the muscles, involved in the conditioning effects. In other words, a ten-second isometric muscle contraction is not likely to require the kind of bodily effort that creates an oxygen debt.

Yet isometrics do have a place in physical conditioning, as one unit of an overall exercise effort that also includes warm-up routines and calisthenics, with perhaps a little running or jogging as well. Briefly, the best way to perform isometric exercises is to inhale deeply just before you start the muscle contraction. Hold your breath while you exert the greatest possible effort in muscle contraction. At that point the muscle should begin to quiver from the strain of the contraction. Hold the contraction for at least five seconds, longer if the exercise requires; use a watch with a sweep second hand for timing. Then relax the muscle and exhale.

Most isometric exercises can be performed with little or no equipment; although special equipment is available for some exercises, many can be performed by using a desk, wall, or door jamb as an immovable object against which you can exert the force of your muscle contractions.

Exercises for Women

Physical conditioning programs for women are essentially the same as for men, although women are more likely to be conscious of bulging muscles that seem to produce bodily proportions they may regard as unattractive. However, there are exercise routines that can have the effect of balancing proportions. Running and cycling, for example, tend to favor development of the muscles from the hips downward. Weight lifting or other exercises designed to develop the muscles from the waist up can be used to advantage by women who want to reshape that part of the body. On the other hand, exercises that tend to develop musculature where it is unwanted can be avoided. Particularly recommended for women who plan to be mothers are exercises that strengthen the abdominal and back muscles. See the illustrations on pp. 1225–1227.

Basic exercises for women include running or jogging, bending and twisting at the waist, situps, and modified pushups, as well as standing on the toes while stretching the arms upward. Special exercises for enhancing the female figure can begin with a series of bustline exercises. One is an isometric press that starts with the palms of the hands facing together, fingers clasped and pointed upward, and arms close to the chest. Inhale deeply and push the hands against each other with maximum effort. Hold the breath while pressing and continue for seven seconds. Then relax, exhale, and repeat the exercise. Two other exercises are performed while lying flat on the floor with a weight in each hand; dumbbells, bricks, or books can serve as weights. Start with weights in hands, arms stretched back over the head with backs of the hands on the floor. Next raise both arms without bending the elbows and move the weights overhead and down to the floor at the hips. While

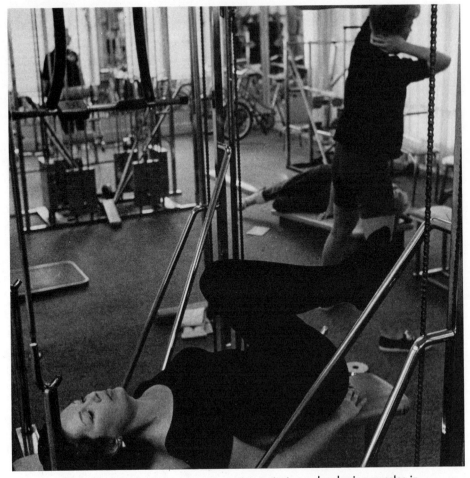

By working out in a gym, women can concentrate on developing muscles in some areas of the body while avoiding unwanted development in others.

counting to yourself for rhythm, return to the original position and repeat the exercise. The second is a variation of the previous exercise, with the weights lifted straight overhead from a starting position of the arms extended sideward at shoulder level. Don't bend the elbows.

Cycle-type exercises and ballet stretches are recommended for hips and thighs. Ballet stretches can be performed from a standing position, with one hand on the hip and the other holding onto a steady object such as a chair. Another exercise for the hips and thighs is patterned after the "cheerleader" position. While kneeling on the floor, hands on hips and back straight, bend backward as far as is comfortable without bending the back or moving the knees. Return to the starting position and begin again.

Among the suggested exercises for calves and ankles is the rocker. With feet together and hands on hips, legs straight, rock back on your heels with toes off the floor. Then rock back with your weight on the toes and the heels off the floor.

WARM-UP EXERCISES

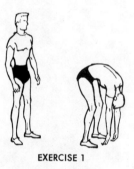

EXERCISE 1

Exercise 1: **Bend and Stretch.** Stand erect, feet shoulder-width apart. *Count 1.* Bend trunk forward and down, flexing knees. Stretch gently in attempt to touch fingers to toes or floor. *Count 2.* Return to starting position. *Note:* Do slowly, stretch and relax at intervals rather than in rhythm.

Exercise 2: **Knee Lift.** Stand erect, feet together, arms at sides. *Count 1.* Raise left knee as high as possible, grasping leg with hands and pulling knee against body while keeping back straight. *Count 2.* Lower to starting position. *Counts 3 and 4.* Repeat with right knee.

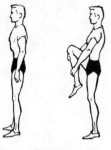

EXERCISE 2

Exercise 3: **Wing Stretcher.** Stand erect, elbows at shoulder height, fists clenched in front of chest. *Count 1.* Thrust elbows backward vigorously without arching back. Keep head erect, elbows at shoulder height. *Count 2.* Return to starting position.

Exercise 4: **Half Knee Bend.** Stand erect, hands on hips. *Count 1.* Bend knees halfway while extending arms forward, palms down. *Count 2.* Return to starting position.

Exercise 5: **Arm Circles.** Stand erect, arms extended sideward at shoulder height, palms up. Describe small circles backward with hands. Keep head erect. Do 15 backward circles. Reverse, turn palms down and do 15 small circles forward.

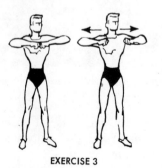

EXERCISE 3

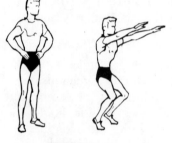

EXERCISE 4

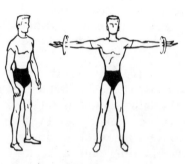

EXERCISE 5

WARM-UP EXERCISES

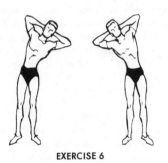

EXERCISE 6

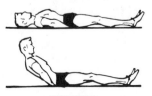

EXERCISE 7

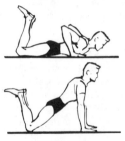

EXERCISE 8

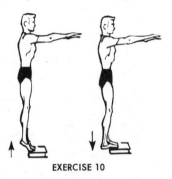

EXERCISE 9

Exercise 6: Body Bender. Stand, feet shoulder-width apart, hands behind neck, fingers interlaced. *Count 1.* Bend trunk sideward to left as far as possible, keeping hands behind neck. *Count 2.* Return to starting position. Counts 3 and 4. Repeat to the right.

Exercise 7: Prone Arch. Lie face down, hands tucked under thighs. *Count 1.* Raise head, shoulders, and legs from floor. *Count 2.* Return to starting position.

Exercise 8: Knee Pushup. Lie on floor, face down, legs together, knees bent with feet raised off floor, hands on floor under shoulders, palms down. *Count 1.* Push upper body off floor until arms are fully extended and body is in straight line from head to knees. *Count 2.* Return to starting position.

Exercise 9: Head and Shoulder Curl. Lie on back, hands tucked under small of back, palms down. *Count 1.* Tighten abdominal muscles, lift head and pull shoulders and elbows up off floor. Hold for four seconds. *Count 2.* Return to starting position.

Exercise 10: Ankle Stretch. Stand on a stair, large book or block of wood, with weight on balls of feet and heels raised. *Count 1.* Lower heels. *Count 2.* Raise heels.

Exercise 11: Toe Touch. Stand at attention. *Count 1.* Bend trunk forward and down keeping knees straight, touching fingers to ankles. *Count 2.* Bounce and touch fingers to top of feet. *Count 3.* Bounce and touch fingers to toes. *Count 4.* Return to starting position.

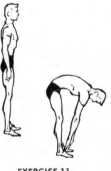

EXERCISE 10

EXERCISE 11

WARM-UP EXERCISES

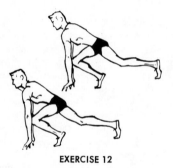

EXERCISE 12

Exercise 12: Sprinter. Squat, hands on floor, fingers pointed forward, left leg fully extended to rear. *Count 1.* Reverse position of feet in bouncing movement, bringing left foot to hands and extending right leg backward — all in one motion. *Count 2.* Reverse feet again, returning to starting position.

Exercise 13: Sitting Stretch. Sit, legs spread apart, hands on knees. *Count 1.* Bend forward at waist, extending arms as far forward as possible. *Count 2.* Return to starting position.

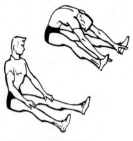

EXERCISE 13

Exercise 14: Pushup. Lie on floor, face down, legs together, hands on floor under shoulders with fingers pointed straight ahead. *Count 1.* Push body off floor by extending arms, so that weight rests on hands and toes. *Count 2.* Lower the body until chest touches floor. *Note:* Body should be kept straight, buttocks should not be raised, abdomen should not sag.

Exercise 15: Situp (Arms Extended). Lie on back, legs straight and together, arms extended beyond head. *Count 1.* Bring arms forward over head, roll up to sitting position, sliding hands along legs, grasping ankles. *Count 2.* Roll back to starting position.

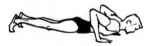
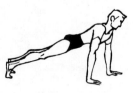

EXERCISE 14

Exercise 16: Leg Raiser. Right side of body on floor, head resting on left arm. Lift left leg about 24″ off floor, then lower it. Do required number of repetitions. Repeat on other side.

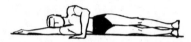

EXERCISE 15

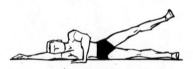

EXERCISE 16

WARM-UP EXERCISES

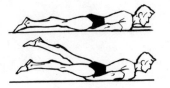

EXERCISE 17

Exercise 17: Flutter Kick. Lie face down, hands tucked under thighs. Arch the back, bringing chest and head up, then flutter kick continuously, moving the legs 8"-10" apart. Kick from hips with knees slightly bent. Count each kick as one.

Exercise 18: Circulating Activities.

Walking. Maintain a pace of 120 steps per minute for a distance of 1 mile. Swing arms and breathe deeply.

Rope. Skip or jump rope continuously using any form for 30 seconds and then rest 30 seconds. Repeat 2 times.

Run in Place. Raise each foot at least 4" off floor and jog in place. Count 1 each time left foot touches floor. Complete the number of running steps called for, then do specified number of straddle hops. Complete 2 cycles of alternate running and hopping.

Straddle Hop. At attention. *Count 1.* Swing arms sideward and upward, touching hands above head (arms straight) while simultaneously moving feet sideward and apart in a single jumping motion. *Count 2.* Spring back to starting position. Two counts in one hop.

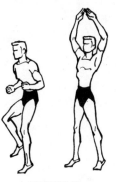

EXERCISE 18

Exercise 19: Situp (Fingers Laced). Lie on back, legs straight and feet spread approximately 1' apart. Fingers laced behind neck. *Count 1.* Curl up to sitting position and turn trunk to left. Touch the right elbow to left knee. *Count 2.* Return to starting position. *Count 3.* Curl up to sitting position and turn trunk to right. Touch left elbow to right knee. *Count 4.* Return to starting position. Score one situp each time you return to starting position. Knees may bend as necessary.

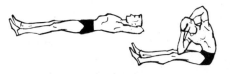

EXERCISE 19

Exercise 20: Situp (Arms Extended, Knees Up). Lie on back, legs straight, arms extended overhead. *Count 1.* Sit up, reaching forward with arms encircling knees while pulling them tightly to chest. *Count 2.* Return to starting position. Do this exercise rhythmically without breaks in the movement.

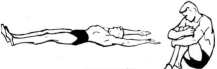

EXERCISE 20

Exercise 21: Sitting Stretch (Alternate). Sit, legs spread apart, fingers laced behind neck, elbows back. *Count 1.* Bend forward to left, touching forehead to left knee. *Count 2.* Return to starting position. *Counts 3 and 4.* Repeat to right. Score one repetition each time you return to starting position. Knees may be bent if necessary.

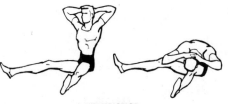

EXERCISE 21

INDOOR EXERCISE PROGRAM

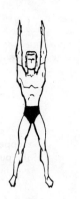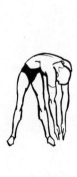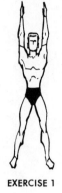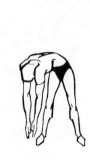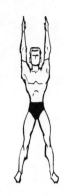

EXERCISE 1

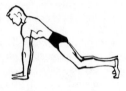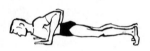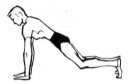

EXERCISE 2

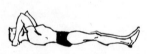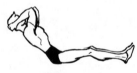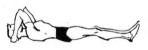

EXERCISE 3

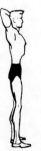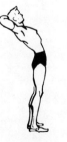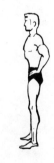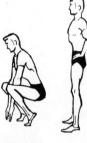

EXERCISE 4   **EXERCISE 5**

INDOOR EXERCISE PROGRAM

TABLE I: PROGRESSION GUIDE

AGE GROUP	LEVEL	EXERCISES					
		1	2	3	4	5	6
17	A	15	18	14	15	15	250
to	B	13	16	13	13	13	235
29	C	11	14	12	11	11	215
30	A	13	14	12	13	13	200
to	B	11	13	11	11	11	185
39	C	9	12	10	9	9	165
40	A	11	11	10	11	11	150
to	B	9	10	9	9	9	135
44	C	7	9	8	7	7	120
45	A	9	8	8	9	9	100
to	B	7	7	7	7	7	90
49	C	5	6	6	5	5	80
50	A	7	6	6	7	7	75
to	B	5	5	5	5	5	70
59	C	3	4	4	3	3	60
60	A	4	5	4	4	4	50
and	B	3	4	3	3	3	40
over	C	2	3	2	2	2	30
Minutes for each exercise		2	1	1	1	2	5

Exercise 1: Side straddle, arms overhead and straight, palms facing. Turn trunk to the left and bend forward over the left thigh, attempt to touch the fingertips to the floor outside the left foot, keep the knees straight. Alternate the movement to the opposite side. • Down and up to one side is one repetition.

Exercise 2: Kneeling front rest, hands shoulder width apart. The weight is supported on the knees and by the arms. Bend elbows and lower body until chest touches the floor. Keeping knees on the floor, raise body by straightening the arms. • Down and up is one repetition.

Exercise 3: Supine position, fingers interlaced and placed behind the head. Maintaining the heels on the floor, raise the head and shoulders until the heels come into view. Lower the head and shoulders until fingers contact the floor and head rests on the hands. • Up and down is one repetition.

Exercise 4: Body erect, feet slightly spread, fingers interlaced and placed on rear of neck at base of the head. Bend the upper trunk backward, raise the chest high, pull the elbows back, and look upward. Keep the knees straight. Recover to the erect position, eyes to the front. • Bending backward and recovery is one repetition.

Exercise 5: Body erect, feet spread less than shoulder width, hands on hips, elbows back. Do a full knee bend, at the same time bend slightly forward at the waist. Touch the floor with the extended fingers, keeping the hands about six inches apart. Resume the starting position. • Down into the touch position and return to the starting position is one repetition.

Exercise 6: Run in place, lift feet 4 to 6 inches off floor. At the completion of every 50 steps do 10 Steam Engines. Repeat sequence until the required number of steps is completed. • Count a step each time left foot touches the floor.

Steam Engines. Lace the fingers behind the neck and while standing in place raise the left knee above waist height, at the same time twist the trunk and lower the right elbow to the left knee. Lower the left leg and raise the right leg touching the knee with the left elbow thus completing the movement to that side. Continue to alternate the movement until the sequence is completed.

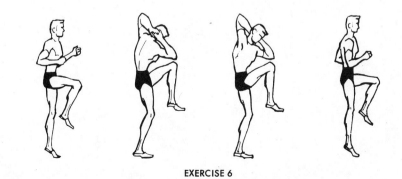

EXERCISE 6

INDOOR EXERCISE PROGRAM

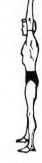
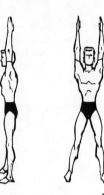
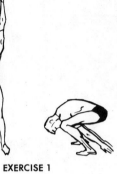

EXERCISE 1

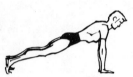

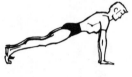

EXERCISE 2

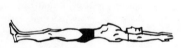

EXERCISE 3

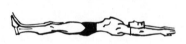

EXERCISE 4

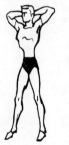
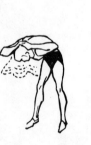
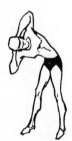
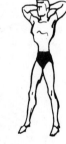

EXERCISE 5

INDOOR EXERCISE PROGRAM

TABLE II: PROGRESSION GUIDE

AGE GROUP	LEVEL	EXERCISES 1	2	3	4	5	6
17	A	17	17	17	9	19	300
to	B	15	15	15	8	17	270
29	C	13	13	13	7	15	245
30	A	15	15	15	8	17	235
to	B	13	13	13	7	15	210
39	C	11	11	11	6	13	190
40	A	13	13	13	7	15	175
to	B	11	11	11	6	13	155
44	C	9	10	9	5	11	135
45	A	11	11	11	6	13	125
to	B	9	9	9	5	11	110
49	C	7	7	7	4	9	100
50	A	9	9	9	5	11	95
to	B	7	7	7	4	9	85
59	C	5	5	5	3	7	75
60	A	6	7	7	4	9	70
and	B	5	5	5	3	7	60
over	C	4	4	4	2	5	50
Minutes for each exercise		1	1	1	1½	1½	6

Exercise 1: Wide side straddle, arms overhead and straight, palms facing. Bend at the knees and the waist, swing the arms down, and reach between the legs as far as possible. Look at the hands. The thighs are parallel to the floor during the bend. Recover to the starting position with a sharp movement. • Down and up is one repetition.

Exercise 2: Front leaning rest position with body straight from head to heels. Bending at the waist and keeping the knees locked, jump forward to a jack-knife position bringing the feet as close to the hands as possible. With the weight on the hands, thrust the legs to the rear resuming the front leaning rest position. • Up into the jack-knife position and return to the front leaning rest position is one repetition.

Exercise 3: Supine position with arms straight overhead, palms facing. With a sharp movement sit up, bringing the heels as close to the buttocks as possible and the knees to the chest. Swing the arms in an arc overhead to a position outside the knees and parallel to the floor. To recover swing the arms overhead keeping them straight. At the same time move the legs forward until they are straight. • Sitting up and returning to the supine position is one repetition.

Exercise 4: Feet spread more than shoulder width apart, fingers laced behind the neck and elbows are back. Bend forward at the waist vigorously, then twist the trunk to the left, then to the right and return to the erect position. Keep the knees locked and back straight. • Bend forward, twist left, twist right, and return to the erect position is one repetition.

Exercise 5: Bend forward at the waist, grasping the right toes with right hand, left toes with left hand, knees are slightly bent. Walk forward retaining this position. • Count a repetition each time a foot contacts the floor.

Figure 6: Run in place, lift feet 4 to 6 inches off floor. At the completion of every 50 steps do 10 Heel Clicks. Repeat sequence until the required number of steps is completed. • Count a step each time left foot touches the floor.

Heel Clicks. Jump upward about 12 inches and bring the heels together. Before landing on the floor, separate the feet 15 to 18 inches. Immediately upon contact with the floor repeat the jump and heel click.

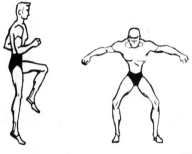
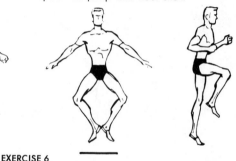

EXERCISE 6

INDOOR EXERCISE PROGRAM

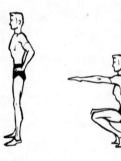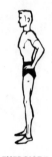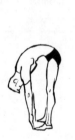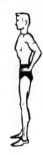

EXERCISE 1

EXERCISE 2

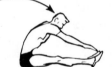

EXERCISE 3

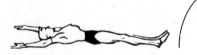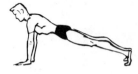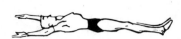

EXERCISE 4

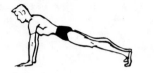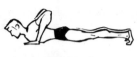

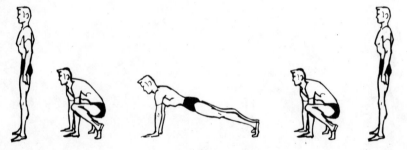

EXERCISE 5

INDOOR EXERCISE PROGRAM

TABLE III: PROGRESSION GUIDE

AGE GROUP	LEVEL	EXERCISES					
		1	2	3	4	5	6
17	A	10	19	19	16	10	350
to	B	9	17	17	15	9	315
29	C	8	15	15	14	8	280
30	A	9	17	17	14	9	270
to	B	8	15	15	13	8	240
39	C	7	13	13	12	7	210
40	A	8	15	15	12	8	200
to	B	7	13	13	11	7	180
44	C	6	11	11	10	6	160
45	A	7	13	13	10	7	150
to	B	6	11	11	9	6	135
49	· C	5	9	9	8	5	120
50	A	6	11	11	8	6	115
to	B	5	9	9	7	5	105
59	C	4	7	7	6	4	95
60	A	5	9	9	7	5	90
and	B	4	7	7	6	4	80
over	C	3	5	5	4	3	70
Minutes for each exercise		1½	1	1	1½	1	6

Exercise 1: Feet spread less than shoulder width apart, hands on hips, elbows back. Do a full knee bend, trunk erect and thrust the arms forward. Recover to the erect position, and with knees locked, bend forward at the waist and touch the toes and recover to the erect position. • Down into the full knee bend, recover, touch toes and recover is one repetition.

Exercise 2: Front leaning rest position with body straight from head to heels. Lower the body until the chest touches the floor, keep body straight. Recover by straightening the arms and raising the body. • Down and touch the floor and recovery to the front leaning rest position is one repetition.

Exercise 3: Supine position, arms overhead, palms facing. With a sharp movement sit up, thrust the arms forward and touch the toes. Keep the legs straight and the heels in contact with the floor. • Sit up, touch toes, and resume the supine position is one repetition.

Exercise 4: Supine position, arms overhead, palms upward. Raise the legs and swing them backward over the head until toes touch the floor. Recover by returning legs to the starting position. • Touch toes overhead and recover to the supine position is one repetition.

Exercise 5: Erect position, feet together. Bend knees and place hands on floor, shoulder width apart. Thrust legs to the rear, body straight from head to heels. Move legs forward assuming squat position, elbows inside of knees. Assume erect position. • Down into full squat, legs to the rear, back to full squat and return to the erect position is one repetition.

Exercise 6: Run in place, lift feet 4 to 6 inches off floor. At the completion of every 50 steps do 10 Knee Touches. Repeat sequence until the required number of steps is completed. • Count a step each time the left foot touches the floor.

Knee Touches. From a stride position, bend the knees and touch the knee of the rear leg to the floor, straighten legs, jump upward and change position of the feet. Again bend knees and touch the opposite knee. Continue alternately touching each knee.

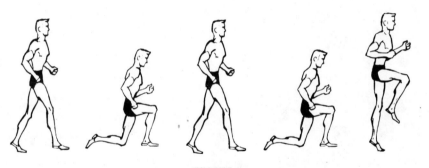

EXERCISE 6

INDOOR EXERCISE PROGRAM

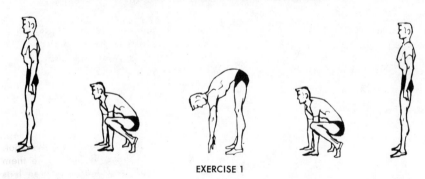

EXERCISE 1

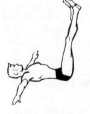
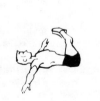
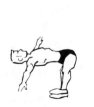
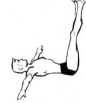
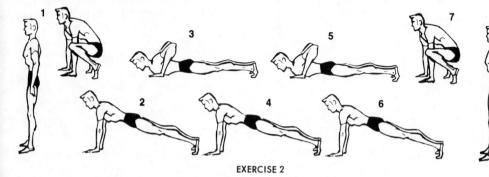

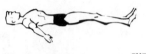
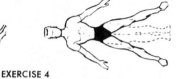

EXERCISE 2

EXERCISE 3

EXERCISE 4

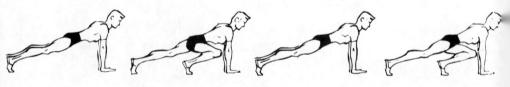

EXERCISE 5

INDOOR EXERCISE PROGRAM

TABLE IV: PROGRESSION GUIDE

AGE GROUP	LEVEL	1	2	3	4	5	6
17	A	12	9	12	24	25	400
to	B	11	8	11	22	23	380
29	C	10	7	10	21	21	360
30	A	11	8	11	23	23	305
to	B	10	7	10	21	21	290
39	C	9	6	9	20	20	275
40	A	10	7	10	20	21	225
to	B	9	6	9	18	18	215
44	C	8	5	8	16	16	205
45	A	8	6	8	16	16	175
to	B	7	5	7	14	14	165
49	C	6	4	6	12	12	155
50	A	6	5	6	13	13	135
to	B	5	4	5	11	11	130
59	C	4	3	4	10	10	120
60	A	5	4	5	10	10	100
and	B	4	3	4	9	9	95
over	C	3	2	3	8	8	90
Minutes for each exercise		1	2	1	1	1	6

Exercise 1: Erect position, hands at sides, feet spread slightly. Bend knees, incline trunk forward, and place hands on floor between legs. Straighten knees, keeping feet in place and fingers touching floor. Again bend knees and resume the first position. Recover to the erect position. • The above sequence is one repetition.

Exercise 2: Erect position, hands at sides, feet together. Bend knees, place hands on floor between legs. Thrust legs to the rear. Execute two complete pushups and then thrust the legs forward bending the knees with arms between the knees. Recover to the erect position. • The completion of all eight counts is one repetition.

Exercise 3: Back position with arms out to sides and legs raised to the vertical. Lower legs to the left, raise legs to the vertical, lower to the right, again raise to the vertical. Keep legs together and the head and hands in contact with the floor throughout the exercise. • The above sequence is one repetition.

Exercise 4: From back position, raise legs with heels 10 to 12 inches from the floor. Spread legs as far as possible, close them together. Continue to open and close legs until required repetitions have been completed. • Opening and closing legs is one repetition.

Exercise 5: Front leaning rest position, body straight from head to heels. Bend the left knee and bring the left foot as far forward as possible, return left leg to original position. Repeat movement with the right leg. Continue exercise alternating left and right legs. • A leg thrust forward and returned to the rear is one repetition.

Exercise 6: Run in place, lift feet 4 to 6 inches off floor. At the completion of every 50 steps do 10 Jumping Jacks. Repeat sequence until the required number of steps is completed. • Count a step each time left foot touches the floor.

Jumping Jacks. Feet spread shoulder width apart, arms extended overhead. Jump upward, bring heels together and at same time squat to a full knee bend position, bring the arms downward and place hands on the floor, elbows inside of knees, directly under the shoulders. Jump to the side straddle and swing the arms sideward overhead.

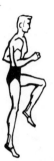
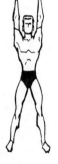
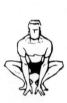
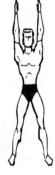
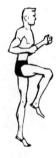

EXERCISE 6

INDOOR EXERCISE PROGRAM

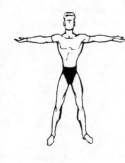
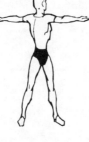
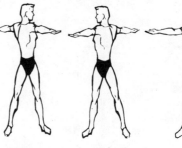

EXERCISE 1

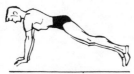
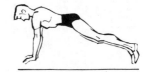

EXERCISE 2

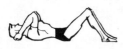

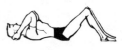

EXERCISE 3

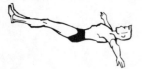

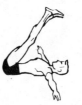

EXERCISE 4

EXERCISE 5

INDOOR EXERCISE PROGRAM

TABLE V: PROGRESSION GUIDE

AGE GROUP	LEVEL	EXERCISES 1	2	3	4	5	6
17	A	14	13	28	14	30	450
to	B	13	12	27	13	28	430
29	C	12	11	26	12	26	410
30	A	12	12	25	12	26	350
to	B	11	11	24	11	24	330
39	C	10	10	23	10	22	310
40	A	11	11	23	11	23	250
to	B	10	10	21	10	21	240
44	C	9	9	19	9	19	230
45	A	9	9	20	9	20	200
to	B	8	8	18	8	18	190
49	C	7	7	16	7	16	180
50	A	7	7	16	7	16	170
to	B	6	6	14	6	14	155
59	C	5	5	12	5	12	140
60	A	6	6	12	6	12	115
and	B	5	5	11	5	10	110
over	C	4	4	9	4	9	105
Minutes for each exercise		2	1	1	2	1	5

Exercise 1: Feet spread more than shoulder width, arms sideward at shoulder level, palms up. Turn trunk to the left as far as possible, recover slightly, repeat to the right and recover slightly. The head and hips remain to the front throughout the exercise. • The above sequence is one repetition.

Exercise 2: Front leaning rest position, body straight from head to heels. Bend the elbows slightly and push with the hands and toes, bouncing the body upward and completely off the floor. In contact with the floor resume the front leaning rest position. • Propelling the body upward and the return to the floor is one repetition.

Exercise 3: Back position, hands interlaced and placed under head, knees bent with feet flat on the floor. Sit up bending the trunk forward and attempting to touch the chest to the thighs. Recover to the back position without moving the feet. • Sit up and recovery to the back position is one repetition.

Exercise 4: On back, arms sideward, feet raised 12 inches from the floor, knees straight. Keeping the legs together, swing legs as far to the left as possible, swing legs overhead, then to the right as far as possible and recover by swinging legs to the front. Legs stop momentarily at each position and do not contact floor until all repetitions are complete. • One repetition is completed when legs make the complete circle.

Exercise 5: From a stride position do a deep knee bend and grasp the right ankle with the right hand, left ankle with the left hand, arms outside knees. Walk forward maintaining the grasp of the ankles. • One repetition is counted each time the left foot contacts the floor.

Exercise 6: Run in place, lift feet 4 to 6 inches off floor. At the completion of every 50 steps do 10 Hand Kicks. Repeat sequence until required number of steps is completed.

Hand Kicks. Stand in place and kick left leg upward, at the same time extend the right arm touching the toe and hand. Repeat with right leg, extending left arm.

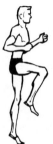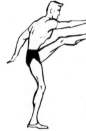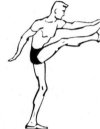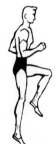

EXERCISE 6

INDOOR EXERCISE PROGRAM

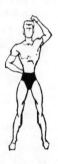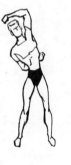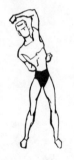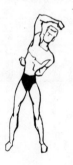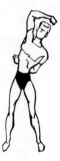

EXERCISE 1

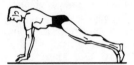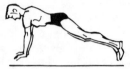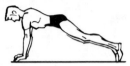

EXERCISE 2

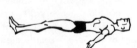

EXERCISE 3

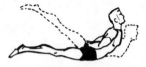

EXERCISE 4

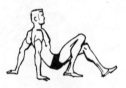

EXERCISE 5

INDOOR EXERCISE PROGRAM

TABLE VI: PROGRESSION GUIDE

AGE GROUP	LEVEL	1	2	3	4	5	6
17	A	17	15	32	32	35	500
to	B	16	14	30	30	33	480
29	C	15	13	28	28	31	460
30	A	15	13	30	30	31	400
to	B	14	12	28	28	29	380
39	C	13	11	26	26	27	360
40	A	13	10	27	27	27	310
to	B	12	9	25	25	25	285
44	C	11	8	23	23	23	265
45	A	11	9	23	23	23	250
to	B	10	8	21	21	21	230
49	C	9	7	19	19	19	210
50	A	9	8	19	19	19	200
to	B	8	7	17	17	17	190
59	C	7	6	15	15	15	175
60	A	8	7	15	15	17	140
and	B	7	6	13	13	15	130
over	C	5	5	10	10	12	120
Minutes for each exercise		2	1	1	1	1	6

Exercise 1: Feet spread shoulder width apart, left fist clenched and overhead, right fist clenched at waistline in rear of body. Simultaneously thrust the left fist as far to the right as possible and the right fist as far to the left as possible. Recover and repeat. Reverse the hands with the right fist above the head and the left in rear at the waistline. Repeat the movement to the opposite side by thrusting the upper body to the left with the arm motion. • The above sequence is one repetition.

Exercise 2: Front leaning rest position. Bend elbows slightly and push with the hands and toes bouncing the body upward and completely off the floor. At the height of the bounce, clap the hands and quickly return them to a position directly under the shoulder to catch the body weight. • Push off the floor, clap hands, and return to the front leaning rest position is one repetition.

Exercise 3: Back position, arms extended to the side at 45 degrees. Raise the legs and the trunk into a V position bringing the trunk and legs as close as possible. Return to back position. • Raising the legs and trunk and recovery to the back position is one repetition.

Exercise 4: Prone position with hands clasped in small of the back. Arch the body, holding the head back and rock forward, relax and repeat the movement. • Arch the body, rock forward, and relax is one repetition.

Exercise 5: From a sitting position lift the hips, supporting the body on the hands and feet. By moving the arms and legs walk on all fours either forward or backward. • A repetition occurs each time the left hand contacts the floor.

Exercise 6: Run in place, lift feet 4 to 6 inches off floor. At the completion of every 50 steps do 10 Pike Jumps. Repeat sequence until required number of steps is completed.
   Pike Jumps. Jump forward and upward from both feet, keeping the knees straight. Swing the legs forward and touch the toes with the hands at the top of each jump.

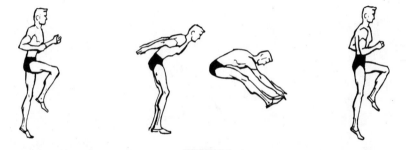

EXERCISE 6

WEIGHT LIFTING

Basic Barbell Exercises

Exercise 1: Squat. 6 repetitions, 50 pounds (commonly called the *flatfoot deep knee bend*). Place the bar upon the shoulders. Stand with feet about 18 inches apart. Keeping the feet flat, lower the body into the low squat position. Come erect and repeat. Exhale as you lower into the squat position and inhale as you come up.

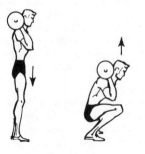

EXERCISE 1

Exercise 2: Waist Bender. 6 repetitions, 40 pounds. Assume the standing position with the bar across the shoulders, feet shoulder-width apart. Bend forward at the waist until the upper body is parallel to the ground; return to the starting position. • Each time you return to the upright position will constitute one repetition.

Exercise 3: Curl. 6 repetitions, 40 pounds. Grasp the barbell with the palms facing to the rear and assume the standing position, feet shoulder width apart. With the barbell held in front of the hips, flex the elbows and lift the weight until the bar touches the upper chest. Lower the barbell back to the hip level position. Inhale deeply with the upward movement and exhale on the downward movement. • Each time the bar touches the chest will constitute one repetition.

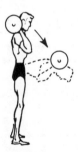

EXERCISE 2

Exercise 4: Side Bender. 6 repetitions per side, 40 pounds. Assume the standing position, feet shoulder width apart, with the bar across the shoulders. Bend to the left as far as possible and return to the starting position. Repeat six times and then execute the same procedure to the right for six repetitions.

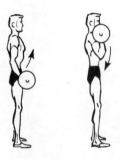

EXERCISE 3

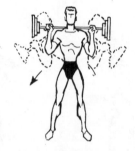

EXERCISE 4

WEIGHT LIFTING

Exercise 5: Standing Press. 6 repetitions, 45 pounds. Grasp the bar with the palms facing forward and assume the starting position. Curl the weight to the upper chest position. Inhale deeply and press the bar upward to an overhead position. Exhale as you lower the bar to the chest position. • Each time the bar is pressed upward constitutes one repetition.

Exercise 6: Upward Row. 6 repetitions, 40 pounds. Grasp the bar, hands close together, palms to the rear, and assume the standing position. Starting with the bar held in front of the hips, flexing the elbows and the shoulder girdle muscles, lift the bar straight up to an overhead position. Inhale deeply as you lift the bar. Exhale as you lower the bar to the hip position. • Each time the bar returns to the hips will constitute one repetition.

Exercise 7: Shoulder Curl. 6 repetitions, 25 pounds. Grasp the bar palms down, and assume the standing position. Keeping the elbows locked, curl the bar, pivoting the arms at the shoulders until the bar is in an overhead position and as far to the rear as possible. Return the bar in the same manner to the hip position. • Each time the bar returns to hip position constitutes one repetition.

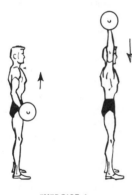

EXERCISE 5

EXERCISE 6

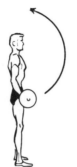
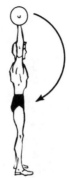

EXERCISE 7

WEIGHT LIFTING

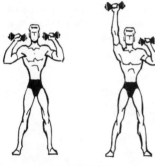

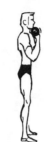
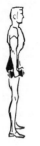

EXERCISE 1

Basic Dumbbell Exercises

Exercise 1: To develop shoulders and the back of the arm. Hold dumbbells at shoulder height. Push bells overhead to a full extension with the palms forward. Lower the bell back to the shoulder. Alternate right and left arm. Inhale as you push weight to full extension. Exhale as you lower the weight to the shoulder. • Repetitions: first week, 8; second week, 10; third week, 12.

Exercise 2: To develop the front of the upper arm. Hold dumbbells at arm's length parallel to the feet. Curl the weight to the shoulder, rotating the bell as the biceps contract. Lower the bell back to the starting position, reversing the rotation. Contract the triceps (back of the arm) to insure a full extension. This is done only after the bell has reached the starting position. Keep the bell under control as you lower it. Alternate right and left arms. Inhale as you curl the weight. Exhale as you lower the weight. • Repetitions: first week, 8; second week, 10; third week, 12.

EXERCISE 2

Exercise 3: Curl weight until forearm is parallel to the floor. Return to the starting position. Repeat required number of repetitions. Curl bells to the shoulders. Lower weight until forearm is parallel to the floor. Return to the shoulder position. Repeat required number of repetitions. Lower bells to the starting position and curl required number of repetitions through full range of movement. Curl both bells at same time. • Repetitions: first week, 4 each movement; second week, 5 each movement; third week, 6 each movement.

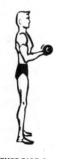

EXERCISE 3

Exercise 4: To develop the back of the upper arm. Hold dumbbells above and back of each shoulder by pointing the elbows up and holding them close to the head. Hold the elbows in place and extend the weight overhead by contracting the triceps. Lower the weight to the starting position. Alternate right and left arm. Inhale as you push weight to full extension. Exhale as you lower the weight to the shoulder. • Repetitions: first week, 8; second week, 10; third week, 12.

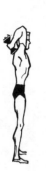
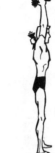

EXERCISE 4

WEIGHT LIFTING

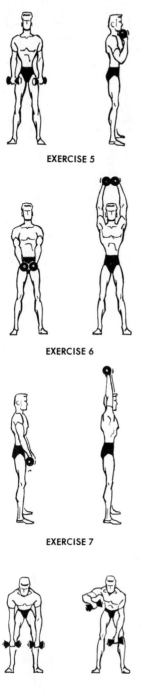

EXERCISE 5

EXERCISE 6

EXERCISE 7

EXERCISE 8

Exercise 5: To develop the shoulders. Use the standing position, holding the bells at arm's length in front of the thighs with the palms to the rear. Raise the bells to the shoulder, keeping the weight close to the body as the elbows go up and out. Lower the weight to the starting position, keeping the weight under control. Inhale as the weight goes up. Exhale as the weight goes down. • Repetitions: first week, 12; second week, 14; third week, 16.

Exercise 6: To develop the shoulders. Use the standing position. Place the feet at shoulder's width apart, bending the knees a little more than usual. Roll the hips back slightly. Hold the bells at arm's length in front of you. Now, raise both bells laterally rotating the arms so the back of the hands come together on completion of the contraction. Keeping the bells under control, lower them to the starting position. Elbows should be slightly bent to avoid strain. • Repetitions: first week, 6; second week, 8; third week, 10.

Exercise 7: To develop the shoulders. Use the standing position holding the bells at arm's length with the palms to the rear. With the elbows slightly out of locked position, raise the bells overhead without rotating the arm. Return to the starting position. Inhale as you raise weight over head. Exhale as you lower weight to starting position. • Repetitions: first week, 6; second week, 8; third week, 10.

Exercise 8: To develop the upper back. Stand with feet at shoulders' width apart. Bend the knees and lean forward until the trunk is parallel to the floor. Hold the bells at arm's length directly below the shoulder. Raise the bells alternately to the shoulder by driving the elbow up and to the rear. Inhale as you pull weight up. Exhale as you lower the weight to the starting position. • Repetitions: first week, 12; second week, 14; third week, 16.

WEIGHT LIFTING

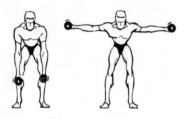

EXERCISE 9

Exercise 9: To develop the upper back. Stand with feet at shoulders' width apart. Bend the knees and lean forward until the trunk is parallel to the floor. Hold the bells at arm's length directly below the shoulders. Extend the arms laterally until they are parallel with the floor. Return to the starting position and repeat. Inhale as the bells are extended laterally. Exhale as the bells are lowered to the starting position. • Repetitions: first week, 6; second week, 8; third week, 10.

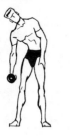
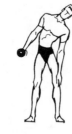

EXERCISE 10

Exercise 10: To exercise the waist. Stand with the feet shoulder width apart. Hold one bell in the right hand at arm's length by the right thigh. Do not bend forward or backward, but lean to the right, lowering the bell below the right knee. Now, lean to the left touching the left hand below the left knee. Repeat the desired number of repetitions. Change the bell to left hand to exercise the right side of the waist. Inhale as weight rises. Exhale as weight goes down. • Repetitions: first week, 15; second week, 20; third week, 25.

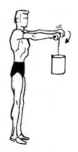
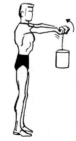

TWIST GRIP

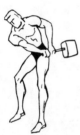
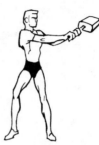
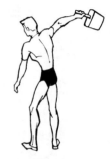

WAR CLUBS

EXERCISES FOR WOMEN

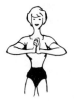

EXERCISE 1

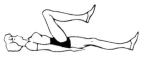

EXERCISE 2

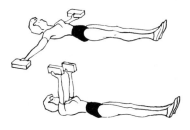

EXERCISE 3

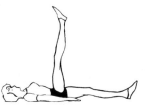

EXERCISE 4

For the Bustline

Exercise 1: The Press. Stand or sit erect. Clasp hands, palms together, close to chest. Press hands together hard and hold for 6 to 8 seconds. Repeat three times, resting briefly and breathing deeply between repetitions.

Exercise 2: Pullover. Lie on back with arms extended beyond head. Hold books or other objects of equal weight in hands. *Count 1.* Lift books overhead and down to thighs, keeping arms straight. *Count 2.* Return slowly to starting position. Repeat 3 to 6 times.

Exercise 3: Semaphore. Lie on back with arms extended sideward at shoulder level. Hold books or other objects of equal weight in hands. *Count 1.* Lift books to position over body, keeping arms straight. *Count 2.* Lower slowly to starting position. Repeat 3 to 6 times.

For the Waist

Exercise 4: Knee Lifts. Lie on back with knee slightly bent, feet on floor and arms at side. *Count 1.* Bring one knee as close as possible to the chest, keeping hands on floor. *Count 2.* Extend leg straight up. *Count 3.* Bend knee and return to chest. *Count 4.* Return to starting position. Repeat 5 to 10 times, alternating legs during exercise. The *double knee lift* is done in the same manner, raising both legs at the same time. Do 5 to 10 repetitions.

Exercise 5: Crossover. Lie on back, arms extended sideward, palms down. *Count 1.* Raise right leg to vertical position and move slowly to left until almost touching floor. Keep arms, head and shoulders on floor. *Count 2.* Return to starting position. *Counts 3 and 4.* Same action to other side. Do 5 to 10 repetitions.

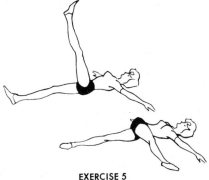

EXERCISE 5

EXERCISES FOR WOMEN

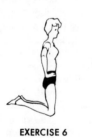

EXERCISE 6

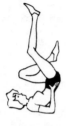

EXERCISE 7

For Hips and Thighs

Exercise 6: Cheerleader. Kneel on floor, back straight, hands on hips. *Count 1.* Bend backward as far as possible, keeping knees on floor and body straight. *Count 2.* Return to starting position. Repeat 10 to 15 times.

Exercise 7: Bicycle. Lie on back with hips and legs supported by hands. Simulate bicycle pumping action with legs. Pump 50-100 times.

Exercise 8: Ballet Stretch. Stand erect with left hand resting on back of chair for support. *Count 1.* Raise right leg sideward as high as possible. *Count 2.* Return to starting position. *Count 3.* Swing right leg forward as high as possible. *Count 4.* Return to starting position. *Count 5.* Swing right leg back as high as possible. *Count 6.* Return to starting position. Do 5 to 10 repetitions, then repeat exercise with left leg.

Exercise 9: Two-Way Stretch. Kneel with hands on floor, back straight. *Count 1.* Arch back, bend head down and bring left knee as close as possible to chin. *Count 2.* Lift head high and extend left leg as far backward and up as possible. Repeat 6 to 10 times with each leg.

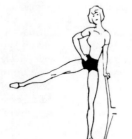
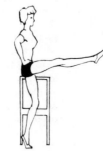
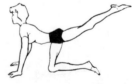

EXERCISE 8

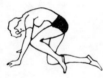

EXERCISE 9

EXERCISES FOR WOMEN

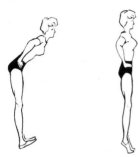

For Calves and Ankles

Exercise 10: Rocker. Stand erect, feet together, hands on hips. *Count 1.* Rock back on heels, keeping legs straight and raising toes off floor. *Count 2.* Rock forward on toes, lifting heels off floor. Repeat 10 to 20 times.

Exercise 11: Hop. Stand erect, feet close together, hands on hips. Hop lightly on both feet 50 times, on the right foot 25 times, on the left foot 25 times, on both feet 50 times.

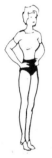

EXERCISE 10

Exercise 12: Stemwinder. Stand erect, left foot lifted clear of floor. Rotate left foot in small circles 20 times. Repeat with right foot.

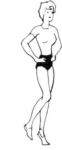

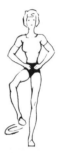

EXERCISE 11

EXERCISE 12

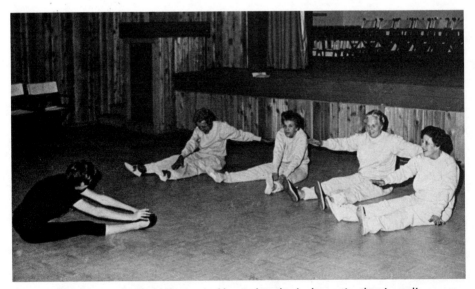

Because people of middle age and beyond tend to be less active than in earlier years, a regular program of calisthenics is especially important for them.

CHAPTER 36

Voluntary Health Agencies

The establishment of over 100 voluntary health agencies since the beginning of this century has been a major factor in the growth of health services to the American public. These agencies, whose activities are made possible by donations of time and money from the public, occasionally augmented by government grants for special projects, have the following objectives: spreading information about various diseases to the professional and lay public; sponsoring research; promoting legislation, and operating referral services on the community level to patients in need of diagnosis, treatment, and financial aid.

Some of these agencies, such as the American Diabetes Association or the Arthritis Foundation, focus on a particular disease; others deal with problems arising from related disorders, such as the National Association for Mental Health and the American Heart Association. Still others, such as Planned Parenthood and the American Social Health Association, have programs vital not only to individuals, but to society as a whole.

To coordinate the activities of these many groups, to promote better health facilities, and to establish standards for the organization and conduct of these agencies, the National Health Council was founded in 1920. Its membership includes government, professional, and community associations, as well as the 19 voluntary health agencies described below, which command a total budget of almost $300 million and involve the services of almost 9 million volunteers.

All of these organizations function on the national, state, and community level. Information and literature may be obtained through local chapters or by writing to the national

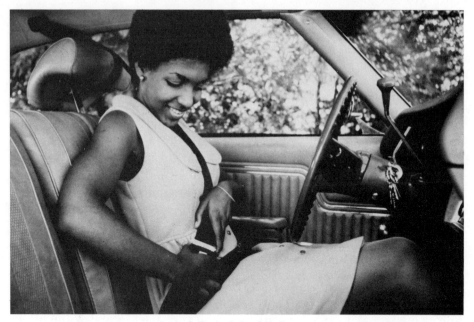

The regular use of seat belts and shoulder harnesses is an important factor in reducing the risk of serious injury in automobile accidents.

office of the organization. Volunteers may offer their services in a variety of ways: as office workers, fund raisers, speakers, and community coordinators.

On the following pages, voluntary health agencies are discussed under the subjects with which they are concerned; the subjects are arranged alphabetically. Other voluntary health agencies are discussed briefly beginning on p. 1247. Due to limitations of space, however, many worthwhile organizations have had to be omitted. The omission of any agency or group should not, therefore, be interpreted as implying any judgment about an omitted organization.

Accident Prevention

The National Safety Council, 444 North Michigan Avenue, Chicago, Illinois 60611, was founded in 1913 to improve factory safety but soon broadened its activities to preventing every type of accident. The Council is now composed of groups and individuals from every part of the population: business, industry, government, education, religion, labor, and law. Its main efforts are devoted to building strong support for official safety programs at the national, state, and community level in specific areas, such as traffic, labor, and home.

The Council believes that practically all accidents can be prevented with the application of the right safeguards. These safeguards include public education and awareness of danger, enforcement of safety laws and regulations, and improved design standards for machines, farm equipment, and motor vehicles.

It maintains the world's largest library of accident prevention materials, distributes a wide variety of safety literature, and issues awards for outstanding safety achievements. It also serves as a national and international clearing house of information about the causes of accidents and how they can be prevented.

In addition to campaigning for increased safety legislation on the national and state level, the Council's current programs include a defensive driving course, which provides effective adult driver training on a mass scale; a safety training institute; and, in cooperation with the American Medical Association, a new approach to the alcohol and driving problem.

Its publication, *Family Safety*, has a record circulation of almost 2 million readers, and its manual called *Fundamentals of Industrial Hygiene* provides more than 1,000 pages of material essential to the safety of factory workers.

For the last few years, the organization has been engaged in a fact-finding project, the Home Safety Inventory, designed to improve building standards and other hazardous environmental factors that contribute to making accidents the fourth leading cause of death in the United States.

Alcoholism

The National Council on Alcoholism, 733 Third Avenue, New York, New York 10017, is the only national voluntary health agency founded to combat alcoholism as a disease by an extensive program on the professional and community level. The Council is completely independent of Alcoholics Anonymous, although the two organizations cooperate fully.

In the more than 70 cities where the Council has branches, alcoholism information centers have been established that provide referral services for alcoholics and their families as well as educational materials for all segments of the community, including doctors and nurses, the clergy, the courts, social workers, and welfare agencies. Local affiliates also help to develop labor-management programs that provide help for employees who suffer from the disease.

The NCA also sponsors research, professional training, legislative action, and treatment centers on the national and local level.

As its national headquarters in New York, the Council maintains the only library in the country devoted exclusively to the subject and study of alcoholism. The collection was begun in 1957 and now consists of over 1,500 books, periodicals, and technical documents on the subject. Its publications department distributes more than 100 different books and pamphlets divided into special categories. Information on this literature as well as on all aspects of the Council's programs is available to anyone who writes to the national headquarters or contacts the nearest local affiliate.

Arthritis

The Arthritis Foundation, 475 Riverside Drive, New York, New York 10027, was established to help arthritis sufferers and their doctors through programs of research, patient services, public health information, and education on the professional and popular level. Its long-term goal is to find the cause,

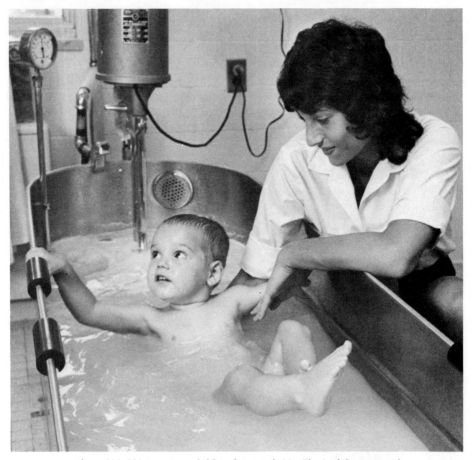

About 250,000 American children have arthritis. Physical therapy and other forms of treatment offer promise of effective rehabilitation.

prevention, and cure for the nation's number one crippling disease.

Two special groups work within the organization: the American Rheumatism Association Section, which governs medical and scientific programs, and the Allied Health Professions Section, which devotes itself to overcoming the shortage of specialized health workers in the field.

The Foundation operates local chapters throughout the United States whose chief concern is the patient who has or might have arthritis. These chapters are centers for in-formation about the disease itself and also serve as referral centers for treatment facilities. In addition, they distribute literature and sponsor forums on the latest developments in research and patient care.

Some chapters support arthritis clinics and home care programs; others provide mobile treatment units that travel to rural communities and work with local doctors and their patients.

A major part of the Foundation's program consists of a network of arthritis clinical research centers which specialize in experiments with new medicines and treatment procedures. The publications distributed by this organization include a wide variety of pamphlets and brochures for the professional reader as well as the interested public.

Cancer

The American Cancer Society, 777 Third Avenue, New York, New York 10017, was established in 1913 by a small group of doctors and volun-

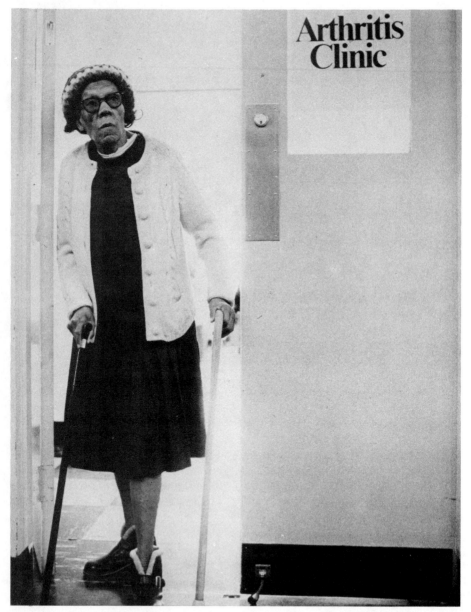

The Arthritis Foundation is working to increase the number of physicians qualified to give the special treatment needed by arthritis patients.

teer workers to inform the public about the possibility of saving lives through the early diagnosis and treatment of cancer. The Society now has 58 incorporated divisions, one in each state plus one in the District of Columbia and seven other metropolitan areas, devoted to the control and eradication of cancer. In addition to the doctors, research scientists, and other professional workers engaged in the Society's activities, over two million volunteers are connected with its many programs.

The ACS conducts widespread campaigns to educate the public in the importance of annual medical checkups so that cancerous symptoms can be detected while they are still curable. Such checkups should include an examination of the rectum and colon and, for women, examination of the breasts and a Pap test for the detection of uterine cancer.

In another of its campaigns, the Society emphasizes the link between cigarette smoking and lung cancer. It also sponsors an extensive program to persuade teen-agers not to start smoking. During its annual April Crusade Against Cancer, the Society distributes approximately 40 million copies of the leaflet listing the seven warning signals of the disease.

On the professional level, the major objective of ACS is to make every doctor's office a cancer-detection center. To achieve this goal, it publishes a variety of literature, offers refresher courses, sponsors seminars, and cooperates closely with local and state medical societies and health departments on the diagnosis and treatment of

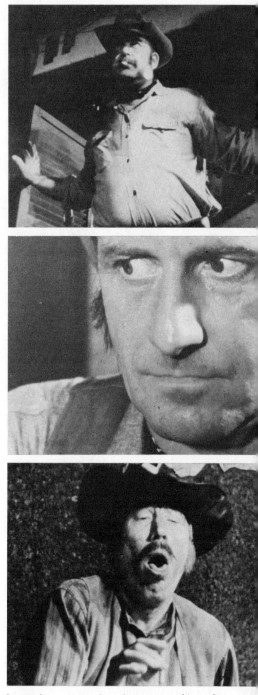

In waging war against cigarette smoking, the American Cancer Society showed a TV commerical in which typical western "bad guys" couldn't draw their six-shooters because smoking doubled them up in fits of coughing.

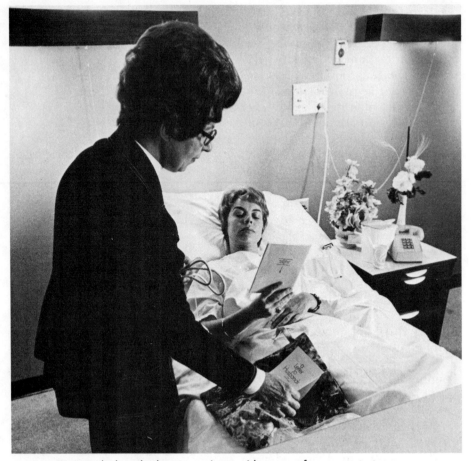

Women who have had mastectomies provide support for new mastectomy patients in the American Cancer Society's volunteer Reach to Recovery program.

cancer. It also arranges national and international conferences for the exchange of information on the newest cancer-fighting techniques, and finances a million-dollar-a-year clinical fellowship program for young physicians.

Among its special services to patients are sponsorship of the International Association of Laryngectomees, for people who have lost their voices to cancer; and Reach to Recovery, a program for women who have had radical mastectomies (breast removal) and who need support and guidance in order to return to normal living. On the community level, ACS operates a counseling service for cancer patients and their families, referring them to the proper medical facilities and social agencies for treatment and care. Through its "loan closets," it provides sickroom necessities, hospital beds, medical dressings, and so on.

Some local divisions of ACS also offer home care programs through the services of the Visiting Nurse Association or a similar agency. Although the Society does not operate medical facilities, treat patients, or pay doctors' fees, some of the chapters support cancer detection programs and professionally supervised rehabilitation services.

Cerebral Palsy

The United Cerebral Palsy Associations, Inc., 66 East 34th Street, New York, New York 10016, founded in 1949 by a small group of concerned parents, now has 301 affiliates across the country where those who are afflicted with the disorder may obtain treatment referral, therapy, and education. The Associations also play an important role in vocational training, job placement programs, and recreational services.

The Research and Educational Foundation of this organization supported the studies that led ultimately to the development of a safe vaccine against rubella, the disease which is responsible for a significant number of birth defects if it occurs during the early months of pregnancy. It is also investigating other possible causes of cerebral palsy in the newborn,

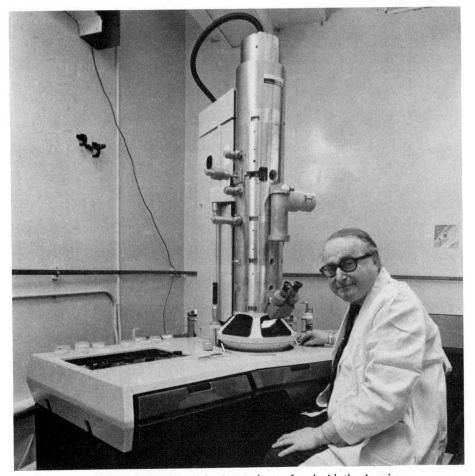

The National Cancer Institute (not to be confused with the American Cancer Society) is a U.S. government agency devoted to cancer research. Here, a scientist prepares to use a powerful electron microscope.

such as the misuse of drugs during pregnancy, and oxygen deprivation during labor and delivery. Grants are also given to universities and medical schools for research into the causes of cerebral palsy and new methods of therapy for treatment of cerebral palsied patients, and also for training medical personnel to deal with this disease.

Cystic Fibrosis

The National Cystic Fibrosis Research Foundation, 3379 Peachtree Road, N.E., Atlanta, Georgia 30326, was organized in 1955 by a group of concerned parents whose children were born with this lung disease. The Foundation now concerns itself with all serious lung ailments of chil-

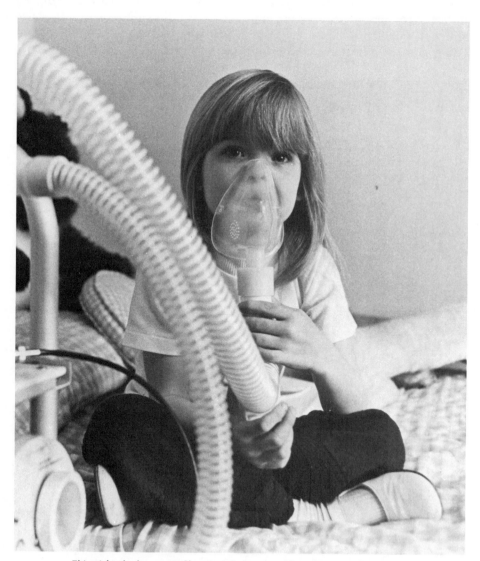

This girl, who has cystic fibrosis, inhales aerosol medications three times a day to liquefy the sticky mucus that blocks the airways of her lungs.

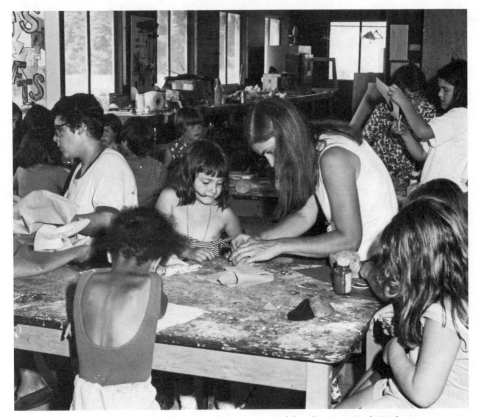

An arts and crafts group at a camp sponsored by the New York Diabetes Association. Such camps are tailored to meet the needs of diabetic children.

dren regardless of their medical names, and it engages in a broad program of research, medical education, public information, and the sponsorship of diagnostic and treatment centers.

The Foundation's 135 local chapters offer advice and information to parents of children with severe lung disease, and have direct connections with the 110 Cystic Fibrosis Centers throughout the country. They refer patients to sources of financial aid, make arrangements for the purchase of drugs at a discount, and lend home treatment equipment to families who cannot afford to buy it.

The national organization makes grants for research activities, con-

ducts professional conferences, and publishes literature for doctors and the general public on various aspects of childhood lung diseases.

Diabetes

The American Diabetes Association, 1 West 48th Street, New York, New York 10020, which was established as a professional society in 1940, has in recent years enlarged its scope so that it currently has 53 affiliated chapters throughout the country which promote the creation of better understanding of diabetes among patients and their families; the exchange of knowledge among physicians and other scientists; the

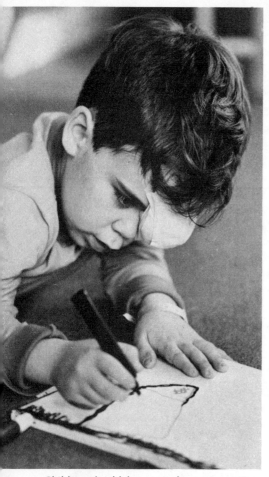

Children should have regular eye examinations beginning early in life, so that any disorders can be promptly corrected.

spreading of accurate information to the general public about early recognition and supervision of the disease; and the sponsorship of basic research.

Since 1948, the ADA has conducted an annual Diabetes Detection Drive supported by widespread publicity in all news media. During this drive, approximately three million testing kits are provided to state and county medical societies to facilitate the early detection and prompt treatment of the disorder.

This annual activity hopes to find the estimated 1,600,000 people who are unaware that they have diabetes.

Among the Association's publications of special interest to diabetics and their families are the *ADA Forecast*, a national magazine that presents news items on research and treatment; *Meal Planning with Exchange Lists*, prepared with the cooperation of the American Dietetic Association and the U.S. Public Health Service; and *A Cookbook for Diabetics*, which contains attractive recipes for meals that can be served to diabetics.

Other activities of the ADA include encouraging the employment of diabetics, and providing special groups such as teachers, police, and social agencies with information on the condition. It has also established a classification of the disease according to its severity. Guidelines on emergency medical care and the scientific journal *Diabetes* are available to doctors.

Drug Abuse

The American Social Health Association, which was organized originally to combat the spread of venereal disease, expanded its program in 1960 to include drug abuse education. For information about its activities in this field, see below under *Venereal Disease*.

Eye Diseases

The National Society for the Prevention of Blindness, 79 Madison Avenue, New York, New York 10016, was founded in 1908 to reduce the number of infants born with impaired sight. In subsequent years, it merged with the American Association for the Conservation of Vision and the Ophthalmological Foundation. The Society is now concerned with investigating all causes of blindness and supports measures and community services that will eliminate them. It also distributes information on the proper care and use of the eyes.

The organization's first and most significant victory was the adoption of laws by almost all states requiring that silver nitrate solution be routinely dropped into the eyes of all newborn babies to counteract the possibility of congenital blindness. This resulted in a dramatic drop in the number of children suffering from eye impairment dating from birth.

For almost half a century, the Society has actively campaigned to reduce the number of people suffering from glaucoma, the second leading cause of blindness in the United States. It has also conducted a national program to educate the elderly in the ease, safety, and advantages of surgery for cataracts, the leading cause of blindness among the aged.

Since 1926, the Society has been conducting preschool vision screening programs administered by teams that travel from big cities to isolated rural communities. Current activities also include research into the cause, treatment, and prevention of eye diseases leading to blindness; assembling data and publishing reports; cooperating with community agencies to improve eye health; promoting conditions in schools and industry to safeguard vision; and advocating eye examinations in early childhood so that disorders can be properly and promptly corrected.

The education division of the Society produces pamphlets, films, and circulating exhibits on all aspects of eye safety and sight preservation. This material is available on request.

Family Planning

Planned Parenthood Federation of America, 810 Seventh Avenue, New York, New York 10019, established in 1961, is the direct result of the birth control clinics originally founded by Margaret Sanger in 1916. The comparatively young organization has quickly grown from a single center in Brooklyn to a nation-wide network of 181 affiliates, with a total of 620 clinics operating in 350 cities. It also assists national family planning organizations in more than 100 countries throughout the world.

Planned Parenthood has five principal goals: to help make information and effective means of family planning—including contraception, voluntary sterilization and abortion—available and easily accessible to all; to educate all American parents in the advantages of limiting the size of their families; to stimulate medical and sociological research; to combat the world population crisis; and to support the efforts of others to achieve these goals in the United States and throughout the world.

Each year, through its clinics, the organization offers family planning information, education, and medically supervised services to over 400,000 men and women of varied social and economic backgrounds at little or no cost. In addition, it conducts clinical research, furnishes and directs professional training of medical and health personnel, and assists city, county, and state governments in developing their own family planning programs.

To meet the increased demand on the part of men for voluntary sterilization, Planned Parenthood has opened 13 vasectomy clinics in various parts of the country. It is also providing migrant workers in more than 20 states with a unique referral program of family planning services. Films and publications on all aspects of the organization's activities are distributed to individuals, community agencies, citizen action groups, schools, and hospitals.

Heart Disease

The American Heart Association, 7320 Greenville Avenue, Dallas, Texas 75231, was founded in 1924 as

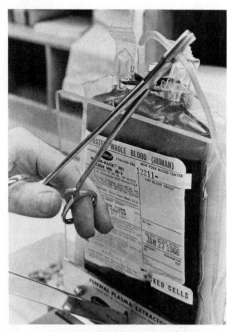

Modern blood bank techniques make quantities of whole blood available to hemophiliacs. Blood can also be fractionated (separated into components).

a professional organization of cardiologists. It was reorganized in 1948 as a national voluntary health agency to promote a program of education, research, and community service in the interests of reducing premature death and disability caused by diseases of the heart and blood vessels. The complex of heart disorders, including atherosclerosis, stroke, high blood pressure, kidney diseases, rheumatic fever, and congenital heart disturbances, is by far the leading cause of death in the United States.

Since its first Annual Heart Fund Campaign in 1949, the Association has contributed more than 150 million dollars to research and has been a major factor in the reduction of cardiovascular mortality statistics. It has spent over two million dollars since 1959 studying human heart transplantation procedures, and has contributed to the development of an artificial heart, plastic heart valves, and synthetic arteries.

Public and professional education programs designed to reduce the risk of heart attack through avoidance of cigarette smoking, obesity, and foods high in cholesterol are conducted on a nation-wide and community level by the Association's affiliates throughout the country. The local chapters are also engaged in service programs for rheumatic fever prevention, stroke rehabilitation, school health, cardiopulmonary resuscitation, and industrial health. In addition, they conduct information and referral services for patients and their families.

The AHA publishes many technical and professional journals as well as material designed for the general public.

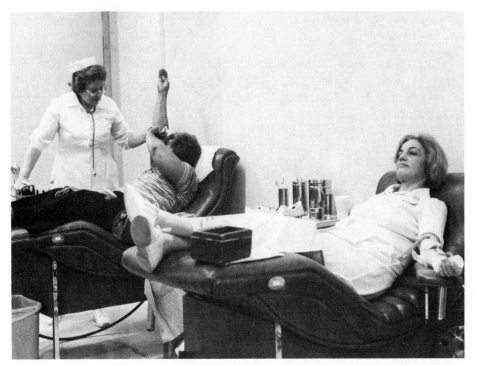

The National Hemophilia Foundation relies on whole blood from donors such as these to supply the clotting factor needed by hemophiliacs.

Hemophilia

The National Hemophilia Foundation, 25 West 39th Street, New York, New York 10018, was established in 1948 to serve the needs of hemophiliacs and their families by insuring the availability of treatment and rehabilitation facilities. It is estimated that there are as many as 100,000 males suffering from what is popularly known as "bleeder's disease," an inherited condition passed from mothers to sons.

The long-term goal of the foundation is to develop a national program of research and clinical study that will provide new information about early diagnosis and effective treatment of the disorder as well as trained professional personnel to administer patient care.

The development in recent years of blood-clotting concentrates is the most important advance to date in the treatment of the disease. This development, supported in part by the Foundation's 53 chapters, makes it possible for patients to have elective surgery and dental work, and to eliminate much of the pain, crippling, and hospitalization of those suffering from hemophilia.

The need for blood supplies from which to extract the clotting factor caused the Foundation to embark on an extensive campaign for blood donations. For this purpose, it has been working closely since 1968 with the American Red Cross and the American Association of Blood Banks. It also maintains close ties with various laboratories and research groups in the development of more powerful concentrates that can be manufactured and sold at the lowest possible cost.

The organization's activities include a national network of facilities with blood banks, clinics, and treatment centers as well as referral services. It has also established a Behavioral Science Department to explore the nonmedical aspects of hemophiliacs' problems, such as education, vocational guidance, and psychological needs.

Kidney Disease

The National Kidney Foundation, 116 East 27th Street, New York, New York 10016, formerly the National Nephrosis Foundation, was organized in 1950 to work toward improved care and treatment for those afflicted with kidney disease through improved methods and services in research, prevention, detection, and diagnosis.

Although the Foundation is growing rapidly, it has scarcely begun to meet the needs of the nearly eight million people who suffer from kidney disorders. However, since its establishment, the number of deaths from nephrosis has been drastically reduced by the use of transplantation from matched donors and the technique of hemodialysis.

Through its 40 affiliates in 35 states, the NKF endorses the wider application of these procedures and supports research, training of professional personnel, construction of facilities, and programs that help to defray the high cost of treatment.

Emphasis is currently being placed on the establishment of screening and diagnostic centers to detect kidney disease as early as possible and to educate the public in recognizing its symptoms. The Foundation distributes many publications on kidney-related subjects to the professional and general public. For the general reader, there are leaflets explaining kidney function and disease, the role of hypertension, and recognition of symptoms of disorder.

Mental Health

The National Association for Mental Health, 1800 N. Kent Street, Rosslyn, Virginia 22209, had its beginnings in 1909, when an ex-mental patient founded the National Committee for Mental Hygiene. In 1950, this group merged with the National Mental Health Foundation and the Psychiatric Foundation to create the organization as it now stands. The purpose of the NAMH is to improve attitudes toward and services for the mentally ill, to work for the prevention of mental illness, and to promote mental health.

Since 1960, the Association's national research program has invested more than one million dollars in studies aimed at finding out more about the causes, treatment, and new ways of preventing mental illness. It has played a significant and pioneering role in the study of schizophrenia.

The NAMH implements its service programs through its chapters in some 1,000 cities, counties, and metropolitan areas throughout the country, and its divisions, which are state associations. In the past few decades, its watchdog efforts have resulted in improved care and treatment in state hospitals, the upgrading of old hospitals and clinics, and

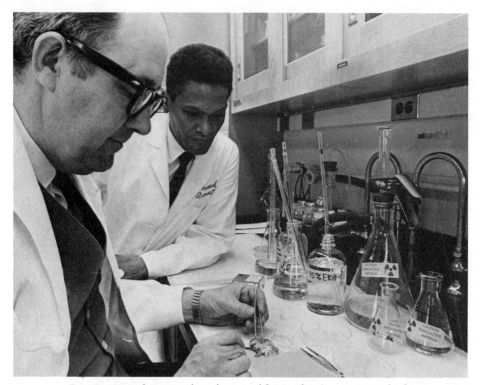

Examinations of tissue and cerebrospinal fluid aid in diagnosing multiple sclerosis. Here a neurologist and his assistant study a tissue specimen.

the erection of better treatment facilities. It constantly provides lawmakers with information about mental illness and the need for a greater number of government-funded resources.

Through widespread campaigning, the Association has helped to focus attention on childhood mental illness and the importance of providing better diagnostic and treatment facilities for young people with serious mental disturbances.

To reduce the number of patients who return to mental hospitals because of inadequate rehabilitation services in their communities, the NAMH has activated local agencies in their effort to help such patients return to normal life and find suitable employment.

Multiple Sclerosis

The National Multiple Sclerosis Society, 205 East 42nd Street, New York, New York 10017, was organized in 1946 with the initial goal of supporting research into the causes and possible cure for this baffling disease of the central nervous system. One of the earliest efforts of the Society was to increase professional and public awareness of the symptoms of multiple sclerosis and the large number of people suffering from it. In addition, a campaign was launched in 1949 for the creation of a new branch of the U.S. Public Health Service to foster and subsidize studies of the disorder. By 1950, the National Institute for Neurological Diseases and Stroke was founded

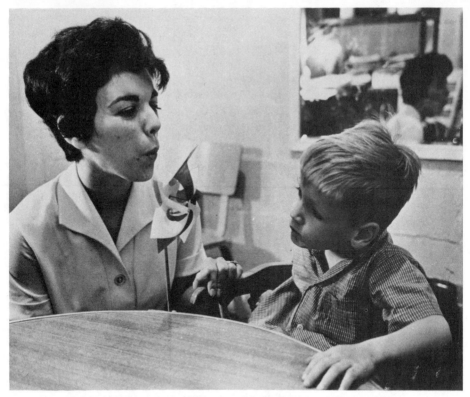

A speech therapist for the National Easter Seal Society uses a pin-wheel as a visual aid in improving her patient's breath control.

as an official government agency. It now spends upwards of three million dollars annually on multiple sclerosis research alone.

Through its more than 200 chapters and affiliated units, the NMSS engages in home and hospital visits, distributes aids to daily living, organizes recreational programs, and supports diagnostic clinics. The local units also arrange educational programs for doctors and rehabilitation and social workers, as well as for patients and their families.

The national office distributes publications for medical personnel and for the interested public, and issues guides for the development of patient services and a quarterly newsletter on research and treat-ment developments. A medical film and two public information films as well as speakers are available for community programs.

Physical Handicaps

The National Easter Seal Society for Crippled Children and Adults, 2023 West Ogden Avenue, Chicago, Illinois 60612, has grown from its pioneering origins in 1919 to a national organization that serves hundreds of thousands of physically handicapped people of all ages. Among its network of over 3,000 facilities are 83 comprehensive rehabilitation centers in 25 states; 131 treatment and diagnostic centers in 28 states; and vocational training workshops, residential camps, special education programs, and transportation services in many different parts of the country.

Because many crippled children and adults in rural areas and small communities are unaware of the services available to them, the Society gives top priority to publicizing its information, referral, and follow-up activities. In recent years, it has also established mobile treatment units in hospitals and nursing homes in rural areas.

Other innovative activities include screening and testing programs to detect hearing loss in newborns and learning disabilities in preschool children, and providing treatment and referral for those who are disabled by respiratory diseases.

The Society collaborates with federal and professional agencies in all programs designed to eliminate architectural barriers to the disabled, and was instrumental in the enactment of legislation making it mandatory that all buildings constructed with government funds be fully and easily accessible to the handicapped. It also initiates and supports significant studies in rehabilitation procedures as well as scientific research in bone transplant techniques.

Extensive literature is distributed to professionals, the public, to parents, and employers. It also assembles special educational packets for parents of the handicapped.

Tuberculosis and Respiratory Diseases

The American Lung Association, 1740 Broadway, New York, New York 10019, is the direct descendant of the first voluntary health organization to be formed in the United States. In 1904, when the National Association for the Study and Prevention of Tuberculosis was organized, this disease was the country's leading cause of death. Since 1975, with the sharp increase in the problems relating to smoking and air pollution, the Association has been known by its present name, which was adopted to reflect the broader scope of its activities.

It now concerns itself not only with the elimination of tuberculosis but with chronic and disabling conditions, such as emphysema, and with acute diseases of the respiratory system, such as influenza. Through its 1,500 affiliates and nation-wide state organizations, it is actively engaged in campaigns against smoking and air pollution.

The early endeavor of the Association to have tuberculosis included among the reportable diseases was accomplished state by state, and since the 1920s, all states have required that every case in the country be brought to the attention of local health officials.

Public awareness of better care and the development of effective drugs have dramatically reduced the number of TB patients, but the Association continues to concern itself with the fact that there are still more than 45,000 new cases each year.

Through its local affiliates, the ALA initiates special campaigns to combat smoking and air pollution, using radio and television announcements, car stickers, posters, and pamphlets, as well as films and exhibits. Educational materials on respiratory diseases are regularly distributed by the national office to

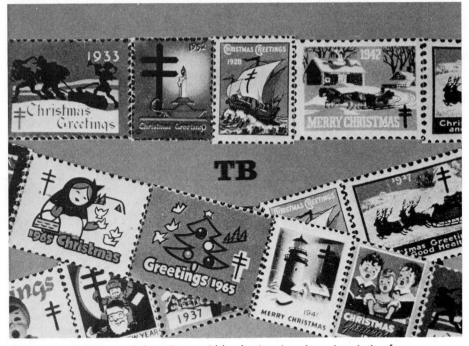

Christmas seals have been sold by the American Lung Association for many years to raise money for research on various respiratory diseases.

doctors, patients, and the general public. Funds raised by the annual Christmas Seal drive also support research and medical education fellowships.

Venereal Disease

The American Social Health Association, 260 Sheridan Avenue, Suite 307, Palo Alto, California 94306, was organized in 1912 to promote the control of venereal disease and to combat prostitution. Since 1960, it has also concerned itself with problems relating to drug dependence and abuse. Although it has no local units, it appoints regional staff members to work with private and public community organizations on special programs related to special health and family life education. For such programs, it provides research and statistical information, educational materials, professional consultation, and plans for voluntary citizen action.

The Association is in close touch with government agencies such as the Public Health Service, the National Institutes of Health, and the various branches of the Armed Forces, as well as the Federal Bureau of Narcotics, the Children's Bureau, and the Office of Education. Through these channels, it promotes its program for VD education in the schools and for research toward the discovery of an immunizing vaccine against syphilis and gonorrhea.

In the drug field, the ASHA is the major national voluntary repository for information and consultation, and maintains the world's most comprehensive collection of source materials on the misuse of narcotics, barbiturates, and the like. It constantly helps communities in diagnosing their problems and produces a number of publications for teachers, guidance counselors, and youth workers.

The agency's original sex education program has been broadened to include all aspects of family life. In literature, lectures, and conferences, it stresses the importance of introducing family life education into the curriculum of elementary and secondary schools and of establishing training programs on this subject in teachers' colleges. These efforts have resulted in the inclusion of family life education in an increasing number of school systems throughout the United States.

Other Voluntary Health Agencies

In addition to those voluntary health agencies which are members of the National Health Council, there are many other organizations which function on a national scale and offer specialized services as well as literature and guidance to professionals, patients, parents, and concerned families. The following is a partial list:

Alcoholics Anonymous, Box 459, Grand Central Annex, New York, New York 10017, is a fellowship of men and women who share their experience and give each other support in overcoming the problem of alcoholism. Chapters exist throughout the country and offer referral services, literature, and information about special hospital programs.

Al-Anon Family Groups, P.O. Box 182, Madison Square Station, New York, New York 10010, is unaffiliated with Alcoholics Anonymous but cooperates closely with it. This organization serves the families and friends of alcoholics, organizing groups for supportive therapy, providing speakers, distributing literature, and offering referral services. There are more than 5,500 such groups in the United States.

Allergy Foundation of America, 801 Second Avenue, New York, New York 10017, was established to help solve all health problems related to allergic diseases by sponsoring research and treatment facilities. It also grants scholarships to medical students specializing in the study of allergy.

American Foundation for the Blind, 15 West 16th Street, New York, New York 10011, is a national research and information center that coordinates the activities of local and regional agencies serving the blind and the deaf-blind. It also records over two million books and magazines each year. Known as The Talking Books, they are produced in cooperation with the Library of Congress and are made available to the blind and other handicapped people free of charge through special libraries throughout the United States.

The Association for Voluntary Sterilization, 708 Third Avenue, New York, New York 10017, was founded in 1937 to inform professionals and the public about the nature and merits of voluntary sterilization as a method of birth control; to encourage family counseling services to include advice on this procedure; and to encourage physicians and hospitals to establish policies that will make this type of surgery

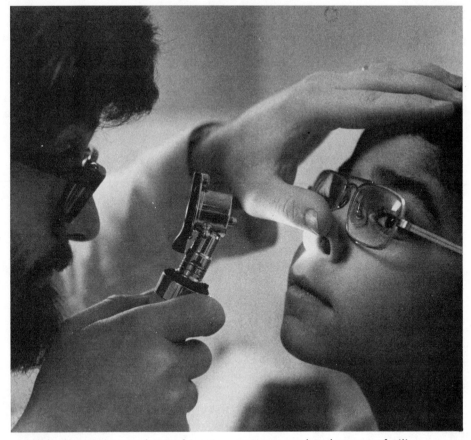

The Allergy Foundation of America sponsors research and treatment facilities for allergic diseases. This patient is being examined for a skin allergy.

available to properly screened applicants. The organization has a roster of 1,600 cooperating physicians in all parts of the United States who accept referrals and perform sterilizations.

The Epilepsy Foundation of America, 1828 L Street, N.W., Washington, D.C. 20036, is the result of a merger in 1967 of two similar organizations. At present, the Foundation has 78 local affiliates which provide information, referral services, and counseling. It conducts a research grant program for medical and psychosocial investigation and distributes a wide variety of literature on request to doctors, teachers,

employers, and the interested public on such subjects as anticonvulsant drugs, insurance, driving laws, and emergency treatment. The national office also maintains an extensive research library and a speakers' bureau.

The Leukemia Society of America, 211 East 43rd Street, New York, New York 10017, was organized in 1950 and now has 69 chapters in 21 states. It supports research in the causes, control, and eventual eradication of the disease which, though commonly thought of as a disorder of the blood, is in fact a disorder of the bone marrow, lymph nodes, and spleen, which manufacture blood. The Society has a continuing program of education through special publications directed to doctors, nurses, and the public. Through its local affiliates, it conducts patient-aid services which provide counseling, transportation, and—to those who need financial assistance—drugs, blood transfusions, and laboratory facilities.

Muscular Dystrophy Associations of America, 810 Seventh Avenue, New York, New York 10019, has as its goal the scientific conquest of muscular dystrophy and all related neuromuscular diseases. Through its 325 chapter affiliates in the United States, the MDAA offers a large number of patient and community services, all of them free. Diagnostic

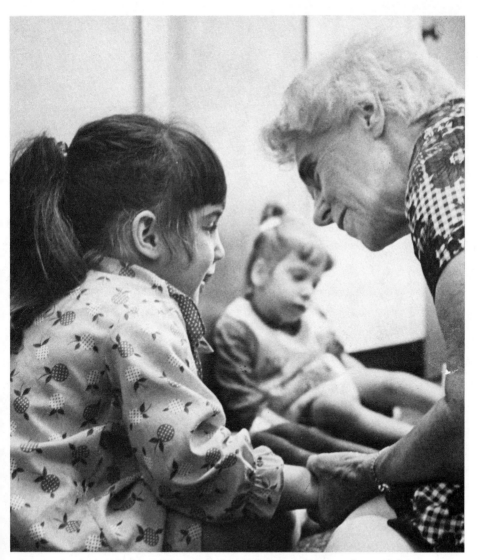

A volunteer working with a young hospital patient. Many service organizations use older volunteers to work with hospitalized or handicapped children.

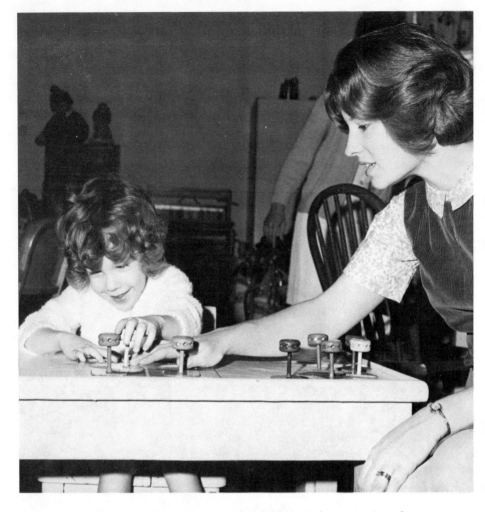

With proper supervision, retarded children can learn a variety of skills that can be developed into occupational goals in adulthood.

workups and tests are available to all those who may, in the opinion of their physician, be suffering from neuromuscular ailments. The local chapters assist in the purchase and repair of such items as walkers and crutches, braces, wheelchairs, and hospital beds when they are prescribed by a doctor.

Other activities include work with elementary and secondary schools for the inclusion of disabled children in existing educational programs and providing recreational programs for these children. Chapters also maintain patient service committees which serve as clearinghouses for information and referral.

The National Association for Retarded Citizens, 2709 Avenue E East, Arlington, Texas 76011, established in 1950, is the only national voluntary agency specifically devoted to promoting the welfare of the mentally retarded of all ages, of whom it is estimated that there are approximately six million in the United States. Through its 1,300 affiliates, it conducts sheltered workshops, encourages employment, supports research, and works for better diagnostic and treatment facilities. Counseling and referral services, as well as extensive literature for professionals and concerned families, are available on request.

The National Foundation-March of Dimes, P.O. Box 2000, White Plains, New York 10602, founded in

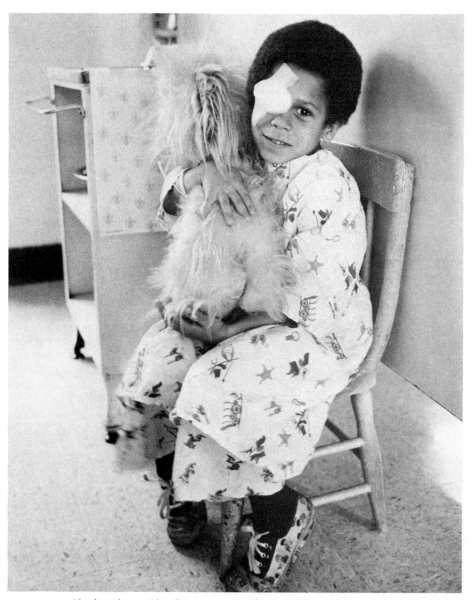

This boy, born with only one eye, is undergoing a series of operations to provide him with an eye socket so that he can wear an artificial eye.

1938 to combat infantile paralysis, is now chiefly concerned with birth defects: finding their causes, most effective treatments, and ways to prevent their occurrence. The Foundation supports 87 medical service centers and 17 research centers which focus on mental retardation of prenatal origin; congenital blindness, deafness, and heart disease; birth malformations such as club feet and cleft palates; and diseases such as diabetes, muscular dystrophy, and cystic fibrosis. The organization has also established the Salk Institute in California, directed by Dr. Jonas Salk, for the purpose of carrying on basic research in the life processes in order to discover what causes the abnormalities associated with birth defects. Since proper prenatal care plays a critical role in the normal development of the fetus, the Foundation enlists the support of every available community service in order to initiate prenatal care programs. Known as PNC clinics, these centers are set up in those parts of the country where they are most needed.

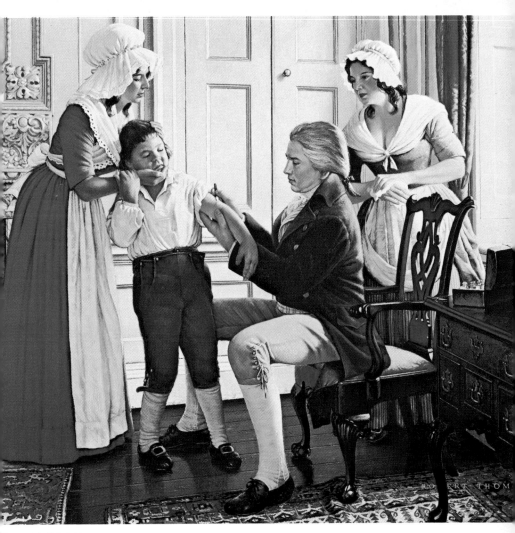

JENNER: SMALLPOX IS STEMMED

The first vaccination against smallpox was performed by Edward Jenner, English rural physician, in his apartment in the Chantry House, Berkeley, Gloucestershire. Exudate from a cowpox pustule on the hand of dairymaid, Sarah Nelmes, was inserted in scratches on the arm of eight-year-old James Phipps, May 14, 1796. The vaccination was effective, for two later attempts to induce infection with smallpox pus were unsuccessful. After proving his discovery, Jenner published his vaccination findings in 1798. Despite opposition, vaccination became accepted practice during Jenner's lifetime.

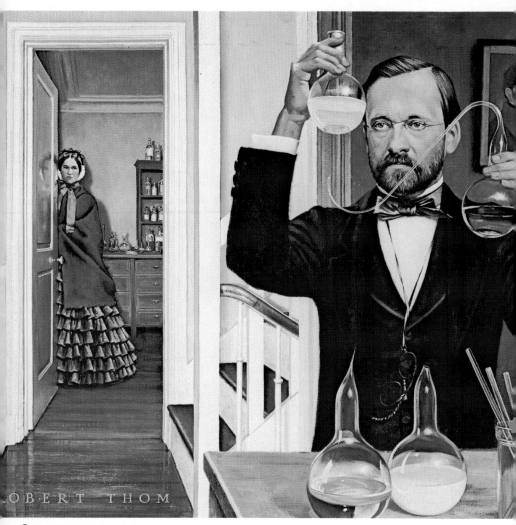

OBERT THOM

PASTEUR: THE CHEMIST WHO TRANSFORMED MEDICINE

Proof that microbes are reproduced from parent organisms, and do not result from spontaneous generation, came from careful experiments in makeshift laboratories of France's famed chemist and biologist, Louis Pasteur (1822-1895), at the Ecole Normale, Paris. Behind him are portraits of his father and mother, which he painted during his youth. Mme. Pasteur waits patiently for him to complete an observation. From basic work in these laboratories came proof of the germ theory of disease, which transformed medical practice; vaccines for virulent diseases, including anthrax and rabies; solution of many industrial biochemical problems; and founding of the Pasteur Institute.

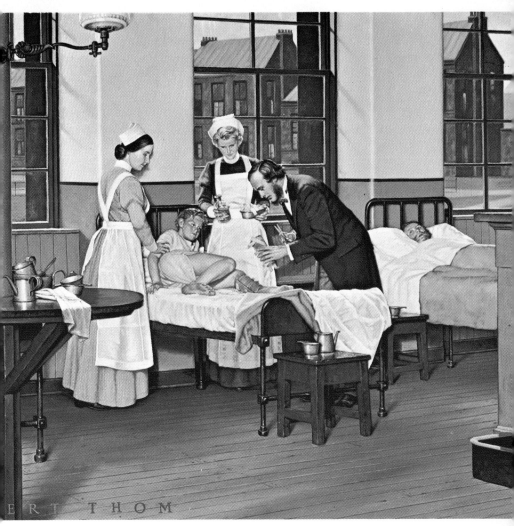

LISTER INTRODUCES ANTISEPSIS

When Surgeon Joseph Lister (1827-1912) of Glasgow Royal Infirmary removed dressings from James Greenlees' compound fracture, the wound had healed without infection—something unheard of before. For six weeks, beginning August 12, 1865, Lister had treated the boy's wound with carbolic acid. Now, Lister had proof of success of his principle of antisepsis—which was to revolutionize methods of treatment and to open new vistas in practice of surgery, of medicine, and of environmental sanitation. Hospitals were turned from "houses of torture and death" to "houses of healing and cure." In 1897, Lister became the first British surgeon to be elevated to peerage.

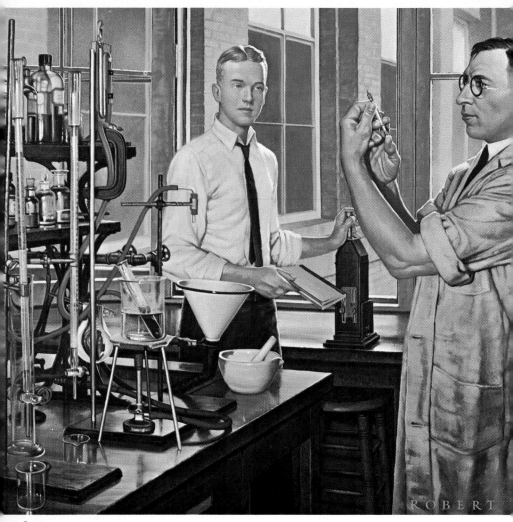

BANTING, BEST, AND DIABETES

During the summer of 1921, Charles H. Best, youthful biologist, and Dr. Frederick G. Banting experimented in laboratories loaned by Professor J. J. R. Macleod of the Physiology Department, University of Toronto. The inexperienced Canadian investigators found what trained research men before them had missed—an extract of the pancreas that controlled the high blood sugar of diabetes mellitus. Proved and reproved on laboratory animals, their extract was tried on a human diabetic in February, 1922. Best developed mass production methods while studying for a medical degree. Banting and Best's discovery of insulin gave hope of life to millions of diabetics who otherwise would have been doomed.

The Ancient Art of Acupuncture

Acupuncture, the Oriental art of inserting needles through the skin for the treatment of physical and mental ailments, is so ancient that its true origin cannot be traced. Some Asian scholars believe that acupuncture may have started during the stone ages; most agree that acupuncture has been used as a form of medical practice for at least 5,000 years. Among the oldest known manuscripts from early Chinese cultures is The Yellow Emperor's Canon of Internal Medicine, written about 400 B.C., which contains a description of the relationships between acupuncture and the religious philosophy of Tao.

Taoism and the Balance of Forces

Taoism teaches that there is a balance of forces in nature. The function of acupuncture in this metaphysical concept of medicine is to restore the balance of forces within the body by either stimulating or calming the organ system that seems to be at the root of the disorder. The two primary forces are the Yin and the Yang, represented by female and male, negative and positive, passive and active, shadow and light, or the earth and the heavens. The two primary forces both oppose and complement each other in a relative manner so that the universe is in harmony when the Yin and the Yang are in balance.

The Taoist concept also recognizes the Five Elements of nature. They are earth, fire, water, metal, and wood. Like Yin and Yang, the Five Elements are interdependent; each has its opposite, and each governs and is in turn governed by another element. Thus, water

1253

creates wood and wood creates fire, but metal overcomes wood and fire overcomes metal, and so on, in a five-sided cycle.

The Law of the Yin and the Yang and the Law of the Five Elements form the basis of traditional Oriental medical practices. Each organ of the body is either Yin or Yang; each organ is also associated with one of the Five Elements. The liver, regarded as the center of metabolic activity that makes life possible, is Yin and is also a wood element. The gall bladder, an anatomical neighbor of the liver, is also a wood element but it is Yang. Wood is the only element of the five that is of an organic nature. In this context, the lungs and the upper digestive tract have functions of supplying oxygen and food for the liver's metabolic activity, the heart helps circulate the metabolic products, and the kidneys and lower digestive tract carry away by-products of metabolism.

When symptoms of a liver disease are revealed by a doctor's diagnosis, the role of acupuncture is to help restore the equilibrium of the organ. If the ailment is associated with a lack of energy, the energy may be restored by pricking the skin with an acupuncture needle at a specific point on the body—a point which may be far removed anatomically from the diseased organ. If the disease is diagnosed as evidence of an excess of energy, a somewhat different application of acupuncture therapy may be prescribed to calm the excess energy flow.

THE FIVE ELEMENTS

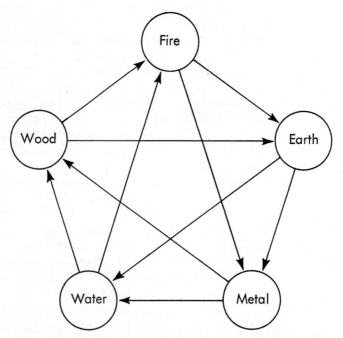

The arrows show how the Five Elements of nature interrelate in various ways, e.g., fire governs metal but is in turn controlled by water.

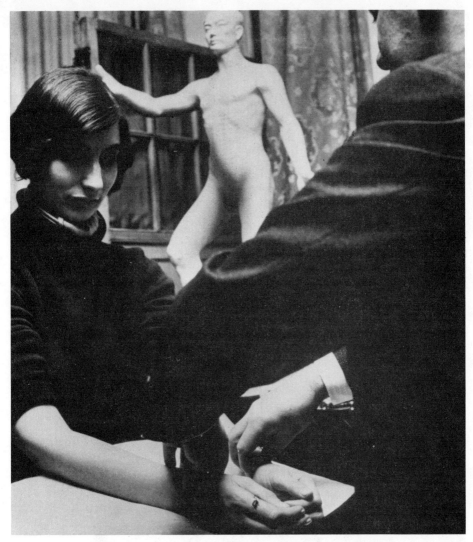

Before any acupuncture needles are inserted, the practitioner takes a series of pulse readings from each of the patient's wrists.

As the reader may have gathered by now, the practice of acupuncture is a complex art that requires a long period of study and training. Even before the first needle is inserted through the patient's skin, the practitioner makes a detailed examination that includes taking 12 pulse readings, six from each wrist at three different points. The examination may also require studying skin col-oration and body odor, palpating the chest and abdomen, and listening to the voice of the patient.

Meridians

After the diagnosis is completed, one or more acupuncture needles are inserted at a point along a *meridian*—the term used to describe a pathway beneath the skin through which

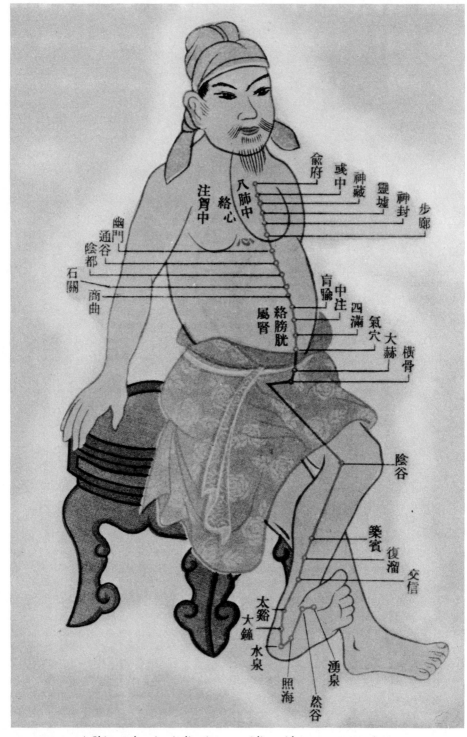

A Chinese drawing indicating a meridian with acupuncture points.

energy flows. Each organ system is associated with a meridian that extends to other areas of the body, which explains the rationale of treating a headache by inserting a needle in a toe. If both parts of the body are connected by a meridian, the energy flow in an organ can be stimulated or calmed by application of a needle to a point along the meridian even though the acupuncture point may be far removed from the site of the organic disorder.

According to traditional Chinese acupuncture texts, there are a dozen meridians and approximately 360 acupuncture points along those meridians. In recent years, practitioners have reported finding additional meridians and many more acupuncture points. A number of efforts have been made to explain the meridians and acupuncture points in terms compatible with scientific medical logic of the western world. It has been pointed out, for example, that meridians frequently follow the pathways of the body's major nerves and blood vessels.

Development of the Embryo

One theory proposed to explain acupuncture suggests that tissues in widely separated parts of the body may be related through the embryonic development of the various organs from three primary tissue layers. The human embryo is composed of an ectoderm (outer tissue layer), mesoderm (middle layer), and endoderm (innermost layer). The muscles and bones are derived from the mesoderm, as are the heart, the urinary organs, and the diaphragm, among other body parts. Also, during development of the embryo, the tiny arms and legs rotate so

that skin and muscles originally on the side facing the body become tissues on the outer surface of the limb, and vice versa. The fact that body tissues migrate and shift positions during embryonic life is thus used to help explain why an acupuncture point on one part of the body might stimulate a seemingly unrelated body area. In other words, it is believed by some acupuncturists that body cells retain throughout adult life a relationship that dates back to the first days of the embryo.

Oval Cells

A recent North Korean report stated that acupuncture points had been examined microscopically and were found to consist of groups of oval cells, surrounded by blood capillaries, just below the skin. The report also said that blood-rich bands of tissues that followed the pathways or meridians also were found. However, the report was not verified by other investigators.

Needles and How They Are Manipulated

The needles used for acupuncture are usually made of stainless steel, although gold and silver needles also are used. The type of metal apparently is not as important as the manner in which the needle is applied. Modern acupuncture practices include such techniques as boiling or otherwise sterilizing the needles, and cleaning the acupuncture point with a small wad of cotton soaked in alcohol. But the medical personnel may or may not provide protection for the skin puncture after the needle is removed: leaving the puncture exposed is part of the method of

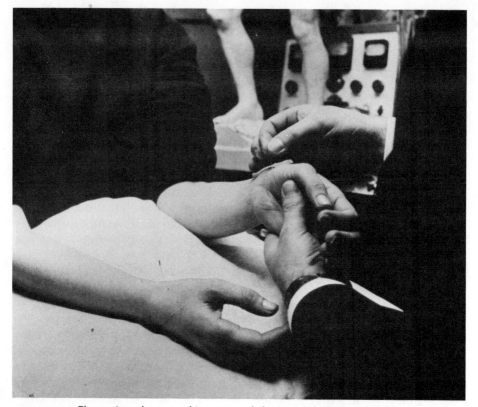

The patient shown on this page and the next is being treated for
sinusitis. Needles are inserted in the hands and the sides of the nose.

treating certain disorders. Extreme
care, however, is taken to avoid
puncturing important blood vessels
or nerve tracts which are near the
acupuncture points. To insert the
needle in skin that is close to the
bone or where there is a minimum of
muscle beneath the skin, the
acupuncturist pinches a fold of skin
between his fingers and aims the
needle at an angle. The needle may
in some cases be inserted at a 45-
degree angle rather than directly
downward into the flesh.

Although the acupuncture needle
usually is inserted only a fraction of
an inch, long needles sometimes are
used to reach points that may be six
inches beneath the skin. The depth

of insertion is measured in *fens*, with
a fen approximating one-tenth of an
inch. In actual practice, the "inch"
measure is based on the length of the
middle bone of the middle finger. If
the patient has a layer of fat beneath
the skin, additional fens of insertion
are applied to get the needle past
the fatty tissue. As a precaution
against the possibility that a needle
will break during insertion, it usually is guided into place by the
fingers of the hand that is not holding
the needle.

Manner of Insertion

The needle is not simply inserted
into an acupuncture point, although
that was a common practice in tradi-

tional Chinese medicine. It is manipulated by moving the needle up and down rapidly while twirling the top between the thumb and fingers. Some acupuncturists manipulate the needle by scratching the needle surface in a rhythmic pattern while it is in place. The modern Chinese method, however, calls for an up-and-down twirling rhythm of about 120 cycles per minute.

A variation of the manual manipulation technique is to attach a source of low-voltage electricity to the needles and allow the electricity to provide a vibratory stimulation at a rate of 120 cycles per minute. The amount of electricity is small, from one-fourth to one-half ampere at six to nine volts. And the frequency of vibration of the needles can with some equipment be varied from 120

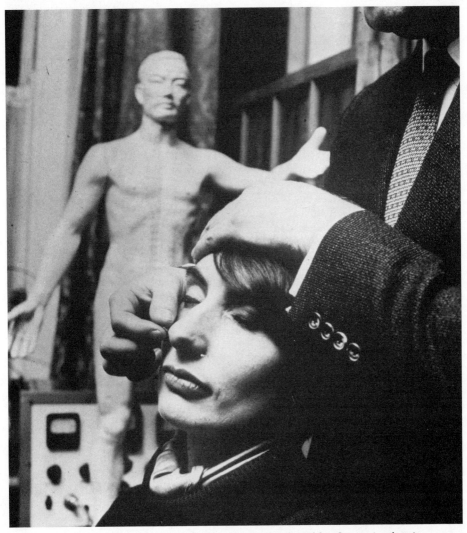

Acupuncture needles are manipulated by the thumb and forefinger. An electric pulsator that sends a weak current through the needles may also be used.

up to 180 cycles per minute if the medical personnel feel that a faster rate will produce certain desired effects. The electrical devices, called *pulsators,* operate on direct current.

Traditional acupuncture methods direct that the practitioner continue to check the various pulses while the needles are in place. They are then removed when the pulses indicate that the meridians are in equilibrium. An acupuncturist's rule-of-thumb is that the pulses will return to normal within a few minutes if the illness is mild, but a serious illness will require a longer period of needling. Even in serious cases of disease the needle seldom is used for longer than a half-hour. Additional treatment may consist of *moxibustion,* or burning a pinch of an herb over an acupuncture point, with the heat providing the extra bit of therapy.

Effectiveness of Acupuncture as Therapy

For reasons less well understood than acupuncture itself, the therapy seems to be more effective for some patients than others. Certain patients reportedly respond to the needle treatment within a few seconds while others appear to receive no benefits from the therapy, even after repeated efforts to reduce the symptoms of an ailment. Some patients find the application of needles painful while others describe the feeling of the needle as similar to an injection of Novacaine ordinarily given by dentists: a numbness about the area of the needle prick.

A review of clinical reports in the *Chinese Journal of Medicine,* an English-language publication of the

People's Republic of China, indicates that acupuncture in government hospitals produces varied results in the treatment of the same ailment. In the treatment of appendicitis in children, for example, acupuncture alone or acupuncture supplemented by antibiotics controlled the symptoms in 87 of 93 of the cases; the patients were pronounced completely recovered and dismissed. In the remaining six cases, acupuncture apparently failed to control the symptoms and surgery was required to complete a cure. Each of the 93 children involved in the study was given acupuncture treatment at the beginning. But if the child continued to appear feverish and his white blood cell count increased, he was taken into the operating room for removal of the appendix by conventional western techniques.

In another report in the official organ of the Chinese Medical Association, a doctor reported on the successful use of acupuncture to treat headache and dizziness side-effects of ten patients who had been given spinal anesthesia during conventional surgical procedures. "This method proved to be much better than routine analgesics because of its simplicity and efficacy," the author reported.

The Use of Acupuncture as a Pain-Killer

Acupuncture has been most successful in the field of anesthesia, and it is probably because of the great strides reported in the use of needling to control pain during surgery that acupuncture has aroused the serious interest of many physicians in the

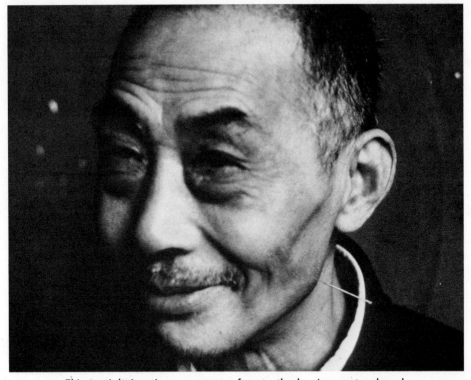

This man is being given acupuncture for a toothache. Acupuncture has also reportedly been successful in treating headaches, including migraine.

western world. The loss of feeling of pain follows the insertion of the fine needles in the arms, legs, ears, nose, or face. It is applied with or without electrical stimulation. In some instances distilled water is injected into the acupuncture points to produce *analgesia,* or loss of pain. American observers of acupuncture anesthesia have reported that in many cases the patient is given a typical western sedative such as pentobarbital (just as he might before a conventional surgical procedure), before the acupuncture needles are applied. The rate of success in achieving analgesia has been reported at around 90 percent by the Chinese when the needles are used to produce anesthesia for operations. It is used in many different kinds of operations, ranging from the mending of broken bones to brain surgery, and including procedures in which the chest is opened to repair a heart defect or to remove a diseased portion of a lung.

According to a recent report in the Chinese *Peking Review,* some 400,000 operations have been performed with acupuncture anesthesia on patients ranging in age from children to adults in their 80s.

Advantages of Acupuncture Anesthesia

One advantage of acupuncture anesthesia reported by Chinese doctors is that in an operation on the eye muscles to correct a defect such as squinting, the patient can move the eyes at the request of the surgeon because he remains fully conscious. The surgeon is thus able to evaluate the results of his work while the patient is still on the operating table. When anesthetic drugs are used, success or failure of the operation cannot be determined until after the drugs wear off and the patient regains consciousness.

Similarly, when acupunctural anesthesia is applied in an operation on the thyroid gland in the throat, the surgeon and patient can talk freely during the operation. This permits the doctor to evaluate vocal functions that might be affected by the throat surgery. During open-chest surgery, the patient can be instructed to maintain abdominal breathing techniques to give the surgeon more freedom in surgical activity that involves the lungs. In orthopedic surgery involving the arms and legs, medical personnel are able to observe the functioning of muscles and tendons of the involved limb while the surgery is in progress.

Origin of Anesthetic Use

According to an official Chinese version of the development of acupuncture anesthesia, a patient in a Shanghai hospital was unable to swallow without pain after his tonsils had been removed by conventional surgical methods. The medical personnel inserted a needle in one of the traditional acupuncture points and the pain stopped immediately. The patient then ate a meal of meat dumplings without difficulty.

The medical workers reasoned that since needling could stop the throat pain of a patient who had just undergone conventional surgery,

perhaps the use of acupuncture could be developed to replace western-type drugs as anesthetics during other tonsil operations. In their enthusiasm, the medical personnel began inserting needles at various acupuncture points in their own bodies to determine various degrees of pain relief. They also started application of acupuncture anesthesia in many kinds of surgery, applying as many as 100 needles at a time at various points in the bodies of patients undergoing lung operations. During that experimental period, according to the Chinese, it was not unusual to see four medical workers employed in an operating room for the sole purpose of manipulating the dozens of needles that had been inserted in the body of one patient.

Gradually, however, the medical personnel found that some acupuncture points were not necessary to produce anesthesia for a particular surgical procedure. The present practice is to use only a few needles, and in some cases only one needle, in key acupuncture points. Also, only one acupunctural anesthetist is required to manipulate the few needles by hand or to control the electric power source when that technique is used.

Although the Chinese themselves cannot offer adequate explanations of how acupuncture works, the procedure apparently has been successful in treating certain kinds of medical and psychiatric cases for many generations. It is perhaps useful to recall that physicians of the western world have prescribed drugs such as aspirin for many years without being able to explain how the chemical is able to relieve pain.

Acupuncture and Modern Medicine

Until the Communist revolution in China, acupuncture was practiced as a kind of folk medicine, mainly by healers in rural areas who lacked the formal training provided by western-type medical colleges. Along with herbal medicine, acupuncture was in fact the only kind of therapy available to perhaps 90 percent of the hundreds of millions of Chinese who live in rural areas. Most of the available medical college graduates practiced in the cities, and the Chinese medical colleges produced only a handful of doctors each year to serve the largest nation on earth. For a period of nearly 40 years before the revolution the Peking Medical College averaged fewer than 30 graduates a year.

Both acupuncturists and herbal practitioners gained respectability in China after the Communist revolution. Chairman Mao Tse-tung directed that both western scientific and traditional Chinese medical techniques be employed as a more effective means of meeting the health needs of the nation. The result has been an interesting blend of modern surgery and pharmaceuticals with acupuncture and herbs. Western observers have reported that each modern hospital in China maintains a large department in which the roots, leaves, and barks of various herb plants are stored and processed. Well-trained teams of pharmacologists, meanwhile, study the ancient herbs for identification of the active ingredients that apparently have therapeutic benefits for the patients. The government, in an effort to protect the patient against reckless experimentation, requires that before a doctor can prescribe acupuncture or herb treatments he must permit the herbs or needling to be applied to his own body.

Although it has been suggested that acupuncture may appear to be a success in the People's Republic of China because of some hypnotic effect related to the enthusiasm of the people for Chairman Mao, the Chinese have pointed out that acupuncture also has been used successfully on dogs, cats, rabbits, and other animals that are not likely to be influenced by the Cultural Revolution or the words of Chairman Mao. Acupuncture has also been employed for some years in Russia, Germany, France, and England, as well as in Taiwan, Japan, and other countries of the Orient, although the precise methods of application vary somewhat. The Russians involved in acupuncture research not only agree with the Chinese that energy flows along the meridians, but claim that it can be detected by electronic instruments. Students of acupuncture outside of China also have reported evidence that when a meridian is severed the flow of energy does not extend beyond the point at which the tissue is cut.

Western-trained physicians who have watched acupuncture as practiced in China seem convinced that it can be effective, particularly as used to produce analgesia in surgery. As reported by American doctors who have visited mainland China, acupuncture anesthesia works better in surgery that involves those parts of the body above the waist, such as the lungs and heart. Other physicians, who were trained in the United States before returning to China to practice, claim that acupuncture has been effective in the treatment of migraine headaches and in controlling irregular heartbeats. Western doctors who have observed the use of acupuncture in the treatment of deafness, a common application of needling in China, reported that they were unable to judge the benefits of such therapy in terms of their own knowledge and experience.

One American doctor who has been trained in the techniques of acupuncture believes the method is compatible with standard western medicine in the treatment of a wide range of ailments. It is not recommended for the treatment of cancer, tuberculosis, or arthritis cases in which the disease has advanced to the point of permanent changes in the body tissues. As for the argument that there is a psychological effect in acupuncture that makes it appear to be more successful than it actually is, the supporters of needle therapy reply that psychology is a factor in the treatment of disease by almost any method.

Questions and Answers

Accidents

Q. Are falls a major cause of death among children?

A. No, less than five percent of falls that result in death involve children 14 or under. Fatal falls are a much more serious problem for old and middle-aged people.

Acetaminophen

See ASPIRIN.

Acne

See SKIN CARE.

Adams-Stokes disease

Q. Does the heart ever really skip a beat?

A. Although the expression is used figuratively about anyone who is excited, "skipping a beat" is something that normal, healthy hearts do not do. The skipping of a beat—the failure of the heart to contract and pump blood on schedule—is a symptom of *Adams-Stokes disease* and is marked by temporary loss of consciousness. Anyone suffering from this symptom should seek medical advice promptly.

Aging

Q. Why is the sense of taste lost in old age?

A. One reason is that taste buds diminish as one gets older until elderly persons have only 20 percent as many taste buds on the tongue as youngsters. Some brain cells also are involved, causing older persons to make more mistakes in identifying specific tastes.

Air travel

Q. Does flying in a jet airplane affect digestion or other body processes?

A. Modern jet aircraft cabins are pressurized to produce a simulated altitude of about 7,500 feet. While normal pressure is maintained, there is no health threat from a lack of oxygen or gaseous expansion in the digestive tract. See also EAR DISCOMFORT.

Albumin (in urine)

See TESTS AND DIAGNOSTIC PRO-
CEDURES/URINE.

Allergy

Q. What is an allergy?

A. An allergy is a sensitivity in an
individual to a substance that is
harmless to others. The sensitivity
may be marked by sneezing, a skin
rash, digestive disturbance, or some
other reaction. Eczema, hives, and
asthma may be allergic reactions.

Q. What is an antibody?

A. An antibody is a substance produced by the body to combat an allergen or foreign substance that has
invaded the body tissues; the antibody may combine with the foreign
substance, neutralize its toxin, or
otherwise render it inactive.

Q. What causes allergic symptoms?

A. In a typical allergic reaction, an
allergen such as pollen or dander
combines with an antibody and triggers the release of histamines. This
in turn results in itching, swelling,
redness, nasal discharge, watery
eyes, or other physical effects.

Q. What are histamines?

A. Histamines are chemicals naturally present in human body tissues;
they dilate blood vessels and render
them more permeable, stimulate certain muscles and glandular secretions, and are actively involved in allergic reactions.

Q. Why do allergic symptoms re-
semble cold symptoms?

A. The eyes, nose, and throat are
"shock organs" for several diseases
transmitted by the atmosphere, including the rhino-virus responsible
for the common cold. As in some allergic reactions, histamines are released by antibody reaction to the
invading virus, causing nasal congestion, nasal discharge, etc.

Q. How can you find out what you
are allergic to?

A. Very dilute solutions of suspected allergens can be applied to
eye or nose membranes or into the
skin of the patient. A sensitive person will react with typical allergic
symptoms; some allergic individuals
may react to a number of possible allergens in skin tests.

Q. What is "hay fever"?

A. Hay fever is a common name for
allergic rhinitis, an allergic reaction
to wind-borne pollens or fungi
marked by nasal discharge, swollen
nasal membranes, coughing, sneezing, and conjunctivitis. It usually is
seasonal and affects about ten percent of the population.

Q. Some people seem to develop
asthma during the Christmas season.
Could they be allergic to Christmas
trees?

A. Allergic reaction to spruce, fir,
or pine trees is not unusual. The
cause may be sensitivity of the person to the odors of evergreen or to
molds commonly found on the trees.
A simple way of avoiding the problem is to use artificial trees instead
of evergreens.

Q. Is it possible to develop a rash
from using perfume or cologne on
the skin?

A. Yes. Some individuals are sensitive to oil of bergamot, a plant product used in colognes and perfumes.
The effect is intensified by exposure
of the perfumed skin to sunlight.

Q. Some people develop a skin
rash after drinking even a small
amount of alcohol. Could this be due
to an allergy?

A. Some individuals experience
allergic reactions similar to asthma
and eczema after ingesting alcohol.
They may be sensitive to alcohol itself or the alcohol may increase sen-

sitivity to other allergens, such as ragweed or certain foods.

Q. Can allergy-caused sinus trouble be cured by moving to an area with a dry climate, like the desert southwest?

A. Many people who have moved to other regions found that a change in climate did not help their sinusitis, possibly because their sinuses were irritated by the dust in the desert atmosphere.

Ambulation
See   HOSPITALIZATION/AMBULATION.

Angina
See HEART DISEASE.

Apoplexy
Q. What is apoplexy?

A. Apoplexy is a rather old-fashioned term for stroke or brain-tissue damage caused by a hemorrhage in the region of the brain.

Arthritis
Q. How common is rheumatoid arthritis?

A. It has been estimated that between two to four percent of the population have this disorder.

Q. At what age do arthritis symptoms first become apparent?

A. In most cases, at about the age of 40.

Q. Is arthritis a disease of old people?

A. Although the disease usually occurs in people 40 or over, it can occur at any age. About five percent of arthritis sufferers are young children.

Q. Are women more often afflicted with this disease than men?

A. Yes, three times as many women have arthritis as men. A common time for the onset of the disease in women is at or shortly after the menopause.

Q. Can arthritis cause a low-grade fever?

A. Some forms of arthritis are associated with a mild fever. But the cause may be an inflammation related to the pain of arthritis and should be checked by a physician.

Q. Are mud baths or mineral baths helpful in treating osteoarthritis?

A. Most of the benefit from so-called "spa" therapy probably is due to rest, relaxation, a change of environment, and diet rather than the baths themselves.

Aspirin
Q. Aspirin can irritate the stomach. Is there a nonprescription pain-killer that can be used instead?

A. Acetaminophen drugs frequently are used to relieve pain in persons sensitive to aspirin. Special aspirin formulations designed to reduce stomach irritation also are available.

Q. Can a patient substitute acetaminophen for aspirin in treating rheumatoid arthritis?

A. No. Acetaminophen has not been found to relieve the inflammation symptoms of rheumatoid arthritis.

Q. Is it safe to pack aspirin around a tooth that aches?

A. The aspirin would do more good if you swallowed it with a glass of water, because aspirin must get into the bloodstream through the digestive tract to be effective.

Q. Is is true that aspirin prevents blood from clotting?

A. Experiments show that it takes several minutes longer for blood to clot in a wound of a person using aspirin. But the effect is not a serious problem except for hemophiliac patients or for those who take large quantities of aspirin over an extended period of time.

Q. Why is it necessary to drink a glass of water every time aspirin is taken?

A. Because aspirin must be dissolved in a watery solution to get into the bloodstream, and a generous amount of water is needed to dissolve the drug properly. Otherwise, the aspirin may irritate the stomach lining while slowly dissolving in whatever fluid is in the stomach.

Asthma
See ALLERGY.

Atherosclerosis
See HEART DISEASE.

Backache
Q. Are men or women more likely to have backache?

A. Backache is common among both men and women.

Q. Are tall, thin people more subject to backache than short people?

A. Generally speaking, taller people, especially if they have long backs, are more likely to develop back trouble than shorter people. Erect posture is more of a strain for them because they lack the stability of shorter people.

Bags under the eyes
See SKIN CARE.

Bilirubin
See TESTS AND DIAGNOSTIC PROCEDURES/BLOOD.

Biopsy
See TESTS AND DIAGNOSTIC PROCEDURES/BIOPSY.

Blood
See TESTS AND DIAGNOSTIC PROCEDURES/BLOOD.

Blood circulation
Q. Are there any exercises that help improve poor blood circulation in the legs?

A. One simple exercise is to lie on your back with your legs raised at a 45 degree angle for a few minutes, draining the blood from your feet. Then sit on the edge of a bed or chair until the blood returns to the feet. Repeat this several times a day.

Blood pressure
Q. Is low blood pressure dangerous?

A. Disorders due to low blood pressure are rare; your blood pressure must be very low before it can be considered a cause for concern.

Q. Sometimes a doctor will check the blood pressure of your right arm and then of your left arm. Isn't the blood pressure the same on both sides?

A. Not always. There are certain disorders in the body that can be detected by comparing the two blood pressure readings. See also TESTS AND DIAGNOSTIC PROCEDURES.

Blood sugar
See TESTS AND DIAGNOSTIC PROCEDURES/BLOOD.

Body odor
See PERSPIRATION.

Body temperature
Q. Is it possible for an otherwise normal person to have a "fever"?

A. Yes. Some people lack the ability to sweat properly and thus are unable to lower their body temperature in a hot, humid environment.

Q. Is a high body temperature serious?

A. Yes. It is a sign that body cells are working faster and breaking down, leading to dehydration. Each degree of fever also increases the work load of the heart and threatens the nervous system. A critical point is 103° F.

Q. Do body temperatures change during the day?

A. Yes, temperatures generally are slightly higher in the afternoon and evening, and lower in the morning. Also, the temperature in women varies with different stages of the menstrual cycle.

Boils
See SKIN CARE.

Brain/speech

Q. Is speech controlled by one hemisphere of the brain? If so, which one?

A. Among right-handed people, who probably make up about 93 percent of the population, speech is almost always controlled by the left hemisphere—the same one that controls their right-handedness. Among left-handed people, about 60 percent also have speech controlled by the left hemisphere in spite of having their dominant hand controlled by the other.

BUN
See TESTS AND DIAGNOSTIC PROCEDURES/BLOOD.

Cancer

Q. What is the leading cause of death from cancer among men?

A. Lung cancer.

Q. Does cigarette smoking increase the chances of getting lung cancer?

A. Men who smoke are ten times more likely to die of lung cancer then men who don't.

Carbuncles
See SKIN CARE

Cats
See TOXOPLASMOSIS.

Chest
See FUNNEL CHEST; PIGEON BREAST.

Children

Q. Some say that soap solutions sold for children's bubble blowing can be harmful to a child. Is this true?

A. Several of the special "soap" bubble preparations have been found to acquire disease organisms when exposed to the environment. Parents should supply freshly prepared solutions made from liquid laundry detergents or "no-tear" shampoos for use in blowing bubbles.

Cholesterol

Q. What level of cholesterol is dangerous?

A. In the U.S., the *average* blood cholesterol level is 245 milligrams (per 100 milliliters—the standard index). Heart disease linked to atherosclerosis (hardening of the arteries) is very high in the U.S. In some other countries, where the average blood cholesterol level is probably about 100–170 milligrams, this type of heart disease is rare. There is no one danger point for every individual, but statistically anyone with a blood cholesterol level over 250 milligrams has a much greater chance—perhaps as much as five times greater—of developing atherosclerotic heart disease than someone with a lower cholesterol level.

Q. Can blood cholesterol levels be reduced through a change in diet?

A. There is evidence that by cutting down on consumption of saturated fats (fatty meats and dairy products) and by increasing the consumption of polyunsaturated fats (vegetable oils, fish, etc.), serum cholesterol levels can be moderately reduced. In any case, it seems wise to take steps along the lines indicated simply to keep your cholesterol level from getting any higher. Adding polyunsaturated fats to the diet, without decreasing the intake of saturated fats, will not lower your serum cholesterol level. See also TESTS AND DIAGNOSTIC PROCE-DURES/BLOOD.

Colds

Q. Are the symptoms of the common cold caused by a single virus?

A. No. About 150 different viruses have been identified as causing common cold symptoms. The fact that so many different viral strains cause the infection precludes the possibility of creating an effective immunizing vaccine.

Q. Is it all right to blow your nose when it's blocked by a cold?

A. If the nose is completely blocked by swollen membranes during a cold, blowing will not open it. Forceful blowing may only spread the infection into the sinuses and Eustachian tubes.

Q. Will nose drops help open a "stuffed" nose?

A. Nose drops should be used cautiously; they give temporary relief which may be followed by greater congestion. Continued congestion may lead to continuous use of nose drops in a vicious cycle.

Contagious diseases
See INFECTIOUS AND CONTAGIOUS DISEASES.

Corneal transplant
See EYE DISEASE.

Cough plate
See TESTS AND DIAGNOSTIC PROCE-DURES.

Crohn's disease

Q. What is Crohn's disease?

A. Crohn's disease, another name for regional enteritis, is an inflammation of the part of the small intestine where the small and large intestines are joined. See also ENTERITIS, RE-GIONAL.

Dandruff

Q. What causes dandruff?

A. Unfortunately, the cause is so far unknown. Theories abound, but no one has been able to prove that bacteria, for example—represented as the cause in one theory—exist in scalps affected by dandruff.

Q. Do any dandruff shampoos or other treatments sold over the counter really help?

A. Yes, some are reasonably effective in controlling dandruff. Certainly, if you have a problem with dandruff, it would pay to experiment with various brands until you find one that works for you. If nothing seems to help, see your physician or ask him to recommend a more effective medication.

Delirium tremens

Q. Is it possible to develop delirium tremens from overuse of tranquilizers?

A. Convulsions, tremors, and other characteristic symptoms of delirium tremens can occur as side effects of certain tranquilizing drugs.

Q. What is the cause of delirium tremens?

A. This is a psychotic disorder marked by delirium, tremors, and vivid hallucinations. It occurs in people who have been chronic alcoholics for several years.

Devil's pinches

Q. What are "devil's pinches"?

A. "Devil's pinches" is a common term for a hereditary disorder marked by the mysterious appearance of bruises on the body. The bruises are essentially harmless and there is no permanent cure for them.

Diabetes

See EYE DISEASE/DIABETIC RETINOPATHY; TESTS AND DIAGNOSTIC PROCEDURES/BLOOD/URINE.

Diagnostic tests

Q. What can a doctor tell about your health by examining spinal fluid?

A. There are at least two dozen physical conditions that can be revealed by study of the spinal fluid, including meningitis, poliomyelitis, brain tumor, lead poisoning, and rabies.

Doctors and patients

The following series of questions and answers relating to doctors and patients is an edited transcription of an interview with Dr. Richard J. Wagman, editor of *The New Complete Medical and Health Encyclopedia*. The interviewer was Sidney I. Landau, managing editor of the Ferguson staff.

Q. Why don't doctors tell the patient more than they do? Why do they often seem so reluctant to tell him what underlies his condition?

A. I think this situation has changed significantly, especially as more and more people are becoming more sophisticated about illness and health. It is extremely foolish for a doctor not to discuss what is going on with his patients. It is far more frightening to the patient to be kept in the dark about his real condition.

Q. Do you think that younger doctors are prone to tell more than older doctors?

A. I think it depends on the individual. I have seen a lot of younger doctors who behave like they are 80, and a lot of older doctors who behave like young people.

Q. What about doctors who do not explain the full reason for performing an operation, for example delivering a baby by Caesarian section?

A. This is the kind of thing that would make me very upset with my doctor, because he would be talking down to me. I am speaking not only as a doctor but as a person who is involved with using doctors. I have a family of my own, after all. I don't like being talked down to. Speaking as a physician, I don't like talking down to people.

Q. Would you tell the truth to someone who was suffering from a terminal illness?

A. I like to tell the truth, and I like to tell the patient as much as I think he can tolerate, if I think the patient wants to know. This is not a yes or no sort of phenomenon; this is picked up by hints, by clues, by innuendos, by the whole approach of the patient to me in terms of the questions he or she asks about his or her illness. I prefer to answer the questions honestly.

If a patient with cancer asks me point-blank, "Do I have cancer?" I will answer yes. I won't necessarily say more. I answer the specific question. If the patient asks more I will go on and answer each specific question and no more.

If you lie to the patient you wind up isolating him, often from his own family, which has to know. At least some responsible member of the family has to know. They may find it difficult to talk to the patient since they are hiding the truth. All of a sudden the patient winds up in an untenable position: he or she has no one to talk to honestly.

This is also predicated on the belief that most patients who are seriously ill know what's going on. They sense the concern of their family and friends. Most people close to the patient are poor liars. I am against isolating the patient like this.

On the other hand, there are some patients who cannot tolerate the truth in this kind of situation, and again I think it is the role of the physician to be sensitive to the clues that the patient gives him.

Q. How should a layman act when visiting someone in the hospital who is gravely ill? Should he pretend he's going to get well? Can you make any blanket rule about this?

A. Two very simple rules. One, the visitor should be himself, and should be friendly and cheerful. Two, he should stay only a short period of time.

House Calls and Telephone Calls

Q. To what extent can the telephone replace office calls and house calls?

A. I am very accessible, and most of my patients do not abuse the privilege of calling. That is, they generally call—not always, but generally—during office hours. A high percentage of the calls can be screened by my nurse, and most of the calls involve problems of anxiety and fear rather than medical emergencies—concerns which are quite legitimate. They often make office visits unnecessary, if it's simply a matter of a patient asking a question about something that has been bothering him.

Q. Why don't doctors make house calls any more?

A. I speak for myself only. I make almost no house calls, and there are a variety of reasons. I say this as a big-city practitioner. There are simply not enough hours in the day. It becomes impossible in terms of getting around. Ninety-nine percent of the house calls are not really and truly necessary. If a patient is seriously ill—for example, someone is having chest pains—he should be seen by a physician, but he also needs to have an electrocardiogram done, for example, and the best place to do this is either in the office or in the hospital. I am very limited in terms of what I can do at a patient's home. I don't carry an electrocardiograph machine in my car. If someone really needs a house call, for instance, in a city like New York, I can arrange for someone to see one of my patients at home and call me and let me know what he has found.

Q. What if a person is too sick to come out?

A. This is nonsense. The question is, must you be seen? And if you have to be seen, then the best place for an X ray or a blood test is the hospital or the office. The trouble is, in order for me to do the greatest good for the greatest number under my care, I have to put the responsibility on the patient to come to the office or, in emergencies, to the hospital.

Q. What if a child has a fever of 105° or something like that?

A. There are emergency measures that can be dealt with on the phone, in terms of the *immediate* care that can be given. In general, pediatric emergencies present another spectrum of disease. The question is, if you have a child who has a high fever or has had a convulsion, must you come out? The answer is, something has to be done immediately—before you can either physically get dressed, get into the car, or what have you. Advice can be given on the phone. That sums up what to do until either you come or one of your delegates comes. I think the patient has to be seen.

Q. What about a bleeding ulcer in an older person?

A. Hospital.

Q. What about heart attacks?

A. The only thing you can do in the case of a heart-attack patient in terms of coming to the house is to give relief of pain. Again, in a big city so much time is lost getting from one end of the city to the other. It is much more sensible to make all the arrangements to get the patient to the hospital. This means that the person is going to be in discomfort or distress no matter what you do, but you are going to get the patient to a place where something can be done as quickly as possible.

Answering Services

Q. How should one deal with an answering service that won't give you your doctor's home phone number?

A. My own attitude with answering services—which leave a great deal to be desired as a general rule—is that you must explain to them that this is an emergency and what you hope for is that they will get either your doctor or whoever is covering for your doctor in his absence. You are not calling directly, but theoretically the answering service should relay the message to the doctor or his substitute who will then call you back.

I tell my patients that if there is something urgent and they have problems with the answering service, that it is their obligation to badger the answering service to impress upon them the urgency of the call. You have to call back if you do not hear from the doctor within a given period of time, depending upon the actual degree of urgency or your anxiety, or both.

Psychosomatic Complaints

Q. In a recent poll of doctors, over 90 percent said their patients suffered from hypochondria and psychosomatic ailments. Have you found this to be true?

A. I can't say 90 percent, but a high percentage of patients who call are troubled with problems in terms of anxiety about their health, including patients who have serious, real illnesses. Usually the reason for the call is something involving fear, fright, worry, or whatever word you want to use.

Q. What about those who come to see you?

A. Also a high percentage.

Q. More pronounced in women than in men? In old people than in young?

A. I can't quote statistics. But higher in women. Women come more freely to doctors than men do anyway.

Q. Older women?

A. Most patients who come to an internist are in the older age group.

Specialists and GPs

Q. How does an internist differ from a general practitioner?

A. The internist is someone who practices only adult medicine. He deals with medical diseases involving, for example, heart, lungs, GI tract, kidneys, blood, the entire gamut of illnesses in adults. He does not practice pediatrics, and he does not deal with surgery, does not deal with obstetrics or gynecology.

The internist as a specialist has really come of age only relatively recently. The internist is rather like the medical counterpart to the surgeon as a specialist.

Q. In what way is the internist a specialist?

A. Internal medicine is considered, at least in most Western countries, as a specific specialty—with special requirements in terms of training. For example, my own training involved a year of internship specifically in medicine. I didn't spend time going through a pediatric service, ob-gyn [obstetrics-gynecology], or surgery. Internists deal entirely with medical problems as an intern, then two or three years of residency, and generally a subspecialty—in my case, cardiology. A general practitioner usually has one to two years of training in postmedical school with a little bit of everything—a little pediatrics, a little bit of surgery, a little bit of ob-gyn, dermatology, etc.

Q. An internist does not have that?

A. That is right.

Q. Is there any need for a general practitioner today?

A. A good GP is worth his weight in gold. He is, in many communities, the family physician—the number one contact for the patient. He may take care of all the individual's health needs or be the one to refer him to the proper specialist. In the big cities, frequently the internist has taken over the role of the family physician.

Q. But isn't it true that often you go to your family doctor, who is an internist, and it seems that he is sort of an agent for leading you on to other doctors who are more specialized in various things? From the point of view of the patient, in purely practical terms, you are paying twice. The temptation is to think twice about going to the doctor at all.

A. There is a lot of truth to that, and I agree with you. This involves, in my opinion, a great deal of responsibility on the part of your—what I call your primary—physician, in this case, the internist. Before he refers you to someone else, he will have to sit back and say, can I handle this myself? Does it need handling by someone else? And this means also he has to realize that this is going to cost the patient money, and consider whether it's really necessary. Unfortunately, I am not sure that everybody does think this way. I think one should.

Q. If your regular doctor is an internist and you want medical advice about digestive troubles, should you go to him or to a GI specialist?

A. I think that is jumping the gun. I think that your internist should be able to handle this very easily. If you have an internist or a GP, one of the things you have to do is have enough faith in him. He is the one who is going to decide when you need a specialist in any field. But don't be afraid to ask him if he thinks a consultation is necessary.

Q. If a doctor you know and respect recommends surgery, is it still advisable to get a second opinion?

A. It depends on how much anxiety you have, how clearcut the situation is, and how much faith and trust you have in the doctor and the doctor's advice. For example, if you have a hernia the treatment is surgical. If you have gallstones, and you had an attack from your gallstones, the treatment is surgical. There are other areas, of course, where the treatment is less clear, such as duodenal ulcer. It all boils down to the old business of whether or not you trust the person who is taking care of you. If you don't, then I think you are in trouble to begin with. You must be able to say to your doctor: I am not sure; let's talk about it.

Q. What is an osteopath?

A. An osteopath is a physician who has graduated from a school of osteopathy. The training is similar to an MD's training but slightly different. There is a bit more orientation towards bones, joints, etc.

Q. Are MD's overqualified? Don't they spend a great deal of time learning more than they have to know in order to do the job they do?

A. If you are asking me is our training too long, yes, because so much of what we learn could probably be taught in shorter form. There are several experiments going on in medical education now—for example, taking people in their final year of medical school and making them interns. At least in my personal experience with people in this program, it is quite successful. So far as medical school goes, I do think it could probably be shortened.

Changing Doctors

Q. What is the best way of finding a doctor if you do not have one?

A. There are many ways: one is by referral from someone in the community who has a doctor he is satisfied with; by calling the county medical society; or by calling the local hospital, if it is a small town, and having them recommend one of several doctors who are near you. This is a very reasonable approach.

Q. How can a patient tell if his doctor is unsatisfactory?

A. I think this is better asked of patients. One way the patient can tell, apart from not getting well, is that the patient can't talk to the doctor. If he is unhappy, he can ask his doctor for a consultation. If the doctor is unwilling, I would raise an eyebrow.

Q. If you do switch doctors, how would you go about obtaining your medical records from your former doctor and making them available to your new doctor?

A. Easily. All you have to do is sign a request slip authorizing your former doctor to release information to your new doctor.

Q. Does he have to release that?

A. It is the customary procedure.

Q. With whom do you sign the release—the old or the new doctor?

A. The new doctor. This is very common; it happens all the time.

Personal Attention

Q. Do doctors nowadays have too many patients to be able to give them enough personal attention? This seems to be one of the major complaints of patients: that doctors just don't spend enough time with them.

A. This is partially true. This depends again on the doctor. One of the reasons that many patients wind up coming to see me is because the previous doctor has not given them enough time. I think that patients have to be able to talk honestly to the doctor and ask questions when they want to. When they arrange for their appointment they can let the secretary or nurse know that they would like a little bit of extra time. This is not unreasonable. At the same time many patients' demands are insatiable in this regard.

Q. In other words, a doctor like any other busy person has to learn to turn people off in a way?

A. Right.

Q. What do you think of doctors calling patients they've just met by their first names?

A. Terrible. This is not a social situation, and I prefer that patients be treated with a certain sense of respect and formality, and feel that this is much better for everybody. I don't like calling patients by their first names.

Fees

Q. Can you give any guidelines on "reasonable" medical fees?

A. No. This is an impossible question. There are guidelines, there are very real guidelines. In fact, most fees are set as a matter of custom, form, and what is "fair" in the area. And this is the kind of thing I cannot discuss in absolute terms and won't, but merely suggest that the patient has to discuss this with the doctor or his delegate, meaning his nurse or secretary.

Q. It's often said that doctors don't mind discussing fees before the examination. But many people have difficulty doing so. How do *you* respond to those who ask about fees?

A. My secretary informs all prospective patients exactly what the charges will be—if the patient asks.

Q. How many of your patients discuss fees with you before being treated? Is this commonplace or an exception?

A. It is common. This raises a very good question, because any time anything that is expensive has to be done I think the patient has to be informed not just that something has to be done, but that it is going to cost money. I also think that many patients have to understand that if something has to be done and is important for their health, even if they can't pay for it now, it has to be done. If they are reasonable people they will accept the necessity of a debt. This can be arranged in terms of any convenient method of payment, even to the extent of $1 to $2 a week. This is not the problem. The point is, I think, that the patient should be informed why something that costs a lot of money is important to him. If this has to be done and the patient can't afford it and you have been taking care of him, then I think it is your obligation to see that he gets into the hands of some facility that can give him either a reduced cost or no cost.

Q. Do doctors have difficulty collecting their fees? If so, who gives them the most trouble—the relatively poor, the middle-class, or the well-to-do?

A. I really don't think that there is any basis for predicting who will not pay. Frequently the very wealthy as well as the very poor don't pay.

Q. Don't pay at all?

A. Right. There is no way to get it. You can sue, but it is hardly worth the effort or trouble. There are a small percentage of people who will not meet their obligations, and I think you just have to write it off as an experience.

Q. When one physician refers a patient to a specialist, does he ever get a cut of the consultant's fee? Is fee-splitting of this sort common?

A. It exists. I have never done it. It is not illegal. It is considered unethical by the profession. My experience with this is zero.

Q. When you as an internist refer someone to a surgeon, do you take into consideration or indicate to the patient how expensive the surgeon is likely to be?

A. I usually mention to a patient that a procedure—especially, for example, open heart surgery—is going to be expensive. At this point, I advise him to discuss the specific fee with the surgeon. If there is a hardship situation I will discuss this with the surgeon myself, quietly and privately.

(This concludes the interview with Dr. Wagman.)

Drug abuse

Q. Why do some addicts give up their habit in their mid-30s?

A. No one knows why, but if addicts manage to survive to their thirties, their need for drugs often moderates or disappears entirely, and they become good subjects for detoxification programs. Some spontaneously give up their addiction at this age without treatment.

Q. Is this true of alcoholics, too?

A. A common pattern of alcoholism is one in which the drug is spontaneously given up for periods of up to several months, but the alcoholic then resumes his former drinking habits with the same compulsion he had before. An alcoholic who "gives up" drinking is by no means cured. Such a period is comparable to a remission in a chronic disease, not a cure.

Ear discomfort

Q. After disembarking from an airplane after flight, some people experience a stuffy feeling in the ears and a temporary loss of hearing. What causes this?

A. Although modern commercial airplanes have pressurized interiors that compensate for changes in atmospheric pressure as the plane lands, some individuals are still sensitive enough to experience the sensations described. The air in the Eustachian tube is forced into the middle ear by the increased external pressure, and is replaced by body fluids. Similar symptoms can be caused by allergy, infection, or enlarged adenoids.

Enteritis, regional

Q. What are the symptoms of regional enteritis?

A. Regional enteritis—inflammation of the intestine—is a chronic disease characterized by abdominal cramps, diarrhea, loss of appetite, fever, lethargy, and sometimes a drop in weight. However, in some cases none of these symptoms appears until the disease has progressed considerably, and most patients experience periods of remission at various times during the course of the illness.

Epilepsy

Q. Is epilepsy ever cured?

A. Drugs can effectively control or reduce the frequency of seizures of the great majority of people with this disease. For unknown reasons, some epileptics eventually become and remain free of seizures while requiring no further medication; these people can be called cured.

Q. In addition to trying to create new medicines for the treatment of epilepsy, what are some of the other areas of epilepsy research?

A. Investigations are under way concerning the surgical removal of the particular brain cells responsible for triggering the convulsive seizures, and the implantation of a brain pacemaker that could act as a circuit breaker in preventing the electrical discharges that precipitate the seizures.

Eye disease/corneal transplant

Q. What is a corneal transplant?

A. A corneal transplant is the procedure in which a clear, healthy cornea provided by an eye bank replaces a cloudy or otherwise damaged one. Approximately 90 percent of such operations are successful in restoring vision.

Q. Does a corneal transplant correct all types of blindness?

A. No. A corneal transplant can correct only those disorders of vision that result from corneal defects caused by injury or disease.

Eye disease/diabetic retinopathy

Q. What is diabetic retinopathy?

A. Diabetic retinopathy, which is one of the leading causes of blindness in the U.S., is a disease of diabetics marked by the formation of new, abnormal blood vessels on the surface of the retina, sometimes protruding into the interior of the eye. They may also bleed.

Q. What causes diabetic retinopathy? Can it be treated successfully?

A. The precise cause of diabetic retinopathy is unknown, but the chance of its occurrence increases with the duration of a patient's diabetes. Current treatment is by a process called *photocoagulation,* in which beams of intense light are flashed into the eye to cause minute burns on the retina. This procedure has reduced the risk of blindness in some diabetics by preventing the proliferation of retinal blood vessels.

Foot care

Q. What is the difference between trench foot and chilblain?

A. Both are caused by prolonged exposure of the feet to cold, short of freezing. But trench foot is more serious, with possible neuromuscular damage. Chilblain is marked by a burning, itching sensation of the skin.

Q. Is it safe to remove corns or calluses with a sharp knife or razor blade?

A. No. The best home remedies are foot baths and corn plasters which soften these horny skin formations on the feet.

Frozen section

See TESTS AND DIAGNOSTIC PROCEDURES/FROZEN SECTION.

Funnel chest

Q. Can someone with "funnel chest" engage in normal physical activities? Is surgery recommended?

A. "Funnel chest," known technically as *pectus excavatum,* is a congenital deformity in which the sternum (the bone to which the ribs are attached, forming the chest wall) is depressed, so that the chest looks hollowed out. It is the opposite of "pigeon breast," in which the chest protrudes. So long as funnel chest does not impair the functioning of the lungs, there is no need to curtail normal physical activity, and no need for surgery. The main problem is usually psychological and social, especially for young people.

Gallstones

Q. Can some gallstones be dissolved medically?

A. Yes. The result of many years of research at the Mayo Clinic and elsewhere is an oral medicine containing a bile acid that dissolves cholesterol gallstones. This new therapy eliminates the need for surgical removal in a large number of cases.

Another alternative to surgery is CDCA (chenodeoxycholic acid) an oral medicine that effectively reduces cholesterol gallstones so that the need for surgery is eliminated in many cases.

Gout

Q. Is there a relationship between gout sufferers and intelligence?

A. Legend has it that gout afflicts the famous more often than ordinary folk. Certainly many gout sufferers have been famous—for example, Benjamin Franklin—but gout can strike anybody, and there does not seem to be any scientific basis for the popular association of gout and fame. Some research suggests, however, a connection between IQ and uric acid, the level of which is elevated in gout patients.

Q. Are men or women more subject to attacks of gout?

A. Men, by an almost ten to one ratio.

Q. Is gout hereditary?

A. Primary gout—that is, gout that is not caused by another disease—is hereditary.

Q. Are attacks of acute gout, as of the big toe, likely to go away without treatment?

A. Yes, usually in one or two weeks, but without treatment you are likely to have recurrences which will eventually cause degeneration of cartilage and deformity. This form of gout, incidentally, is called *acute gouty arthritis*.

Q. Are any other diseases often associated with gout?

A. Kidney stones are a frequent complication of gout. The excess of uric acid that causes gout can also result in uric acid stones occurring in the kidneys.

Growth, stunted

Q. Do stunted children show an abnormal growth pattern in their early years?

A. Yes. Stunted children can usually be identified even at an early age because instead of growing a normal two or three inches each year, their stature increases by only about one inch.

Q. When a stunted growth pattern becomes apparent, is there any possible treatment for it?

A. Yes. If the cause of the child's stunted stature is determined to be a deficiency of growth hormone, the child may be given injections of pituitary hormone. This treatment is called pituitary replacement therapy.

Guthrie test

See TESTS AND DIAGNOSTIC PROCEDURES/GUTHRIE TEST.

Hair

See UNWANTED HAIR.

Handedness

Q. What percentage of people are left-handed?

A. An estimated seven percent are left-handed. See also BRAIN/SPEECH.

Hansen's disease

Q. What is Hansen's disease?

A. Hansen's disease is the preferred designation for leprosy. G. H. A. Hansen was a Norwegian physician and scientist who was the first to identify the bacterial organism that causes the disease.

Hardening of the arteries (atherosclerosis)

See HEART DISEASE.

Headache

Q. Can emotional tension lead to a migraine headache?

A. In those subject to migraine headaches, emotional stress may precipitate a migraine episode.

Q. Should migraine sufferers avoid certain foods, such as chocolate?

A. Chocolate is a common offender in migraine headaches. Some individuals also suffer headaches due to allergies to milk, eggs, corn, legumes, cinnamon, and cola drinks.

Q. Does reading under a dim light cause headaches?

A. You are more likely to get a headache from reading under a light that is too bright and glaring than under one that is not bright enough. Of course, if you are tired to begin with, reading under a dim light may cause headache from general fatigue. The eyes, however, operate like a camera, and are not strained or otherwise damaged by use under a dim light.

Q. Can air or noise pollution cause headaches?

A. Some people apparently are sensitive to air pollutants and develop headaches after traveling from rural to industrialized urban areas. Loud noises can be painful; they also can aggravate headaches caused by stress.

Q. What is a "caffeine-withdrawal" headache?

A. Caffeine causes a constriction of the blood vessels in the head, an effect that inhibits headaches. When a person who drinks large amounts of coffee or other caffeine beverages suddenly stops using the beverage, the arteries become dilated. This stretches nerve endings in the arteries, causing a headache.

Heart attack

Q. Are heart attacks the leading cause of death?

A. In western society, among the 30-to-65-year-old age group, yes. They are more common among men than women, and are by far the commonest cause of sudden death; about 90 percent of sudden deaths are caused by heart attack.

Q. Are both left and right halves of the heart equally vulnerable to heart attack?

A. Myocardial infarction, the medical term for the death of heart tissue, usually strikes the left ventricle, the most muscular portion of the heart, which pumps the blood through the arteries to blood vessels throughout the body. Infarction of the right ventricle or atrium is much less common.

Heartburn

Q. What happens to cause heartburn?

A. Heartburn is a burning sensation in the lower esophagus—the tube that conducts swallowed food from mouth to stomach. It is caused by a flow of gastric juices from the stomach back into the esophagus. It can be caused from eating or drinking too much; it is also common in the aftermath of gastric surgery and in the later stages of pregnancy. It has nothing to do with the heart, but the burning sensation may be felt in the region of the heart.

Q. What can be done to relieve heartburn at night?

A. Avoid spicy or other foods that may irritate the digestive system, especially during the evening meal, and learn to sleep with the upper part of the body elevated.

Heart disease

Q. Can emotional stress trigger an attack of angina?

A. Yes, angina is often precipitated by extreme emotional excitement. Physical exertion and cold weather are also common precipitating factors, especially in combination.

Q. What causes angina?

A. The most common cause is atherosclerosis, a narrowing and hardening of the blood vessels that supply blood and oxygen to the heart. Thus, when the supply is inadequate to meet stepped-up needs, such as after a heavy meal or during strenuous activity, an angina attack may result.

Q. What is the relationship between atherosclerosis and heart disease?

A. Atherosclerosis describes a condition in which the interior of the blood vessel walls hardens and in which a deposit of various substances builds up, thus narrowing the opening in the vessel. Blood flow is therefore slowed. If it is slowed too much, angina may develop. If the

flow of blood is blocked entirely, a clot may break off and be carried by the bloodstream to the heart, where a blockage could trigger a heart attack. See also CHOLESTEROL.

Q. How common is congenital heart disease?

A. About two to five percent of all heart disease after infancy is congenital—that is, it existed at birth.

Q. What do heart valves do and what can go wrong with them?

A. The purpose of heart valves is to permit a free flow of blood in one direction only, either from the atria (or auricles) to the ventricles during diastole, or from the ventricles to the great vessels during systole. Essentially, two problems can develop:

(1) The valve can narrow, a condition known as *stenosis,* thus permitting an insufficient flow of blood; or

(2) The valve can close imperfectly or too slowly—i.e., it leaks—thus permitting a backward flow of blood, called valvular *regurgitation, insufficiency,* or *incompetence.*

Q. Can both stenosis and regurgitation exist in the same valve at the same level?

A. Yes, they can and frequently do.

Q. What is mitral stenosis?

A. A narrowing and hardening of the mitral heart valve, which regulates the flow of blood from the left atrium to the left ventricle.

Q. Does mitral stenosis occur equally often in men and women?

A. No, it is much more common in women. The reasons for this are obscure. See also ADAMS-STOKES DISEASE.

Heart pacemaker

Q. How many people use pacemakers to control the rate of heartbeat?

A. In 1976, there were about 45,000 persons in North America wearing permanently implanted heart pacemakers.

Q. What is the purpose of a heart pacemaker that is implanted in the body?

A. The artificial pacemaker replaces or supplements a natural pacemaker in the heart that normally generates electric signals to make the heart muscles contract. In some diseases, the natural pacemaker fails to produce a proper series of signals needed to make the heart pump blood at a normal pace. Unless corrected, as with an artificial pacemaker, ·the patient faces disability or death.

Q. Where is a permanent pacemaker implanted in a patient's body?

A. A pacemaker generally is implanted under the skin in an area below the collarbone. It is connected to the heart tissue by a wire running through a vein from the heart to the shoulder area.

Q. Is an operation for implanting a heart pacemaker dangerous?

A. Permanent pacemaker implantation is a very safe operation, even in elderly patients, and generally results in relieving symptoms of heart distress.

Q. Is a general anesthetic used during implanting of a heart pacemaker?

A. A general anesthetic is required if the wires for a pacemaker are connected directly to the heart muscle. However, pacemaker wires sometimes can be inserted via a catheter in a vein, in which case a local anesthetic may be used.

Q. Is a heart pacemaker heavy?

A. The average heart pacemaker, including power source, transistors, and other components, weighs about six ounces.

Q. Can the pacemaker generator malfunction after it is implanted?

A. Failure of pacemaker components, except for batteries, is rare. But some electrical equipment such as electric razors, microwave ovens, and even automobile ignitions can interfere with pacemaker activity.

Q. How long do batteries for heart pacemakers last?

A. Pacemaker batteries usually last from three to five years before they must be replaced.

Q. How can a doctor check up on a heart pacemaker after it is implanted in the body?

A. By studying X-ray pictures which will show if wires are in place, if the batteries are still good, etc. Newer model pacemakers have special markings designed to reveal important information on X-ray pictures. Wires have a special coating to make them show up better on X-ray film.

Q. Can pacemakers be powered by nuclear energy without harm to the patient?

A. Since 1970, more than 1,600 nuclear-powered pacemakers have been implanted. They have an expected life of 20 years but are still being studied for possible complications before wider use is approved.

Hernia, hiatus

Q. What is hiatus hernia?

A. It is hernia, or "rupture" of the muscle barrier between the stomach and esophagus that permits a backflow of the stomach's gastric acid into the esophagus.

Q. What is the treatment for hiatus hernia?

A. The best results can be

achieved by following a careful diet, wearing loose-fitting clothing around the abdominal area, and sleeping with the upper part of the body elevated. Surgery may be recommended if conservative measures fail to improve the condition.

Herpes

Q. Is the herpes virus that causes "cold sores" responsible for any other disorders?

A. Yes. The most serious disorder caused by the herpes simplex virus is an infection of the cornea that may result in scar tissue and impairment of sight. The infection is called *herpes simplex keratitis.*

Hirschsprung's Disease

Q. What is Hirschsprung's disease?

A. Hirschsprung's disease is a congenital disorder of childhood in which the colon becomes enlarged as a result of a defect in part of the nervous system that controls bowel movement. In this disorder, the colon never completely evacuates its contents into the rectum. Cases that do not respond to medical treatment may require surgical correction.

Hirsutism

See UNWANTED HAIR.

Hospitalization/ambulation

Q. Why do hospitals have people out of bed and walking about so soon after an operation?

A. Primarily to prevent the development of blood clots that might spread to the lungs. This therapy actually began by necessity during World War II when an acute doctor-and-hospital-bed shortage made it necessary to get patients physically out of the hospital earlier. The results convinced doctors that early ambulation was more effective than traditional confinement to bed. It presented fewer complications.

Hypertension

Q. What is meant by "essential hypertension"?

A. "Essential" means without a known cause. Essential hypertension refers to a group of symptoms including elevated blood pressure and progressive damage to the blood vessels.

Immunization

Q. Are there some parts of the U.S. where immunization requirements must be complied with before a child can enter a public school?

A. Yes. In many parts of the United States, local city and county departments of health require immunization against diphtheria, polio, measles, and rubella (German measles) before a child is permitted to attend school.

Immunology/SCID

Q. What is the meaning of SCID?

A. SCID stands for Severe Combined Immune Deficiency. It is a congenital disease in which a child is born with an inability to fight off infectious organisms and other foreign cells or substances that enter the body.

Q. What happens to a child diagnosed as having SCID?

A. Until recently, the condition has been fatal if untreated unless the child was kept in an isolation room which is germfree. Such rooms do exist in some hospitals.

Q. Is there any possible treatment for SCID?

A. The ideal treatment for SCID is transplantation of bone marrow from a sibling whose tissues are compatible with those of the patient. Such a donor is available in only about 15 percent of all cases.

Q. Is any progress being made in treating SCID?

A. Recent research indicates that the disorder in some patients is due to a lack of a crucial enzyme called adenosine deaminase which is found in normal red blood cells and is essential for the manufacture of antibodies. Periodic transfusions of small amounts of washed and irradiated red blood cells have corrected the SCID syndrome in a few cases.

Indigestion

Q. Is it all right to take a laxative to get rid of a stomach pain?

A. No. In fact, if the pain continues for more than an hour or so, and if it is severe, it would be wise to call your doctor. The cause could be appendicitis or another serious condition.

Q. What is the cause of stomach gas following a meal?

A. Most of the "gas" in the stomach is caused by swallowing air during a meal.

Q. Can indigestion be caused by a lack of gastric acid in the stomach?

A. Yes. There is a wide range of acid levels in normal individuals, and while some people are troubled by too much gastric acid, others can suffer from too little stomach acid.

Infectious and contagious diseases

Q. What is the difference between "infectious" disease and "contagious" disease?

A. Contagious in general means "spread by contact from one person to another person." An infectious disease involves an invading organism, whether it be bacteria or virus. In general, there is more of a tendency to think of infection in an isolated setting within the individual himself as opposed to someone else.

Q. But are most infectious diseases also contagious?

A. Not necessarily. Cystitis is a bacterial infection of the bladder. This is infectious within the given individual but not contagious, meaning that others are not going to catch it because they are in the same room.

Ingrown toenails

Q. How can you avoid ingrown toenails?

A. By wearing shoes that provide enough room for toes and nails, and by trimming the nails carefully—not too short—and by rounding them only slightly at the corners. See also NAILS.

Injury

Q. Why do some persons experience a severe chill after an injury?

A. Some people react to a painful injury or cramp with a brief chill of several minutes. The effect seems to be a reaction to pain.

Jet lag

Q. Is jet lag a serious health problem?

A. Jet lag is a popular term used to describe a disturbance in a person's normal day-night cycle caused by rapidly moving into a different time zone. It is not serious, but the human body usually needs two to four days to adjust to a new schedule for eating and sleeping. See also AIR TRAVEL.

Lipids

Q. What are lipids?

A. Lipids are fatty substances that are essential to living cells. An excess of some lipids, especially cholesterol, is believed to be a factor in contributing to heart disease. Other lipids which are the products of normal metabolism accumulate in the bodies of people who are the victims of rare hereditary disorders grouped together as "lipid storage diseases."

Q. What are the lipid storage diseases?

A. Among the lipid storage diseases are Tay-Sachs disease, Gaucher's disease, fucosidosis, and metachromatic leukodystrophy. All are at present incurable.

Q. Is the cause of lipid storage diseases known?

A. In each case, the particular lipid storage disease is caused by the lack of a single enzyme among the many thousands of enzymes produced by the body for the normal chemical processes of metabolism.

Q. Do all lipids storage diseases have the same symptoms?

A. No. Symptoms vary from disease to disease. Some cause mental retardation, one causes blindness, another results in kidney failure. Practically all of the inherited lipid storage diseases result in early death.

Q. Is there any way of finding out whether an unborn child may inherit one of the lipid storage diseases?

A. Yes. Through genetic counseling, it is possible to identify carriers of the faulty genes that transmit some of these diseases.

Liver spots
See SKIN CARE.

Medical insurance

Q. Does medical insurance ever provide coverage for a second or third expert opinion on whether to have elective surgery?

A. Yes. In an attempt to curb some unnecessary nonemergency surgery, some health insurance plans provide compensation for charges incurred for a second and sometimes a third consultation.

Mg.%
See TESTS AND DIAGNOSTIC PROCEDURES.

Migraine
See HEADACHE.

MLNS

Q. What do the initials MLNS stand for?

A. A children's disease known as mucocutaneous lymph node syndrome in which the symptoms of fever, rash, swollen hands and feet, and bright "strawberry" tongue are self-limiting. However, in about two percent of all cases, a heart involvement occurs that is fatal.

Moles
See SKIN CARE.

Munchausen's syndrome

Q. What kind of disease is Munchausen's syndrome?

A. This is not a real disease but an assortment of make-believe complaints used by some people, otherwise normal, who want to obtain medical care or hospitalization.

Nails

Q. What causes a fingernail to loosen or fall off?

A. A number of things, among them fungus infections, bacterial or

yeast infections, psoriasis, or hemorrhage such as that caused by hitting a
finger with a hammer.

Q. Does nail polish injure the
nail?

A. Nail polish protects the nails
except in rare cases of allergic reaction. Nail polish remover can injure
the nails if too much is applied, because the drying effect of polish removers can split the nails.

Narcolepsy

Q. What is narcolepsy?

A. Narcolepsy is a neurological
syndrome in which an abnormality
of the brain results in the disorganization of sleep and the components
of sleep. It is estimated that this
chronic and disabling sleep disorder
affects about 250,000 Americans of
all ages.

Q. What are the symptoms of narcolepsy?

A. There are four main symptoms
of narcolepsy; a narcoleptic can have
one of the symptoms, all four of
them, or any combination. The first
symptom is known as sleep attacks
—falling asleep at unsuitable times
and having an exhausted feeling
most of the time. The second symptom is catalepsy—a total collapse of
muscle tone usually triggered by
some strong emotion, particularly
surprise, anger, or great pleasure.
The third is hallucinating immediately before sleep, and the fourth
is a feeling of paralysis or immobility
immediately after waking up or just
as one falls asleep.

Q. How is true narcolepsy diagnosed?

A. Narcolepsy is diagnosed by observation of the symptoms described
and by measurements of the patient's sleep patterns.

Neuropharmacology

Q. What is neuropharmacology?

A. Neuropharmacology is the
study of the effects of drugs such as
amphetamines, barbiturates and the
like on the chemistry of the brain.
Compare PSYCHOPHARMACOLOGY.

Nevus, junction
See SKIN CARE.

Newborns

Q. Is there a kind of doctor who
specializes in the care of newborn
babies?

A. Yes, a perinatologist is a pediatrician who specializes in providing
intensive care before, during, and
after birth to the newborn baby,
especially to one born prematurely
or with congenital defects requiring
surgery.

Nurse-Midwife

Q. Why aren't nurse-midwives
considered as respectable in the
United States nowadays as they are
in Europe?

A. They are. In 1971, the American College of Obstetricians and
Gynecologists officially stated that
"in medically directed teams, qualified nurse-midwives may assume
responsibility for the complete care
and management of uncomplicated
maternity patients."

Q. How do nurse-midwives qual-
ify for their profession?

A. A nurse-midwife begins her
training by attending a three- or
four-year nursing school and becoming a registered nurse. She then
affiliates with a hospital in order to
get one year of experience in obstet-
rical nursing. Student nurse-midwives must also observe and assist at
about 50 labors and deliveries, and

under supervision they are required to manage a minimum of 20 deliveries on their own.

Osgood-Schlatter disease

Q. What is Osgood-Schlatter disease?

A. Degeneration of the protuberant upper end of the tibia just below the knee joint. It usually occurs in adolescents during periods of rapid growth. In most cases the affected bone tissue eventually regenerates.

Osteoarthritis

See ARTHRITIS.

Pacemaker, artificial

See HEART PACEMAKER.

Perspiration

Q. Is there really such a thing as breaking out in a "cold sweat"?

A. Yes. Normally, the eccrine glands that secrete sweat respond only to exercise or heat—except for those on the palms and soles and under the arm, which also respond to emotional excitement, such as fear, sexual stimulation, etc. But under extreme conditions, emotional stimulation can make the eccrine glands over the whole body respond, even when the body has not been warmed from physical effort. The evaporation of this sweat results in a chill, or "cold sweat."

Q. What causes body odor?

A. The aprocrine glands, much less numerous than the eccrine glands which secrete sweat, respond to emotional stimulation by secreting a fluid that acts on the sweat, especially under the arms, where perspiration cannot easily evaporate, to multiply bacteria already present on the skin; the proliferation of such bacteria produces body odor.

Q. What is the purpose of the apocrine glands?

A. They have no known purpose. One theory suggests that, since these glands develop only with sexual maturity and decline with age—which is why children and the elderly do not have the characteristic body odor—the odor once served as a sexual attraction to the opposite sex. Many other animals utilize body scents in this way.

Q. What's the difference between a deodorant and an antiperspirant?

A. A deodorant is designed to suppress or mask body odor. Many deodorants therefore contain antibacterial ingredients and are also pleasantly scented. An antiperspirant is designed to reduce perspiration, although many antiperspirants also have antibacterial properties.

Q. Isn't stopping sweating unhealthy?

A. No antiperspirant can suppress all perspiration; at most it is reduced by about half. Sweating is not, as commonly believed, a way to dispose of body waste. The purpose of sweating is to help regulate body temperature.

Q. Won't one build up an immunity to deodorants or antiperspirants and have to switch?

A. No, this is a misconception. You do not build up an immunity to deodorants or antiperspirants. On some occasions they may not seem to work well enough, but they have not lost their effectiveness; you have just lost your confidence in them.

Q. Why do men need a stronger deodorant than women do? Do they sweat more?

A. Men don't need a stronger deodorant than women do. The secretion from the body-odor-causing apocrine glands is about the same for both sexes. However, the fact that most women shave under their arms probably gives them an advantage, since hair serves to encourage bacteria growth.

Q. Are allergic responses to underarm deodorants very common?

A. You certainly may be allergic to a deodorant, but you should also suspect other causes, such as irritation from clothing or, in the case of women, from shaving. When drying under the arms, you should pat the area gently; hard rubbing can cause irritation to the sensitive skin there.

Physical fitness

Q. Can someone who has had a heart attack ever engage in strenuous physical activity, such as tennis?

A. Every case is different. There are many former heart patients who have, under a doctor's care, resumed their physical activities in sports such as tennis. However, it is imperative to resume such activities only after consulting your physician, and then in gradual stages of increased participation.

Pigeon breast

Q. Can pigeon-breasted people engage in normal physical activities?

A. "Pigeon breast," known technically as *pectus carinatum*, is a congenital deformity in which the sternum (the bone to which the ribs are attached, forming the chest wall) protrudes. It is the opposite of "funnel chest," in which the chest is depressed. There is usually no need to curtail normal physical activity. The chief problem is usually a cosmetic one, i.e., the psychological effect on one's social life and self-image, which can be very severe, especially for young people. Corrective surgery, however, would be extensive and complicated, and is not usually recommended in the absence of physical problems.

Prader-Willi syndrome

Q. What is Prader-Willi syndrome?

A. Prader-Willi syndrome refers to a bizarre eating disturbance whose victims, chiefly children between the ages of two and five, are afflicted with an insatiable desire for food. The disorder, which is named for the two doctors who first described it in 1956, is not inherited, nor does it appear to be related to emotional stress. Present studies indicate that it is the result of a neurological disturbance caused by malfunction of the hypothalamus of the brain.

Psoriasis

Q. How common is psoriasis?

A. About two percent of people in the United States have psoriasis.

Q. Does it affect one sex more than the other?

A. No, it affects men and women equally.

Q. At what age does it first appear?

A. Usually between the ages of 15 and 30.

Q. Is psoriasis contagious?

A. No, not at all. It is probably an inherited disorder.

Psychological counseling

Q. How does group therapy work?

A. Group therapy is the general term for a wide variety of therapeutic situations in which the participants try to find more satisfactory ways of living their lives through honest self-examination and the expression of their authentic feelings. Mutual respect, support, and trust are the principles on which the effectiveness of group therapy is based. The group may be led by a professional psychiatrist, a lay analyst, or a psychiatric social worker, or the leadership of each session may rotate among the participants.

Q. What are encounter groups?

A. An encounter group is a form of group therapy in which people are encouraged by each other and by a trained counselor to get in touch with their suppressed feelings of fear, rage, anger, shame, etc., by means of unrestrained verbalization and physical contact.

Psychopharmacology

Q. What kind of research is done by psychopharmacologists?

A. Psychopharmacologists are scientific specialists who study the actions of drugs such as LSD or tranquilizers on the mind. Compare NEUROPHARMACOLOGY.

Puberty

Q. Are middle-class American girls reaching sexual maturity at a younger age with each succeeding decade?

A. No. The average age at which girls begin to menstruate is 12.8 years, and this figure has remained the same over the last 30 years.

Raynaud's disease

Q. What is Raynaud's disease?

A. Raynaud's disease is a condition in which the arteries in the fingers and toes experience spasms, usually after exposure to cold. The tips of fingers and toes become bluish (cyanotic) or ashen, then sometimes red.

Q. What causes this condition?

A. It can be a complication of rheumatoid arthritis, a connective tissue disease, neurological disease, etc. It can also result from piano playing or other occupations in which the fingertips are struck or jarred repeatedly. (In such cases, the condition is usually known as *Raynaud's phenomenon*.) But Raynaud's disease is frequently not secondary to any known underlying condition. Its cause in such cases is unknown. It is known that emotional states can trigger an attack of finger and/or toe spasms, but this certainly does not preclude physiological causes.

Q. Who is most likely to get Raynaud's disease?

A. Women, by a five to one ratio, are more commonly afflicted than men.

Q. How is it treated?

A. In most cases, the condition will stay the same or improve with age (usually at about age 40). Patients subject to Raynaud's disease should definitely not smoke and should take care to avoid exposure to cold. Mild sedatives may be prescribed by a physician if spasm episodes are frequent or severe.

Reye's syndrome

Q. What is Reye's syndrome?

A. Reye's syndrome is a complication that may follow a number of different kinds of viral infections, including influenza and chicken pox. The disorder, which is extremely rare, affects mainly children and involves primarily the liver, interfering with that organ's ability to help remove poisonous substances from the bloodstream. The resulting buildup of toxic wastes in the blood results in damage to the liver, the brain, and the kidneys. Symptoms include mental confusion, severe nausea and vomiting, hyperactivity and excitability, followed by convulsions and finally coma. Because the disorder frequently is fatal if not treated at an early stage, immediate medical attention is required.

Q. How is it treated?

A. The patient is closely watched on an around-the-clock basis so that any serious complication, such as a buildup of pressure on the brain, can be immediately counteracted with drugs or by other means. Treatment may include transfusions of fresh blood to replace the patient's blood containing the toxic agent.

Q. Is there a cure for Reye's syndrome?

A. No, but the disease is believed to be self-limiting. Treatment is directed at enabling the patient to survive during the critical period in which the disease is running its course.

Rickettsial diseases

Q. What causes typhus and is there a "shot" you can get as protection against typhus?

A. Typhus is a debilitating, frequently fatal disease caused by a tiny organism called a rickettsia. The rickettsia usually is transmitted to humans through the bite of a body louse. A vaccine is available and is recommended for travelers to some underdeveloped countries of the world.

Q. Is Rocky Mountain spotted fever a disease you can get only in the Rocky Mountains?

A. No, this rickettsial disease was discovered in the Rocky Mountains but occurs in other areas as well, particularly in the eastern U.S. It is transmitted by wood ticks.

SCID
See IMMUNOLOGY.

Serum sickness

Q. What is serum sickness?

A. Serum sickness is an immunological reaction to the introduction of serum (the clear fluid portion of the blood), as an animal serum used as an antitoxin, into the body. The reaction may be acute and severe. It is a form of allergic shock or anaphylaxis, and can be avoided by always having a skin test to check for reaction before a serum is introduced into the body.

SGOT
See TESTS AND DIAGNOSTIC PROCEDURES/BLOOD.

Shaving
See UNWANTED HAIR.

Skin cancer

Q. Is skin cancer more common in the South than in the North?

A. Yes, skin cancer is about ten times more common in the South than the North because of increased exposure to sunlight in the South.

Q. Are dark-skinned people less likely to develop skin cancer than fair-skinned people?

A. Yes, blonds and redheads are more subject to skin cancer than dark-skinned people.

Skin care

Q. What is the cause of "liver spots" on the skin?

A. The brownish areas of discoloration that may appear on the skin in later life have nothing to do with the liver but sometimes indicate a minor systemic disorder. A general physical examination usually is needed to pinpoint the exact cause.

Q. Please explain why dark circles sometimes appear under the eyes.

A. Because the skin of eyelids is thin, blood in veins beneath the skin may make the area seem darker and bluer than surrounding skin. During menstruation or illness, this discoloration may become more obvious.

Q. What causes "bags" under the eyes?

A. As a person ages, tissues that normally hold the skin of the eyelids firmly become weak, and subcutaneous fat pushes the skin outward. Plastic surgery is the only cure for this effect. Puffiness of the eyelids may be a sign of fluid accumulation due to kidney or heart disease.

Q. What is a junction nevus?

A. A junction nevus is a darkly pigmented tumor, resembling a common mole, that develops at the junction of the two layers of the skin, the dermis and epidermis.

Q. Can a mole or junction nevus become a skin cancer?

A. While unusual, a mole or junction nevus can darken and enlarge into a precancerous tumor. It is wise to have a physician remove the growth before the change can occur.

Q. What is the difference between a boil and a carbuncle?

A. The main difference is that a carbuncle is bigger than a boil and involves two or more hair follicles.

Q. What is dermabrasion and will it remove acne scars?

A. Dermabrasion is a technique of rubbing away the outer layer of skin to get rid of scars. The skin is covered with bandages to control bleeding and infection and a new skin layer replaces the old in about a month.

Q. Are warts contagious?

A. Yes. They are caused by a virus and are likely to develop on moist areas of the skin or areas that have been injured.

Q. What are the medical treatments for warts?

A. Some warts can be removed by freezing them with supercooled liquids. Warts also are treated with X rays, medicines applied to the skin, and by surgical excision.

Q. Can warts be "charmed" away by suggestion?

A. There is no scientific basis for this notion; when warts disappear after hexing, the wart is regressing because of other factors and the apparent "charm" effect is coincidental.

Q. What is the cause of skin wrinkling?

A. It is not completely known why skin wrinkles, although heredity apparently is one factor. Others are loss of weight, exposure to wind and sun, and loss of supporting tissue beneath the skin as a part of aging.

Sleep

Q. During the onset of sleep, one occasionally has the sensation of falling or floating. Is this effect a symptom of a serious disorder?

A. No. The sensation of falling or floating while drifting off to sleep is a not unusual hypnagogic illusion, or hallucination. It occurs in a semi-dreamlike state but is not a true dream. Some people experience visual illusions—faces, landscapes, or geometric shapes—while falling asleep.

Q. Sometimes while sleeping the entire body may jerk for no apparent reason. Is this normal?

A. The sudden incoordinate jerking of a part or the whole body, called nocturnal jerking, is a natural occurrence during light sleep. The phenomenon is believed to result from a sudden release of muscle tension by a nervous system impulse in the cerebral cortex of the brain. Usually no harm is done and the event is quickly forgotten. Pet owners are well aware that this phenomenon is not restricted to humans. Dogs and cats also jerk reflexively during light sleep.

Q. What is REM sleep?

A. REM sleep is a phase of sleep during which there are bursts of rapid eye movements—abbreviated REM. This phenomenon, originally reported in 1953, coincides with a state of intense physiological activity. In addition to the rapid eye movements, the heartbeat quickens, blood pressure rises, and the rate of electrical impulses in the brain increases. The rapid eye movements are also associated with dreaming.

Q. What is NREM sleep?

A. NREM sleep (non-REM sleep) is qualitatively different from REM sleep. It seems to be a restful and recuperative state. Approximately 75 percent of all sleep time is spent in NREM sleep.

Q. Does the sleeper first experience one kind of sleep and then the other, and then wake up?

A. No. Sleep occurs in cycles: a period of about 90 minutes of NREM sleep precedes the onset of the first REM period, which lasts from 5 to 15 minutes. This alternation occurs throughout the night, with the REM phases getting somewhat longer toward waking. The NREM-REM alternation is sometimes called the *sleep-dream cycle* because dreams occur more often and more dramatically in REM sleep than they do in NREM sleep.

Speech
See BRAIN/SPEECH.

Stimulant drugs

Q. Can stimulant drugs affect the growth of children?

A. It has been found that two types of drugs (Dexedrine and Ritalin) used to treat hyperactive children seem to retard the normal gains in height and weight when administered in large doses over long periods of time.

Stitch

Q. What causes a stitch in the side?

A. A stitch—or sudden ache in the upper left or right part of the abdomen—is associated with vigorous activity, often occurs after eating, and is aggravated by cold weather. Its cause is not known, but it is believed to be linked to a decreased supply of oxygen in the blood circulating to the diaphragm.

Suicide

Q. What are the two main causes of death among young people in the United States?

A. Accidents are the leading cause of death among young people in the United States. The second leading cause is suicide.

Q. Are young people in the highest risk age group for suicide?

A. No. The highest risk age group is the elderly, who account for one-fourth of all suicides in the United States.

Sweat
See PERSPIRATION.

Tests and diagnostic procedures

Q. On some laboratory reports, test results are written as numbers followed by mg.%. Please explain.

A. Mg.% is a scientific notation that means the number of milligrams of a substance found in 100 milliliters of blood. See below under BLOOD.

Q. On your physical exam sheet, you may see something like "BP 130/74." What does this mean?

A. It means your blood pressure (BP) was 130 (systolic) over 74 (diastolic) as measured in millimeters of mercury. See also BLOOD PRESSURE.

Biopsy

Q. What is a biopsy?

A. A microscopic examination of the tissue cells from a lump, nodule, ulcer, or hard mass. The procedure is commonly used to determine if an abnormal growth may be cancer.

Q. What is meant by needle biopsy?

A. A sample of tissue cells from an organ is taken through a long needle inserted into the body—an alternative to using surgery to examine tissue from the liver, kidney, or other organs.

Blood

Q. What does BUN on a laboratory report mean?

A. BUN is an abbreviation for blood urea nitrogen; it is a measure of the health of the kidneys. The normal range is 10–20 mg.%

Q. Why is cholesterol measured in blood tests?

A. The cholesterol level of the blood indicates possible premature hardening of the arteries. A normal level is 150–300 mg.%

Q. On a copy of a blood test from the laboratory there may be a reference to SGOT. What does this mean?

A. This is medical shorthand for serum glutamic oxaloacetic transaminase; sometimes it is called simply transaminase. It is an enzyme which in abnormal quantities could indicate liver disease or coronary heart disease.

Q. Is there a blood test for diabetes?

A. Yes. An abnormally high level of sugar in the blood suggests diabetes.

Q. What is bilirubin and what does its presence in the blood tell a doctor?

A. Bilirubin is a pigment that colors the bile. An abnormally high level in the blood could mean the patient has liver or gall bladder disease.

Q. What does it mean if one's blood sugar is below normal?

A. It could indicate a tumor of the pancreas or an overactive production of insulin.

Cough Plate

Q. What is a cough plate?

A. It is a sterile plate used to collect bacteria from a patient for study. The patient coughs onto the plate. The test may be used, for example, in the diagnosis of whooping cough.

Frozen Section

Q. What is a frozen section?

A. A suspicious lump of tissue is frozen quickly with carbon dioxide gas, and a thin slice cut from the tissue is stained with a dye for study under a microscope. The test usually is done during surgery in order to determine quickly if the tissue should be removed or if it is relatively harmless.

Guthrie Test

Q. What is a Guthrie test?

A. This is a special method of examining a urine sample in order to determine if a patient may have phenylketonuria (PKU), an inherited metabolic disease.

Urine

Q. Does sugar in the urine mean one has diabetes?

A. Generally, yes. It is one test for diabetes. However, it is possible to have the disease without a significant level of sugar in the urine.

Q. Why is a urine sample tested for albumin?

A. The presence of albumin in urine would suggest an abnormal functioning of the kidneys, perhaps due to a disease such as nephritis.

Q. Why does the lab technician check the color of a urine sample?

A. Normal urine is clear or amber in color. If it is tinged with red, the cause could be bleeding in the urethra, bladder, kidneys, prostate (in men), or elsewhere in the urinary tract. A brown coloration could indicate liver disease.

Tetanus

Q. How often should you get a tetanus booster?

A. Every ten years, assuming that you haven't sustained a wound, especially a puncture-type wound, that might be infected with tetanus germs. In that event, you should have a booster if you haven't had one in a year's time.

Q. What should someone who is not immunized do when he sustains a wound that may be infected with tetanus germs?

A. He should seek medical assistance immediately. He will be given tetanus toxoid and may also be given an antitoxin—either a human antitoxin or one from a horse or cow.

Tic douloureux

Q. Can a young person have "tic douloureux," or trigeminal neuralgia?

A. These severe facial pains can occur at any age after puberty, but usually do not begin to appear before the age of 50.

Tourette's disease

Q. What is Tourette's disease?

A. Named for the French neurologist, Gilles de la Tourette, this disease is marked by violent muscular jerking of the head and shoulders, as well as of the extremities, along with grunting, explosive obscenities uttered by the victim.

Toxoplasmosis/cats

Q. Can people catch diseases from cats?

A. Yes. Cats are the chief source of a disease called toxoplasmosis, which is caused by a parasite to which cats as well as other animals are the host.

Q. Is toxoplasmosis a serious disease?

A. Not in most cases. Animals themselves may harbor the infectious organism without showing symptoms, and probably half the adult population has been infected by the "toxo" parasite at one time or other without knowing it. In some people, the infection runs a course similar to mononucleosis; in others, it may cause inflammation of the retina. However, the disease is very dangerous if contracted by a pregnant woman. While symptoms usually bypass the mother, prenatal infection of the fetus can cause irreversible brain damage, blindness, or death.

Typhus

See RICKETTSIAL DISEASES.

Ulcers

Q. Are peptic ulcers caused by too much stomach acid?

A. Not necessarily; some individuals have high levels of stomach acid but never develop ulcers. However, oversecretion of stomach acid can aggravate an existing ulcer.

Q. What are some of the signs of a bleeding ulcer?

A. The patient may vomit blood or, more commonly, the blood will travel through the intestine and cause the patient's stools to be colored black.

Q. Will a stomach ulcer eventually become a stomach cancer?

A. A stomach ulcer may occasionally develop into a cancerous growth. A person with a peptic ulcer should be examined regularly by a doctor who can watch for possible precancerous changes.

Unwanted hair

Q. Is excessive hair in women caused by too much male hormone production?

A. Women with excessive facial hair are entirely feminine, and tests usually do not indicate an elevated production of the male hormone. It is normal for those of each sex to produce both male and female hormones; women normally produce about two-thirds as much of the male hormone as do men.

Q. Does shaving make hair grow faster than before?

A. No. Shaving has no effect on the rate of growth of hair. However, since short hair is thicker and less flexible than long hair, a trimmed beard may give a denser appearance than untrimmed facial hair.

Q. Why is it better to shave hair when it is wet?

A. Hair can absorb a great deal of water, making it softer and much easier to cut. The best time to shave body hair is after a bath or shower.

Urine & urinalysis
See TESTS AND DIAGNOSTIC PROCEDURES/URINE.

Warts
See SKIN CARE.

Weight problems

Q. Is exercising a good way to lose weight?

A. No. Exercising is beneficial for other reasons, such as maintaining good muscle tone, but it is not an efficient way to lose weight. The only way to lose weight is to diet so that your body is taking in fewer calories than it is consuming.

Wrinkling
See SKIN CARE.

X Rays

Q. How often should a dentist take a full set of X rays?

A. Unless there is some special problem, a full set of X rays—16 to 18 pictures of an adult patient's teeth—need not be conducted more often than every three to five years. Some authorities feel that a full set of dental X rays need not be made more than every six to ten years.

Measures and Weights

U.S. SYSTEM

LENGTH

Unit	Metric Equivalent
inch (in.)	2.54 centimeters
foot (ft.) = 12 inches	30.48 centimeters or 0.3048 meter
yard (yd.) = 3 feet or 36 inches	0.9144 meter
rod (rd.) = 5.5 yards or 16.5 feet	5.0292 meters
furlong = 220 yards or 40 rods or ⅛ mile	201.168 meters
mile (mi.) = 5,280 feet or 1,760 yards or 8 furlongs	1.6093 kilometers

AREA

Unit	Metric Equivalent
square inch (sq. in.)	6.452 square centimeters
square foot (sq. ft.) = 144 square inches	0.093 square meter or 929.03 square centimeters
square yard (sq. yd.) = 9 square feet	0.836 square meter
square rod (sq. rd.) = 30.25 square yards	25.293 square meters
acre (A.) = 160 square rods or 4,840 square yards or 43,560 square feet	0.4047 hectare or 4,047 square meters
square mile (sq. mi.) = 640 acres	259.00 hectares or 2.590 square kilometers

LIQUID MEASURE

Unit	U.S. Equivalent in Cubic Inches	Metric Equivalent
gill (gi.) = 4 fluid ounces	7.219	0.118 liter
pint (pt.) = 4 gills	28.875	0.473 liter
quart (qt.) = 2 pints	57.75	0.946 liter
gallon (gal.) = 4 quarts	231	3.785 liters

The British imperial gallon (4 imperial quarts) = 4.546 liters or 277.42 cubic inches. The U.S. gallon is approximately ⅚ of the British imperial gallon.

APOTHECARIES' FLUID MEASURE

Unit	U.S. Equivalent in Cubic Inches	Metric Equivalent
minim (min.)	0.0038	0.0616 milliliter
fluid dram (fl. dr.) = 60 minims	0.225	3.697 milliliters
fluid ounce (fl. oz.) = 8 fluid drams	1.805	29.573 milliliters
pint (pt.) = 16 fluid ounces	28.875	0.473 liter

DRY MEASURE

Unit	U.S. Equivalent in Cubic Inches	Metric Equivalent
pint (pt.)	33.600	0.551 liter
quart (qt.) = 2 pints	67.200	1.101 liters
peck (pk.) = 8 quarts	537.605	8.810 liters
bushel (bu.) = 4 pecks	2,150.42	35.239 liters

CUBIC MEASURE

Unit	Metric Equivalent
cubic inch (cu. in.)	16.387 cubic centimeters
cubic foot (cu. ft.) = 1,728 cubic inches	0.028 cubic meter
cubic yard (cu. yd.) = 27 cubic feet	0.765 cubic meter
cord (cd.) (for cordwood) = 128 cubic feet	3.625 cubic meters

AVOIRDUPOIS WEIGHT

Unit	Metric Equivalent
grain (gr.)	0.0648 gram
dram (dr.) = 27.34 grains	1.772 grams
ounce (oz.) = 16 drams or 437.5 grains	28.349 grams
pound (lb.) = 16 ounces or 7,000 grains	453.59 grams or 0.453 kilograms
hundredweight (cwt.) = 100 pounds	45.36 kilograms
ton = 2,000 pounds	0.907 metric ton or 907.18 kilograms

TROY WEIGHT

Unit	Metric Equivalent
grain (gr.)	0.0648 gram
pennyweight (dwt.) = 24 grains	1.555 grams
ounce (oz. t.) = 20 pennyweight or 480 grains	31.103 grams
pound (lb. t.) = 12 ounces or 240 pennyweight or 5,760 grains	373.24 grams or 0.373 kilogram

APOTHECARIES WEIGHT

Unit	Metric Equivalent
grain (gr.)	0.0648 gram
scruple (s.) = 20 grains	1.296 grams
dram (dr.) = 3 scruples or 60 grains	3.888 grams
ounce (oz.) = 8 drams or 480 grains	31.103 grams
pound (lb.) = 12 ounces or 5,760 grains	373.24 grams or 0.373 kilogram

SYMBOLS

#	pound(s)
'	foot, feet
"	inch(es)

Apothecaries' Measure

℔	pound(s)	℥	ounce(s)
ℨ	dram(s)	℈	scruple(s)
♏, ♏, ♏	minim		

METRIC SYSTEM

LENGTH

Unit	Equivalent in Meters	U.S. Equivalent
millimeter (mm)	0.001	0.03937 inch
centimeter (cm) = 10 millimeters	0.01	0.3937 inch
decimeter (dm) = 10 centimeters	0.1	3.937 inches
meter (m) = 10 decimeters or 100 centimeters or 1,000 millimeters	1	39.37 inches or 3.28 feet or 1.09 yards
decameter (dkm) = 10 meters	10	32.81 feet or 10.93 yards
hectometer (hm) = 10 decameters	100	328.08 feet or 109.36 yards
kilometer (km) = 10 hectometers	1,000	0.6214 mile or 1,093.6 yards or 3,280.8 feet

AREA

Unit	Equivalent in Square Meters	U.S. Equivalent
square millimeter (sq mm, mm²)	0.000001	0.00155 square inch
square centimeter (sq cm, cm²) = 100 square millimeters	0.0001	0.155 square inch
square decimeter (sq dm, dm²) = 100 square centimeters	0.01	15.5 square inches
square meter (sq m, m²) or centare (ca) = 100 square decimeters or 10,000 square centimeters or 1,000,000 square millimeters	1	10.76 square feet or 1.196 square yards
square decameter (sq dkm, dkm²) or are (a) = 100 centares	100	119.60 square yards or 0.0247 acre
square hectometer (sq hm, hm²) or hectare (ha) = 100 ares	10,000	2.47 acres
square kilometer (sq km, km²) = 100 hectares	1,000,000	0.386 square mile or 247.105 acres

VOLUME (LIQUID MEASURE)

Unit	Equivalent in Liters	U.S. Equivalent
milliliter (ml)	0.001	0.034 fluid ounce
centiliter (cl) = 10 milliliters	0.01	0.338 fluid ounce
deciliter (dl) = 10 centiliters	0.1	3.38 fluid ounces
liter (l) = 10 deciliters or 100 centiliters or 1,000 milliliters	1	1.05 liquid quarts or 33.814 fluid ounces or 0.908 dry quart
decaliter (dkl) = 10 liters	10	2.64 gallons or 0.284 bushel
hectoliter (hl) = 10 decaliters	100	26.418 gallons or 2.838 bushels
kiloliter (kl) = 10 hectoliters	1,000	264.18 gallons

CUBIC MEASURE

Unit	Equivalent in Cubic Meters	U.S. Equivalent
cubic centimeter (cc, cu cm, cm³) = 1,000 cubic millimeters	0.000001	0.061 cubic inch
cubic decimeter (cu dm, dm³) = 1,000 cubic centimeters	0.001	61.023 cubic inches
decistere (ds)	0.1	3.53 cubic feet
cubic meter or stere (s) = 1,000 cubic decimeters or 1,000,000 cubic centimeters	1	1.308 cubic yards
decastere (dks)	10	13.1 cubic yards

MASS OR WEIGHT

Unit	Equivalent in Grams	U.S. Equivalent in Avoirdupois Weight
milligram (mg)	0.001	0.0154 grain
centigram (cg) = 10 milligrams	0.01	0.1543 grain
decigram (dg) = 10 centigrams	0.1	1.543 grains
gram (g) = 10 decigrams or 100 centigrams or 1,000 milligrams	1	15.43 grains or 0.03527 ounce
decagram (dkg) = 10 grams	10	0.3527 ounce
hectogram (hg) = 10 decagrams	100	3.527 ounces
kilogram (kg) = 10 hectograms	1,000	2.2046 pounds
quintal (q) = 100 kilograms	100,000	220.46 pounds
metric ton (t or MT) = 10 quintals or 1,000 kilograms	1,000,000	1.1 tons or 2,204.6 pounds

A metric carat (car.) (used in weighing gems) = 200 milligrams or 3.086 grains avoirdupois.

Other metric prefixes occasionally used are: micro- (one-millionth of), myria- (10,000 times), mega- (1,000,000 times) (a unit).

SYMBOLS

t	10^{12} times (a unit); tera-	c	10^{-2} times (a unit); centi-
g	10^{9} times (a unit); giga-	m	10^{-3} times (a unit); milli-
m	10^{6} times (a unit); mega-	μ	10^{-6} times (a unit); micro-
k	10^{3} times (a unit); kilo-	n	10^{-9} times (a unit); nano-
h	10^{2} times (a unit); hecto-	p or $\mu\mu$	10^{-12} times (a unit); pico- or micromicro-
dk	10 times (a unit); deka-	Å, λ	Angstrom unit
d	10^{-1} times (a unit); deci-	$\mu\mu$	micromicron
		μ	micron

Glossary

The *Glossary* consists of approximately 3,000 definitions. Entries are alphabetized letter by letter rather than by separate words. For example, *corpuscle* precedes *corpus luteum*. Entries listed in inverted order, such as *epiphysis, slipped,* are alphabetized as if they were one word. The slant bar (/) is used to separate synonyms, such as *auditory nerve/acoustic nerve*. In such entries, only the portion before the slant bar is considered in the alphabetization. Some entries have more than one synonymous term. Because of the relatively large number of synonyms used in medicine, it was felt that the repetition of synonyms at the place of definition would be valuable to the reader and serve to avoid possible confusion.

All cross-references are introduced by *see* or *see under* followed by a colon. For example: **acoustic nerve** see: auditory nerve. A word or phrase in italic type within a definition means that additional information can be found by looking up that word. For example, the entry for CAT scanner reads:

> **CAT scanner/body scanner** computerized X-ray machine used in *CAT scanning*

The reader is directed to look up *CAT scanning* for information that will make clear what a CAT scanner is.

Abbreviations used are: *esp.* for especially; *usu.* for usually; *n.* for noun; *adj.* for adjective; *v.* for verb; *sing.* for singular; *pl.* for plural. Irregular plural or singular forms are given in parentheses following the entry, e.g., **fungus** (*pl.* fungi).

Some entries have more than one meaning. Separate meanings are individually numbered. Occasionally, a cross reference will be made to a particular definition of another entry. In such cases the appropriate definition number immediately follows the referent word.

Since this glossary was based primarily on the text of THE NEW COMPLETE MEDICAL AND HEALTH ENCYCLOPEDIA, it is extremely up to date and, in comparison with other glossaries of medical terms for the general public, comprehensive in coverage. It is hoped that this glossary will answer any questions the reader may have about terms used in the text.

A

a- (prefix) not, as in afebrile, not feverish

abdomen in human beings, the cavity between the diaphragm and the floor of the pelvis, in which the stomach, intestines, liver, and other organs are located

THE ABDOMINAL AREAS

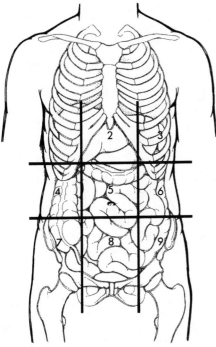

1. right hypochondriac area
2. epigastric area
3. left hypochondriac area
4. right lumbar area
5. umbilical area
6. left lumbar area
7. right iliac area
8. hypogastric area
9. left iliac area

To help identify particular regions of the abdomen, the abdominal region has been divided into nine areas. These areas have been superimposed over the internal organs of the abdomen.

abortion the expulsion of a nonviable fetus prior to term, either induced or involuntary (miscarriage or spontaneous abortion)

abortion, spontaneous see: miscarriage

abrasion scraped place on the skin, as from a fall

abscess collection of pus in a body cavity formed by tissue disintegration, and often accompanied by painful inflammation

absence attack or seizure see: petit mal

absorption assimilation by means of the digestive process

accommodation the thinning or thickening of the lens of the eye in order to adjust the focus of vision at different distances

acetabulum the hip socket

achalasia failure of a sphincter muscle to relax, causing, in the case of the cardiac sphincter, abnormal dilation of the esophagus

Achilles tendon the thick tendon that connects the muscles at the back of the calf of the leg to the bone of the heel

acid any of various chemical compounds that in a water solution are sour in taste, turn blue litmus paper red, and are capable of reacting with another compound (a base) to form a salt

acidosis chemical imbalance in the blood marked by an excess of acid, sometimes affecting diabetics and leading possibly to diabetic coma

acidotic having or marked by acidosis

acinous cell cell in the pancreas that secretes digestive juice, as distinguished from the cells of the islets of Langerhans

acne common eruptive skin disorder due to clogging or inflammation of the sebaceous glands

acoustic nerve see: auditory nerve

acromegaly disorder of the pituitary gland characterized by enlarged head, hands, feet, and most body organs

acrophobia compulsive or persistent fear of heights

ACTH/adrenocorticotrophic hormone hormone secreted by the anterior lobe of the pituitary gland which stimulates the growth and function of the adrenal cortex

acupuncture the Oriental art of traditional medicine in which needles are inserted at specific points through the skin to treat disease and induce anesthesia

acupuncturist one skilled in acupuncture

acute sudden and severe, as a disease

Adams-Stokes disease temporary loss of consciousness caused by the heart's missing a beat, i.e., its failure to contract and pump blood on schedule

addiction the compulsive habitual use of a drug for other than medical reasons

Addison's anemia see: anemia, pernicious

Addison's disease chronic hypofunction (underfunctioning) of the adrenal cortex, characterized by weakness, loss of body hair, and increased skin pigmentation

adenocarcinoma carcinoma involving epithelial tissue of a gland

adenoid enlarged lymphoid growth behind the pharynx

adenoidectomy surgical removal of the adenoids

adenoma benign tumor which can cause hyperfunction of the parathyroid glands

adenopathy any glandular disease characterized by swelling of the lymph nodes

adenotonsillectomy/T and A operation surgical removal of the adenoids and tonsils

adipose of or pertaining to fat; fatty

adipose tissue body fat

adrenal cortex the outer part of the adrenal gland, which produces several hormones that affect metabolism of foods, secondary sex characteristics, skin pigmentation, and resistance to infection

adrenalectomy surgical removal of an adrenal gland

adrenal gland either of two small ductless glands situated above each kidney

adrenaline/epinephrine adrenal hormone which acts to stimulate the heart, dilate the blood vessels, and relax bronchial smooth muscles

adrenal medulla inner part of the adrenal gland

adrenocorticotrophic hormone see: ACTH

aerobic occurring or capable of living only in air or free oxygen, as certain bacteria

aerobics exercises that involve a workout for the lungs and heart as well as the muscles

affect emotion, as distinguished from thought or perception

affective reaction see: manic-depressive reaction

afferent applied to nerves, receiving sensations; sensory

afferent nerves see: sensory nerves

aflatoxin toxic substance produced by a fungus that develops typically in stored grains or legumes such as peanuts and that is associated with cancer of the liver

African trypanosomiasis see: sleeping sickness

afterbirth the placenta: so called when expelled from the uterus after the birth of a baby

agoraphobia fear of open spaces

agranulocytosis acute disease characterized by almost total disappearance of neutrophils from the blood, and often following the use of certain drugs

AHF see: antihemophilic factor

ailurophobia fear of cats

airway 1. passageway for air 2. plastic breathing tube for administering artificial respiration from rescuer's mouth to victim's mouth

albino organism with deficient pigmentation. In human beings, skin is usu. milky or translucent, hair is white, and eyes appear pink

albumin any of a class of protein substances found in the blood

albuminuria the presence of protein in the urine

alcohol colorless, flammable liquid distilled from fermented grains, fruit juices, and starches

alcohol, denatured ethyl alcohol made unfit to drink, used industrially and as a disinfectant

alcohol, ethyl see: ethyl alcohol

alcohol, grain see: ethyl alcohol

alcoholic one suffering from alcoholism

alcoholism disease characterized by excessive and compulsive use of alcoholic beverages

alcohol, methyl see: methyl alcohol

alcohol, wood see: methyl alcohol

aldose a kind of sugar

algophobia fear of pain

alimentary tract or canal/gastrointestinal tract or canal passageway for food utilized in the digestive process, extending from the mouth to the anus, and including the esophagus, stomach, intestines, and rectum

alkali any of various chemical compounds that neutralize acids and turn litmus paper blue

alkaloid organic substance containing nitrogen and having a powerful toxic effect on animals and man, as morphine or strychnine

alkalosis chemical imbalance in the blood marked by an excessive alkali content

allergen substance or material capable of causing an allergic reaction

allergenic having the properties of an allergen

allergic pertaining to or caused by allergy

allergic rhinitis/hay fever annually recurring inflammation of the mucous membranes of the nose and eyes caused chiefly by the pollen of certain plants

allergic shock/anaphylactic shock violent shock reaction, often accompanied by a rash, due to an oversensitized reaction to a foreign substance transmitted by an insect bite

allergist/allergologist physician specializing in the diagnosis and treatment of allergies

allergologist see: allergist

allergology the branch of medical science dealing with the diagnosis and treatment of allergies

allergy condition of heightened susceptibility to a substance that in similar amounts is innocuous to others

allograft see: homograft

alopecia see: baldness

alopecia areata see: baldness, patchy

alveolar bone either of the bones of the upper and lower jaws that include sockets for the teeth

alveoli (*sing.* alveolus) air sacs situated in the lungs

Alzheimer's disease see: presenile dementia

amalgam mercury and silver compound, often used to fill teeth

amblyopia dimness of sight not due to refractive error or disease

ambulation act of walking or moving about

ambulatory able to walk

amenorrhea absence or cessation of menstruation

amenorrhea, acquired see: amenorrhea, secondary

amenorrhea, primary failure of menarche (the onset of menstruation) to occur

amenorrhea, secondary/acquired amen- orrhea cessation or interruption in the occurrence of menstruation

American trypanosomiasis see: Chagas' disease

amino acid any of a group of compounds that form an essential part of the protein molecule

amnesia loss or impairment of memory, sometimes temporary

amniocentesis/prenatal diagnosis procedure for determining whether a fetus is afflicted with an inherited disorder by sampling the amniotic fluid of a pregnant woman

amniocentesis, saline see: saline amniocentesis

amnion/amniotic sac membranous sac enclosing the embryo in mammals, birds, and reptiles

amniotic fluid/bag of waters the fluid within a membrane surrounding an embryo in the uterus of a pregnant woman

amniotic sac see: amnion

amoebic dysentery form of dysentery caused by an amoeba

amphetamine/Benzedrine/pep pills any of a class of drugs that stimulate the central nervous system, used medically to treat depressive mental disorders and sometimes to retard appetite, and used illicitly to induce a state of abnormal alertness and excitement

Amphotericin B antibiotic substance used to treat histoplasmosis and other deep-seated fungus infections

ampulla (*pl.* ampullae) any dilated part or sac, as the base of each of the semicircular canals of the inner ear

amputate to remove surgically by cutting, as a gangrenous limb

amyotrophic lateral sclerosis see: sclerosis, amyotrophic lateral

anabolism the process by which nutrients are built up into the living organism; constructive metabolism. Compare *catabolism*

anaerobic occurring or capable of living without air or free oxygen, as certain bacteria

anal fissure crack, split, or ulceration in the area of the two anal sphincters that control the release of feces

analgesia incapacity to feel pain

analgesic drug that lessens or eliminates the capacity to feel pain

anal sphincter the ring of muscle fibers surrounding the anus and controlling the passage of wastes from the body

anaphylactic shock see: allergic shock

androgen any of various hormones found in males which control the appearance and development of masculine characteristics, also present although in smaller amounts in females

androsterone an androgen secreted in the urine

anemia deficiency in the amount or quality of red blood corpuscles or of hemoglobin in the blood

anemia, hemolytic form of anemia caused by an abnormally high rate of breakdown of red blood cells, exceeding the capacity of the bone marrow to replace them with new cells

anemia, hemophilic anemia caused by bleeding into joint cavities in advanced hemophilia

anemia, iron-deficiency anemic condition caused by insufficient iron in the diet

anemia, pernicious/Addison's anemia anemia characterized by the enlarged size and reduced number of red blood cells, caused by the body's inability to absorb vitamin B$_{12}$

anemia, sickle-cell see: sickle-cell anemia

anesthesia loss of sensation

anesthesiologist physician specializing in the study and administration of anesthetics

anesthesiology the branch of medical science that deals with the study and administration of anesthetics

anesthetic drug, gas, or other substance or procedure that produces anesthesia

anesthetic, general anesthetic, usu. in the form of gas, that produces anesthesia by rendering the patient unconscious

anesthetic, local anesthetic applied locally, usu. by injection, to produce regional anesthesia

anesthetic, regional anesthetic applied locally to produce anesthesia in a region of the body

anesthetic, spinal local anesthetic usu. applied by injection to the tissues surrounding the spinal cord and affecting spinal nerves below the point of injection

anesthesic, topical anesthetic applied locally to a body surface to produce regional anesthesia

anesthetist person trained to administer anesthetics

aneurysm localized dilation of the wall of an artery, forming a pulsating sac and usu. accompanied by pain due to abnormal pressure

angina pectoris condition causing acute chest pain because of interference with the supply of oxygen to the heart

angiocardiography visualization by X ray of the heart and its major blood vessels after injection of an opaque fluid

angioedema swelling of the subcutaneous tissues

angiogram X ray of a blood vessel obtained by the injection of an opaque liquid material into the blood vessels

angiography visualization of the blood vessels

angiology the branch of medical science dealing with the blood vessels and lymph vessels

ankylosing spondylitis see: spondylitis, rheumatoid

ankylosis the stiffening or fixation of a joint, as by disease or surgery

annular having the shape of a ring

anorexia loss of appetite

anorexia nervosa emotional disturbance, esp. of young women, characterized by aversion to food and resulting emaciation

anovulatory without ovulation

anoxemia deficiency of oxygen in the blood

anoxia oxygen deficiency of the body tissues

antacid any alkaline substance that can neutralize stomach acidity caused by gastric juices, often prescribed in ulcer diets

anterior toward the front

anterior lobe hypophysis the anterior part of the pituitary gland that produces growth hormones and hormones that stimulate other glands

anterior urethra the meatus, or external opening, of the urethra in the penis

anthelmintic drug used to expel or destroy parasitic worms

anthrax malignant, infectious disease of sheep, cattle, and other animals, caused by a bacillus and sometimes transmitted to humans

anti- against; opposed to; opposite to

antibiotic any of a large class of substances, such as penicillin and streptomycin, produced by various microorganisms and fungi that have the power to destroy or arrest the growth of other microorganisms, including many that cause infectious diseases

antibody substance produced by the body to counteract infection and in response to specific antigens

anti-clotting compound see: anticoagulant

anticoagulant substance that retards clotting of the blood

anticonvulsant medicine used to control epileptic seizures

antidepressant drug that stimulates physiological activity, thereby tending to alleviate depression

antidiuretic hormone see under: vasopressin

antidote anything that neutralizes or counteracts the effects of a poison

antigen any of several substances, including toxins, enzymes, and proteins, that cause the development of antibodies when introduced into an organism

antihemophilic factor/AHF substance that causes clotting and stops bleeding in hemophiliacs

antihistamine any of a number of drugs that counteract the nasal engorgement and vasoconstrictor action of histamine in the body, often used in the treatment of hay fever

antimetabolite chemical that interferes with cell metabolism

antiperspirant astringent preparation which acts to diminish or prevent perspiration

antitoxin antibody produced in response to the presence of a specific toxin, which it neutralizes

antivenin antitoxin to venom or serum prepared to counteract the effects of venom

anuria inability to urinate

anus the opening at the lower extremity of the alimentary canal

anvil/incus the middle of the three ossicles of the middle ear, the bone between the hammer and the stirrup

anxiety reaction neurosis characterized

chiefly by anxiety unrelated to any apparent cause

aorta the large artery originating from the left ventricle of the heart that forms the main arterial trunk from which blood is distributed to all of the body except the lungs

aortic valve the membranous valve between the left ventricle of the heart and the aorta

Apgar system system of rating the health of newborn babies

aphasia partial or total loss of the power of articulate speech due to a disorder in the cerebrum of the brain

aplasia arrested development or congenital absence of a part or organ of the body

aplastic marked by aplasia; underdeveloped

apnea cessation or interruption of breathing

apoplexy see: stroke

appendectomy surgical removal of the vermiform appendix

appendicitis inflammation of the vermiform appendix characterized by pain in the right lower abdomen, nausea, and vomiting

appendicular skeleton see under: skeleton

appendix vermiformis see: vermiform appendix

appetite, loss of see: anorexia

aqueous humor the clear, limpid alkaline fluid that fills the anterior chamber of the eye from the cornea to the lens

arachnoid the middle of the three membranes that envelop the brain and spinal cord

areola the dark circular area around the nipple of a breast or around a pustule

arrest slow or stop the progress of, as a disease

arrhythmia variation from the normal heartbeat

arterial having to do with or carried by the arteries

arteriogram X-ray picture of an artery

arteriography technique of injecting an opaque substance into the coronary arteries and observing the material by X ray as it runs its course through the heart muscle

arteriole small artery, esp. one that leads to a capillary

arteriosclerosis thickening and hardening of the walls of an artery, with impairment of blood circulation

arteritis inflammation of an artery

artery any of a large number of muscular, tubular vessels conveying blood away from the heart to all parts of the body

artery, pulmonary artery that delivers oxygen-poor blood from the heart to the lungs

arthritis inflammation of a joint, characterized by pain, swelling, and tenderness

arthritis, chronic gouty see: gouty arthritis, chronic

arthritis, gonorrheal complication of gonorrhea affecting the joints

arthritis, hemophilic painful swelling and bleeding into joint cavities

arthritis, hypertrophic see: osteoarthritis

arthritis, pyrogenic form of arthritis characterized by fever

arthritis, rheumatoid see: rheumatoid arthritis

arthropathy any disease of the joints

articulate form a joint, as one bone with another

artificial pneumothorax see under: pneumothorax

artificial respiration artificial maintenance of respiration in someone who has ceased to breathe, esp. mouth-to-mouth resuscitation

ascaris see: roundworm

ascorbic acid/vitamin C white, odorless, crystalline compound found in citrus and other fresh fruits and green leafy vegetables, and also made synthetically, that prevents scurvy

asepsis prevention of infection by the maintenance of sterile conditions

aseptic free from disease-causing microorganisms

aseptic meningitis see: meningitis, aseptic

asphyxiation loss of consciousness caused by too little oxygen in the blood, generally as a result of suffocation by drowning or the breathing in of noxious gases

aspirate withdraw by suction

aspiration act or process of aspirating

aspiration, vacuum see: vacuum aspiration

aspirin analgesic drug that has fever-reducing properties, widely used to treat symptoms of the common cold, rheumatoid arthritis, and many other conditions

assimilation the process by which digested food is made an integral part of the solid parts or fluids of an organism

asthenia lack or loss of strength; weakness

asthma chronic respiratory disorder characterized by recurrent paroxysmal coughing caused by spasms of the bronchi or diaphragm, and due in many cases to an allergic reaction

astigmatism distorted vision caused by an uneven curvature of the cornea

asymptomatic having no observable symptoms of a disease

ataxia absence or failure of muscular coordination

atherosclerosis hardening of the inner walls of the arteries, resulting in a loss of elasticity, and accompanied by the deposit of fat and by degenerative tissue changes

athetosis derangement of the nervous system in which the hands and feet, esp. the fingers and toes, keep moving or twitching

athlete's foot ringworm of the foot, caused by a parasitic fungus

atopic see: ectopic

atrioventricular block disruption of normal transmission of signals between the upper and lower chambers of the heart, as from scar tissue, that may affect blood flow to the brain and cause blackouts or convulsions

atrium (*pl.* atria)/**auricle** one of the two upper chambers of the heart, which receive blood from the veins and transmit it to the ventricles

atrophy the wasting or withering away of the body or any of its parts, as from disease or lack of use

atrophy, bone see: decalcification

attenuated weakened in strength, as a microorganism for use in a vaccine

audiologist one who specializes in the treatment of those with hearing problems

audiometer device that measures hearing

auditory canal/auditory meatus either of two passageways, the external auditory canal leading from the outer ear to the tympanic membrane or eardrum, and the internal auditory canal passing through the temporal bone to the brain

auditory meatus see: auditory canal

auditory nerve/acoustic nerve nerve consisting of the cochlear nerve and the vestibular nerve and connecting the inner ear with the brain, conveying the sense of hearing and of equilibrium

aura subjective, momentary sensory perception of an unusual nature that occurs just before the onset of an epileptic convulsion

Aureomycin trade name for the antibiotic tetracycline

auricle see: atrium

auscultation diagnostic procedure of listening, as to sounds in the chest with a stethoscope

autism mental disorder of children, marked by lack of response to external activities

autistic suffering from or pertaining to autism

autograft tissue graft taken from one part of a patient's body for transplanting in another part

autonomic nervous system network of nerves originating in the spinal column, and including the sympathetic and parasympathetic nervous systems, that control and stimulate the functions of body tissues and organs not subject to voluntary control, such as the heart or stomach

autopsy post-mortem examination of a body, as to determine the cause of death

avulsion a tearing or wrenching away, as a structure or part of the body, as a result of an accident or by surgery

axial skeleton see: skeleton, axial

axilla the armpit

axillary pertaining to or in the region of the armpit

axon cylindrical fiber in neurons carrying impulses away from the cells

B

Babinski reflex reflex of the toes, normal in infants, in which the large toe is extended upward and the other toes splayed when the underside of the foot is stroked, an indication in adults of neurological disease

baby teeth/deciduous teeth/milk teeth/

primary teeth the first temporary set of human teeth, 20 in all, which begin to appear about the age of six months and are usu. complete by the end of the second year

bacillary dysentery a usu. acute form of dysentery caused by bacilli

bacillus (*pl.* bacilli) any of a class of straight, rod-shaped bacteria having both beneficial and disease-causing effects

backbone see: spinal column

bacteria (*sing.* bacterium) one-celled microorganisms that come in three varieties—bacillus, coccus, and spirillum—and that range from the harmless and beneficial to the virulent and lethal

bacterial endocarditis see: endocarditis, bacterial

bacteriophobia fear of germs

bag of waters see: amniotic fluid

baldness/alopecia common hereditary condition of males marked by a gradual loss of hair on the crown of the head until only a fringe remains around the sides and in the back, often called male pattern baldness

baldness, patchy/alopecia areata sudden but usu. temporary loss of hair in patches

barber's itch see: sycosis

barbiturate any of a class of drugs derived from barbituric acid that depress the central nervous system, used medically as sedatives and sleeping pills and in the treatment of epilepsy and high blood pressure

barium metallic element used in compounds, esp. barium sulfate, in radiography of the gastrointestinal tract because it is radiopaque—impervious to X rays

barium enema enema in which a barium mixture is used to visualize the inner walls of the large intestine by X ray, used to detect cancer and other diseases

barium meal liquid containing barium taken orally for the visualization of the upper gastrointestinal tract by X ray

barium sulfate an insoluble barium compound used to facilitate X-ray pictures of the stomach and intestines

barium swallow X-ray examination of the esophagus as the patient swallows a liquid containing barium

baroreceptors/barostats sensitive nerve

cells that respond to changes in blood pressure and may help to regulate it

barostats see: baroreceptors

Basal Body Temperature/BBT accurate measure of body temperature taken under uniform conditions, used to determine a woman's day of ovulation

basal ganglia group of nerve cells embedded in the cerebral hemisphere, the largest part of the human brain

basal metabolism the minimum energy, measured in calories, that the body needs to maintain essential vital activities when it is at rest

basal thermometer thermometer marked in tenths of degrees instead of fifths, used by women to determine the time of ovulation

BBT see: Basal Body Temperature

bedwetting see: enuresis

belladonna plant with purple-red flowers whose leaves and roots yield a number of poisonous alkaloids used in medicine

Bell's palsy facial paralysis due to lesion of the facial nerve

bends see: decompression sickness

benign mild or nonmalignant, and responding to treatment

Benzedrine see: amphetamine

beriberi disease of the peripheral nerves characterized by partial paralysis and swelling of the legs, caused by the absence of B complex vitamins

bicuspid/premolar one of the four upper or four lower cusped teeth located between the cuspids (or canine teeth) and the molars

bile bitter, viscid alkaline fluid used in digestion, esp. of fats, that is secreted by the liver and stored in the gallbladder

bilharziasis see: schistosomiasis

biliary tract duct that conveys bile

bilirubin pigment found in bile

biodegradable capable of being broken down, as a chemical compound, by microorganisms

biodegrade break down (a substance) chemically by the action of microorganisms

biological death death of the brain, following clinical death

biomicroscope see: slit lamp microscope

biopsy excision of tissue or other material from a living subject for clinical and diagnostic examination

birth canal passageway formed by the cervix and vagina through which a fetus passes in the birth process

birth control the regulation of conception by employing preventive methods or devices

birthmark mark or stain existing on the body from birth

birthmark, vascular see: hemangioma

bite, improper see: malocclusion

black cancer see: melanoma

black fever see: kala-azar

black lung disease form of pneumoconiosis common in coal miners and caused by constant exposure to coal dust

bladder elastic membranous sac near the front of the pelvic cavity, used to store urine temporarily

bladder, infection of see: cystitis

bladder, inflammation of see: cystitis

bleb blister formed in the epidermis

bleeder see: hemophiliac

blepharoplasty surgical technique to correct congenital defects in the eyelids or to alter their size or shape, including the removal of "bags" under the eyes

blister small rounded sac, esp. on the skin, containing fluid matter, often resulting from injury, friction, or scalding

blister, blood blister containing blood from broken capillaries, often resulting from a pinch or other injury

blood count examination of blood components, used in diagnosis. A complete blood count (CBC) reveals the size, shape, and number of white and red cells and platelets in a cubic millimeter of blood. A differential blood count determines the percentage of leukocytes and other cells.

blood group/blood type classification of the blood, commonly designated AB, A, B, and O, based on the specific generic differences in the composition and chemical properties of the blood

bloodletting see: phlebotomy

blood poisoning/septicemia introduction of virulent bacteria into the bloodstream, usu. from a local infection such as a boil or wound, and marked by chills, fever, and fatigue

blood pressure pressure of the blood on the walls of the arteries, varying with the resilience of the blood vessels and with the heart's contraction (systole) or relaxation (diastole), usu. represented by two numbers, the systolic pressure followed by the diastolic pressure

blood pressure, high see: hypertension

blood serum the watery, clear portion (serum) of blood

blood sugar see: glucose

blood type see: blood group

blue baby infant born with cyanosis (imperfect oxygenation of the blood) resulting from a congenital heart defect

body scanner see: CAT scanner

body scanning see: CAT scanning

Boeck's sarcoid see: sarcoidosis

boil/furuncle abscess of the skin caused by bacterial infection of a hair follicle or sebaceous gland

bolus lump or mass of food that has been chewed and softened with saliva

bone hard tissue of which the skeleton of a vertebrate animal is largely composed

bone atrophy see: decalcification

bone, inflammation of osteomyelitis

bones, brittle see: osteogenesis imperfecta

bone, softening and thickening see: Paget's disease 1

botulism poisoning caused by eating spoiled or improperly prepared or canned food and characterized by acute gastrointestinal and nervous disorders

bowel, large see: intestine, large

Bowman's capsule dilated structure surrounding a glomerulus as part of the nephron of a kidney

brain cage see: cranium

brain damage tissue destruction of the brain caused by an injury before, at, or after birth

brain damage, minimal see: minimal brain dysfunction

brain death see: biological death

brain, "lesser" see: cerebellum

brain scan procedure of injecting a radioactive substance into the brain tissue or fluid and recording its movement by X rays

brain scanning CAT *scanning* of the brain

brain stem all of the brain except the cerebellum, cerebrum, and cerebral cortex; the midbrain

brain surgeon see: neurosurgeon

brain waves, recording of see: electroencephalography

breast enlargement see: mammoplasty

breast reduction see: mastoplasty

breathalyzer device for measuring the concentration of alcohol in the bloodstream of drivers of motor vehicles

breath, bad see: halitosis

breech presentation birth with the baby positioned to present the buttocks first instead of the head first

bridge a mounting for holding false teeth, attached to adjoining teeth on each side

Bright's disease see: nephritis

bromidrosis perspiration odor

bronchi (*sing.* bronchus) the two forked branches of the trachea

bronchial asthma see: asthma

bronchial tree the bronchi and bronchial tubes

bronchial tubes the subdivisions of the trachea conveying air into the lungs

bronchiole minute subdivision in a bronchial tube

bronchitis inflammation of the bronchial tubes, characterized by coughing, chest pain, and fever

bronchitis, acute short, severe attack of bronchitis, often brought on by exposure to cold or breathing in of irritating substances, including pollutants

bronchitis, chronic recurring attacks of bronchitis after periods of quiescence

brucellosis/Malta fever/undulant fever persistent infectious disease caused by a bacterium (*Brucella*) transmitted to humans from infected animals, as goats, cattle, or swine, and marked by recurrent fever, sweating, weakness, and generalized aches and pains

bruxism habit of grinding the teeth during sleep or when otherwise under strain

bubo inflammatory swelling of a lymph gland, esp. in the groin or armpit

bubonic plague form of plague characterized by buboes

buccal pertaining to the cheek or mouth cavity

Buerger's disease circulatory disorder associated with cigarette smoking

bulbar pertaining to a bulb, esp. the bulb of the medulla oblongata of the brain

bunion painful swelling of the foot, usu. at the outer side of the base of the big toe

Burkitt's lymphoma malignant lymphoma affecting the jaw, found esp. among children in Africa

bursa any of the fluid-filled sacs within the body that tend to lessen friction between movable parts

bursitis inflammation of a bursa

bursitis, calcific painful condition characterized by calcium deposits in the shoulder tendon or calcification in a bursa at the shoulder

byssinosis/white lung disease lung disorder caused by inhaling cotton dust

C

cadaver dead human body, esp. one intended for dissection

Caesarian section surgical delivery of a baby by cutting through the abdominal wall into the uterus

caffeine chemical found in the leaves and berries of coffee, used as a stimulant and diuretic

caisson disease see: decompression sickness

calcification the degenerative hardening of tissue due to the deposit of calcium salts

calcinosis see under: interstitial calcinosis

calcitonin hormone secreted by the parathyroid glands, important in regulating the amount of calcium in the body

calculus collection of hard material, as a deposit in an organ or duct or on the teeth

callus 1. tough, thick skin, as on the soles of the feet, formed from continuing friction or pressure
2. the new bony tissue between and around the fractured ends of a broken bone that is in the process of reuniting

calorie unit of heat used esp. to express the heat or energy-producing content of foods

calyx (*pl.* calyces) cup-shaped recess in the kidney pelvis which serves as a collecting point for urine

canalization formation of new channels or ducts within tissues

canals of Schlemm ringlike vein in the sclera of the eye that helps maintain a proper balance of aqueous humor

cancer any of various diseases that prob-

ably have different causes and originate in different tissues, but which all involve neoplasms that spread by metastasis, resulting in progressive tissue degeneration

candidiasis see: moniliasis

canine tooth see: cuspid

canker sore small ulcerous lesion in the mouth near the molar teeth, inside the lips or in the lining of the mouth

cannabis hashish or marihuana

Cannabis sativa the Indian hemp plant, from whose flowering tops are derived marihuana and hashish

cannula narrow tube inserted into a body cavity or vessel, as to extract a substance or introduce a medication

capillary any of a network of microscopic blood vessels connecting the arteries with the veins

caput succedaneum swelling under a newborn baby's scalp soon after birth, that usu. dissolves in a few days

carbohydrate any of a group of compounds, including sugars, starches, and cellulose, that contains carbon combined with hydrogen and oxygen, essential in the metabolism of plants and animals

carbolic acid/phenol powerful caustic poison distilled from coal tar oil and used as a disinfectant

carbon monoxide colorless, odorless gas that is highly poisonous when inhaled since it combines with the hemoglobin in the blood and thus excludes oxygen

carbon tetrachloride colorless liquid that can be poisonous if inhaled over a long period, often used as a fire extinguisher or cleaning fluid

carbuncle painful, extensive inflammation of the skin, marked by hardness and the discharge of pus

carcinogen carcinogenic substance

carcinogenic causing cancer or increasing the incidence of cancer in a population

carcinoma malignant tumor that arises in the tissue that lines body cavities and ducts (epithelial tissue)

cardia the opening between the esophagus and the stomach

cardiac of or relating to the heart

cardiac arrest a stopping of the heartbeat

cardiac catheterization the advancing of a catheter, or thin tube, through the veins to the heart chamber, in order to detect abnormalities and obtain blood samples

cardiac insufficiency see: insufficiency

cardiac massage/cardiovascular pulmonary resuscitation/CPR emergency procedure consisting of the application of rhythmic pressure on the chest in order to compress the heart and start it beating after cardiac arrest

cardiac muscle the striated but involuntary muscle of which the heart is composed

cardiac sphincter ring of muscle at the entrance of the stomach, or cardia, that opens to allow food to enter from the esophagus

cardiac X-ray series chest X rays taken after the patient has swallowed an opaque liguid such as barium sulfate

cardiogram 1. record produced by a cardiograph
2. electrocardiogram

cardiograph 1. instrument for recording the force of the movements of the heart
2. electrocardiograph

cardiologist physician specializing in the diagnosis and treatment of heart disease

cardiology the branch of medical science dealing with the heart, its physiology and pathology

cardiovascular pertaining to the heart and blood vessels

cardiovascular disease/heart disease disorders affecting the heart and blood vessels

cardiovascular pulmonary resuscitation see: cardiac massage

cardiovascular specialist physician specializing in the diagnosis and treatment of diseases of the heart and blood vessels

caries decay of a bone or tooth (*dental caries*)

cariogenic causing caries, or tooth decay

carotene orange or red crystalline pigment converted to Vitamin A in animal metabolism

carotid artery either of two major arteries of the neck supplying blood to the head

carpal pertaining to the bones of the carpus, or wrist

carpus the wrist

carrier person who is immune from infection of specific disease-causing bacteria that his body carries and that can be transmitted to others who are not immune

cartilage tough, elastic supporting tissue

cartilage plate/epiphysis extremity of a long bone, originally separated from it by cartilage but later consolidated with it by ossification

cast bit of tissue, often microscopic, having taken the shape of a vessel or cavity in which it was formed, that is found in excretions and may indicate the presence of disease

CAT computerized axial tomography. See: CAT scanning

catabolism the destructive aspect of metabolism, in which living matter breaks down nutrients into simpler substances. Compare *anabolism*

catalepsy abnormal condition characterized by lack of response to stimuli and by muscular rigidity, often associated with a psychological disorder

catalyst substance or agent that causes a chemical reaction while remaining stable, such as an enzyme or hormone in the human body

cataract 1. the gradual clouding and opacity of the lens of the eye, leading to impaired passage of light
2. an opaque area of the lens of the eye caused by this condition

cataract, senile cataract affecting elderly people due to degenerative changes in the lens

catatonic schizophrenia see: schizophrenia, catatonic

cathartic medicine for purging bowels

catheter slender tube for drawing off fluid from a body cavity, esp. urine from the bladder

catheterization the introduction of a catheter into the body

CAT scanner/body scanner computerized X-ray machine used in *CAT scanning*

CAT scanning/body scanning/computerized axial tomography procedure for producing a cross-sectional, computer-generated, composite X-ray picture of the body or an organ, as the brain, by rotating about a site and taking a series of radiographs directed to it

caudal situated at the tail end or bottom; posterior

caudal anesthesia/caudal/caudal block

form of anesthesia in which the patient is injected in the region of the lower spinal cord (sacral canal) to block pain in the pelvic area

caul membrane (amnion) surrounding the fetus if it is unruptured and intact about the baby's head at delivery

cautery, chemical see under: chemosurgery

cavities see: dental caries

CBC complete blood count; see under: blood count

cc cubic centimeter

cecum blind pouch or cavity open at one end, esp. the cavity below the ileocecal valve that forms the first section of the large intestine

celiac pertaining to the abdomen

celiac disease see: malabsorption syndrome

cells, taste see: taste bud

cellular therapy treatment for the process of aging in which a person is injected with cells from healthy embryonic animal organs with the idea that the animal cells from the particular organ injected will then migrate to the same organ in the aging body and reactivate it

cementum the layer of body tissue developed over the roots of the teeth

central nervous system the portion of the nervous system that contains the brain and spinal cord and controls voluntary action and movement

centrifuge 1. (*n.*) rotary machine employing centrifugal force to separate substances having different densities, as the constituents of blood
2. (*v.*) subject to a whirling motion to separate component parts, as of blood, that have different densities

cephalhematoma swelling under a newborn baby's scalp that usu. dissolves within a few weeks

cerebellum large section of the brain located below and behind the cerebrum, consisting of a central lobe and two lateral lobes, and which coordinates voluntary muscle movements, posture, and equilibrium

cerebral arteriogram an X-ray picture of the brain used to investigate brain damage, esp. after a hemorrhage or stroke, and made by injecting opaque dye into the blood vessels serving the brain and X-raying them

cerebral arteriosclerosis degenerative changes in the arteries of the brain

cerebral cortex the cells and fibers that look like a convoluted layer of gray matter and that cover the cerebral hemisphere of the brain.

cerebral hemisphere one of the two halves into which the brain is divided

cerebral hemorrhage hemorrhage into the cerebrum of the brain or within the cranium

cerebral palsy inability to control movement caused by nonprogressive brain damage resulting from a prenatal defect or birth injury

cerebrospinal fluid/CSF/spinal fluid the clear, colorless fluid that surrounds the brain and spinal cord

cerebrospinal meningitis inflammation of the membranes that cover the brain and spinal cord

cerebrovascular of or relating to the vessels supplying blood to the brain

cerebrum the upper anterior part of the brain, consisting of two hemispherical masses which constitute the chief bulk of the brain in man, assumed to be the seat of thought and will

cervical 1. pertaining to the cervix of the uterus
2. pertaining to the neck or any neck-like part

cervical cap contraceptive device made usu. of soft plastic which fits over the cervix

cervical spine see: cervical vertebrae

cervical vertebrae/cervical spine the top seven vertebrae of the backbone, which are located in the neck and support the head

cervicitis inflammation of the cervix of the uterus

cervix neck of the uterus

Cesarian section see: Caesarian section

cestode see: tapeworm

chafing inflammation of two opposing skin surfaces, caused by warmth, moisture, or friction

Chagas' disease/American trypanosomiasis disease of Central and South America, a form of trypanosomiasis, caused by certain protozoa and spread by the bite of the assassin bug, characterized by fever, edema, and chronic heart disease

chancre lesion resembling a sore with a

hard base, the primary syphilitic lesion

chancre, soft see: chancroid

chancroid/soft chancre venereal disease that produces a soft chancre

change of life see: menopause

chapping condition in which skin is irritated, cracked, or roughened, more common in wintry weather

character disorder see: personality disorder

charas resin obtained from the Cannabis sativa (marihuana) plant

chemical diabetes see: diabetes, chemical

chemosurgery medical technique which utilizes chemistry, surgery, and microscopic analysis, esp. used in the treatment of skin cancers

chemotherapy medical technique used in the prevention or treatment of disease by chemical disinfection of affected organs and tissues, esp. through the use of synthetic drugs whose action is specific against certain pathogenic microorganisms

chest cavity/thoracic cavity body cavity corresponding to the chest, enclosed by the ribs

chest/thorax the part of the body enclosed by the ribs

chest X ray X-ray photograph of the chest cavity that may reveal various abnormalities of the heart, blood vessels, or lungs

chicken pox contagious viral disease, esp. of children, marked by a rash

chilblains localized inflammation of the skin, usu. on the extremities or face, causing itching, swelling, and redness

childbirth, natural childbirth regarded as a natural and relatively painless function in which the prospective mother is encouraged to participate consciously

chin, plastic surgery on see: mentoplasty

chiropodist see: podiatrist

chiropody see: podiatry

chiropractic method of therapy based on the theory that disease is mainly due to nerve malfunction, which may be corrected by manipulation of bodily structures, esp. the spinal column

chloasma see: liver spots

chlordiazepoxide see: Librium

Chloromycetin brand name of an antibiotic used to treat typhoid

chloroquine drug used in the treatment of gout and other conditions

chlorpromazine see: Thorazine

chocolate cyst see: cyst, chocolate

cholecyst see: gall bladder

cholecystitis inflammation of the gall bladder

cholecystogram visualization of the gall bladder by X ray

cholera acute, infectious, chiefly epidemic bacterial disease characterized by diarrhea, vomiting, prostration, and dehydration

cholesterol fatty crystalline alcohol derived principally from the bile and present in gallstones, the blood, and in brain and nerve tissues

chondromalacia the softening of a cartilage, as under the kneecap

chondrosarcoma form of cancer originating in the cartilage at the end of a bone

chorea/St. Vitus's dance disease of the nervous system characterized by involuntary muscular twitching

choroid the middle, vascular coat of the eyeball

chromosome one of the rod- or loop-shaped bodies, usu. paired, found in the nucleus of every cell and containing genes

chronic continuing for an extended period of time, as a disease

chronic gouty arthritis see: gouty arthritis, chronic

chyme partly digested food, in semiliquid form, as it passes from the stomach to the small intestine

cilia (*sing.* cilium) tiny hairs in the nose and breathing passages that help filter out foreign particles that enter the body

ciliary muscles the set of muscle fibers, attached to ligaments, which support the lens of the eye

circulatory shock see: shock

cirrhosis condition associated with excessive drinking in which there is an abnormal formation of connective tissue and a wasting of the tissue of the liver

clap vernacular name for *gonorrhea*

claudication see: intermittent claudication

claustrophobia compulsive or persistent fear of enclosed places

clavicle the bone connecting the shoulder blade and breastbone; the collarbone

cleft lip/harelip genetic defect in which the upper lip is not completely joined

cleft palate genetic defect in which the hard palate is not completely joined

climacteric, female see: menopause

climacteric, male in men, the psychological equivalent of the menopause, characterized by forgetfulness, depression, and declining sexual interest

clinical pertaining to or based on the actual process or symptoms of a disease as observed, as distinguished from those described as typical from a statistical or theoretical point of view

clinical death cessation of respiration and heartbeat

clitoris small, erectile organ of the female in the front part of the vulva

clonic of or characteristic of clonus

clonic phase the period during a grand mal epileptic convulsion when spasms of rigidity and relaxation (or jerking) occur in rapid succession

clonic spasm see under: spasm

clonus muscular spasm characterized by rapid alternation of contraction and relaxation

closed bite form of malocclusion, a severe overbite in which upper teeth extend far over lower teeth when the jaws are together

closed fracture/simple fracture/complete fracture fracture in which bone is completely broken, but without accompanying break in the skin

coagulation clotting, as of blood

coarctation stricture or contraction, as of a cavity or blood vessel

coated tongue condition in which the tongue is coated with a whitish substance, consisting of food particles and bacteria, which can indicate fever, illness, or a temporary lack of saliva

cocaine white, bitter, crystalline alkaloid used as a local anesthetic and a narcotic

co-carcinogen substance which is not cancer-producing but reacts with other substances to produce cancers

coccidioides fungus fungus, the spores of which can cause coccidioidomycosis

coccidioidomycosis/desert rheumatism/ valley fever infectious disease caused by fungus spores and characterized by symptoms resembling pneumonia and tuberculosis and the formation of reddened bumps

coccyx the tail end of the spinal cord

cochlea spiral-shaped structure of the inner ear containing the essential organs of hearing, including the organ of Corti

cochlear nerve the part of the auditory nerve leading from the cochlea of the inner ear to the brain, conveying the sense of hearing

codeine white, crystalline alkaloid, derived from morphine and used in medicine as an analgesic and to suppress coughing

coitus see: sexual intercourse

coitus interruptus contraceptive method in which the male withdraws before he ejaculates

cold, common viral infection of the respiratory tract

cold sores/fever blisters/herpes simplex small blisters, usu. about the mouth, that often accompany a cold or fever, caused by the herpes simplex virus

colitis inflammation of the colon; see also ulcerative colitis

collagen fibrous protein that forms the chief constituent of the connective tissues of the body, such as cartilage, skin, bone, and hair

collapsed lung see under: pneumothorax

collarbone see: clavicle

colon the part of the large intestine extending from the cecum to the rectum and divided into the ascending colon, transverse colon, descending colon, and the sigmoid

colon, ascending the section of the colon extending up from the cecum along the right side of the abdomen

colon, descending the section of the colon leading from the transverse colon and extending down the left side of the abdomen

colonoscope speculum used to examine the colon

color blindness/achromotopsia inherited vision defect consisting of the total or partial inability to discriminate between certain colors, usu. red, green, and blue

colostomy the formation of an artificial opening in the colon through which solid wastes can pass

colostrum the creamy, yellowish, milk-like substance rich in proteins, that is produced by a mother's breasts the first few days after having given birth

colposcopy microscopic technique for visual examination of the cervix and vagina

coma prolonged loss of consciousness

comminuted fracture fracture in which bone is splintered or crushed

common bile duct duct formed by the juncture of the hepatic and cystic ducts, and carrying digestive enzymes from the liver, pancreas, and gall bladder to the duodenum

complete blood count see under: blood count

complete fracture see: closed fracture

compound fracture/open fracture fracture accompanied by an open wound, often exposing bone that is completely broken

compulsion urgent need to perform certain ritualistic acts, often irrational, a symptom of certain neuroses

computerized axial tomography see: CAT scanning

conception union of spermatozoon and ovum, first step in the birth process; fertilization

concussion violent shock to the brain, typically caused by a blow to the head, as in a fall, that impairs the functioning of the brain, usu. temporarily

condom membranous sheath for the penis which serves as a contraceptive device

condyloma acuminatum see: venereal wart

cone one of many photosensitive cone-shaped bodies in the retina of the eye, sensitive to color and daylight vision

congener natural product of fermentation found in small amounts in all alcoholic beverages

congenital acquired prior to or at birth, or during development as a fetus, as fetal abnormality due to the mother's contraction of rubella

congenital heart disease deformity of the heart or of major blood vessels existing from birth

congestion excessive accumulation of blood or fluid in an organ or tissues

conjunctiva mucous membrane on the inner part of the eyelid and extending over the front of the eyeball

conjunctival sac the small sac at the inner corner of the eye between the eyeball

and the lower lid that serves as a collecting pool for tears

conjunctivitis inflammation of the conjunctiva

connective tissue the fibrous tissue that binds together or supports the parts of the body, as cartilage, tendons, and ligaments

conscience see: superego

conservative of or involving procedures or treatment intended to preserve function of diseased or injured parts, utilizing established therapeutic methods

constipation inactivity of the bowels resulting in difficult, infrequent, or incomplete evacuation

constrict become narrower, as a blood vessel

contact dermatitis see: dermatitis, contact

contact lens one of a pair of glass or plastic lenses fitted directly over the cornea of each eye to correct vision defects

contagion communication of disease by contact, direct or indirect

contagious (of a disease) transmitted by direct or indirect contact

continuous positive airway pressure procedure in which high-oxygen air is forced into the lungs of newborns suffering from respiratory difficulty

contraception the prevention of conception

contraceptive device or substance designed to prevent conception

contraceptive, oral/the pill the birth control pill, which is composed of synthetic hormones that suppress ovulation and thus prevent pregnancy

contraindication symptom or sign that makes a particular course of treatment inadvisable

conversion hysteria see: conversion reaction

conversion reaction/conversion hysteria neurosis characterized by manifestation of physical symptoms, such as blindness or deafness, without organic cause, as an expression of psychic conflict

convulsion/seizure spontaneous violent and abnormal muscular contraction or spasm of the body

Cooley's anemia see: thalassemia

corium see: dermis

corn horny thickening of the cuticle,

common on the feet

cornea the transparent lens surface of the eye

coronary encircling or crowning, such as the two arteries branching from the aorta and encircling the heart

coronary arteries and veins the network of arteries and veins that nourishes the muscle and tissue of the heart

coronary artery disease fatty obstructions in the coronary vessels that nourish the heart, impairing adequate delivery of oxygen to the heart

coronary insufficiency insufficient blood circulation through the coronary arteries

coronary occlusion closure of the coronary artery, due to buildup of fatty deposits or coronary thrombosis

coronary thrombosis interference with the blood supply to the heart muscle because of a blood clot in the coronary artery

corpus callosum fibrous tissue connecting the two hemispheres of the cerebrum of the brain

corpuscle one of the cells that make up blood, either a red corpuscle (erythrocyte) or a white corpuscle (leukocyte)

corpus luteum mass in the ovary formed by the rupture of a Graafian follicle that releases an ovum during each menstrual cycle

corpus luteum cyst see: cyst, corpus luteum

cortex the outer layer or covering of an organ or part, as of the cerebrum or cerebellum of the brain (called gray matter), of the adrenal glands, or of the kidneys

corticoids any of the hormones manufactured in the adrenal cortex

corticosteroid 1. any of the steroids secreted by the cortex of the adrenal gland 2. any steroid hormone resembling in its effects the steroids secreted by the adrenal gland

corticosterone steroid hormone of the adrenal cortex associated with blood sugar levels and other metabolic functions

Corti, organ of see:: organ of Corti

cortisone powerful hormone extracted from the adrenal cortex and also made synthetically

coryza inflammation of the mucous membranes in the nose and connecting si-

nuses, with discharge of mucus, characteristic of a head cold

cosmetic surgeon physician specializing in cosmetic surgery

cosmetic surgery plastic surgery concerned with improving the appearance of parts of the body

costal pertaining to or near a rib or ribs

cough expel air or phlegm from the lungs in a noisy or spasmodic manner

cowpox live calf lymph virus, used in smallpox vaccinations

coxa the hip or hip joint

coxa vara deformity of the hip joint caused by curvature of the femur toward the joint, thus shortening the affected leg and causing a limp

Coxsackie virus any of a group of viruses causing various diseases in humans, including a form of meningitis

CPR cardiovascular pulmonary resuscitation. See: cardiac massage

cradle cap disease of the scalp, esp. in babies, marked by yellowish crusts

cranial nerves the twelve pairs of nerves that originate within the brain

cranioplasty surgical correction of the skull, as to repair a congenital defect

craniotomy any surgery involving an opening in the skull

cranium the part of the human skull that encloses and protects the brain

cresol compound obtained by destructive distillation of coal, beechwood, or pinewood, used as an antiseptic and disinfectant

cretinism condition associated with thyroid deficiency during early development, marked by physical deformities, dwarfism, and mental retardation

crib death see: sudden infant death syndrome

crossed eyes/crosseye strabismus characterized by a tendency of the eyes to turn inward toward the nose

crosseye see: crossed eyes

cross-match intermix constituents of the blood of a prospective donor with that of a prospective recipient to check blood compatibility

croup spasm of the trachea, esp. the larynx, occurring in children and marked by difficulty in breathing and a barking cough

crown the part of a tooth exposed beyond

the gum and covered with enamel

cryosurgery type of surgery in which extremely low temperatures are employed either locally or generally to destroy tissue, as in malignant skin lesions

cryotherapy inducement of peeling by freezing the skin with carbon dioxide to improve appearance of flat acne scars and shallow wrinkles

cryptorchidism/cryptorchism failure of the testicles to descend normally

cryptorchism see: cryptorchidism

CSF see: cerebrospinal fluid

culdoscopy technique for examining the female reproductive organs within the abdominal cavity

culture the development of microorganisms or living cells in a special medium, as gelatin, often as a means of analyzing a body fluid or tissue for the presence of disease

cupula structure within each of the semicircular canals of the inner ear, communicating changes in motion

curettage the scraping of a cavity with a curette, as to remove morbid matter or obtain tissue for diagnosis

curette surgical instrument, usu. resembling a spoon or scoop with sharpened edges, used in curettage

Cushing's syndrome excess of hormones secreted by the adrenal cortex, characterized by weakness, purple streaks in the skin, and a moon face

cusp 1. one of the projections or points on the crown of a tooth
2. one of the triangular flaps of a heart valve

cuspid/canine tooth/eye tooth one of the two upper or two lower sharp, pointed teeth located between the incisors and the bicuspids

cutaneous pertaining to, affecting, or on the skin

cuticle 1. epidermis
2. crescent of toughened skin around the base of a nail

cyanosis disordered circulatory condition due to inadequate oxygen supply in the blood and causing a livid bluish color of the skin

cyanotic bluish in color due to cyanosis

cyclamate synthetic nonnutritive sweetener, usu. of sodium or calcium

cycloid see: cyclothymic

cyclothymic/cycloid describing a personality disorder in which the individual is subject to sharply defined moods of elation or depression

cynophobia fear of dogs

cyst saclike mass containing liquid or semisolid material

cyst, chocolate ovarian cyst formed from misplaced endometrial tissue growing on the ovary

cyst, corpus luteum ovarian cyst formed from a fluid produced by the corpus luteum

cystectomy 1. surgical removal of the gall bladder or of the urinary bladder
2. surgical removal of a cyst

cyst, follicular/retention cyst ovarian cyst formed from the contents of a Graafian follicle

cystic duct duct that carries bile from the gall bladder to the juncture with the hepatic duct, where the common bile duct is formed

cystic fibrosis hereditary disease of infants and young children marked by cysts, excessive fibrous tissue, and mucous secretion

cystitis inflammation of the bladder, characterized by a burning sensation when voiding, frequent need to urinate, and sometimes blood in the urine

cystocele hernia in which part of the bladder protrudes through the wall of the vagina

cystoscope device used to view the interior of the bladder after being inserted in the urethra

cystoscopy the technique of viewing the interior of the bladder by means of a cystoscope

cystostomy the making of an artificial outlet from the urinary bladder

cyst, retention see: cyst, follicular

D

D and C see: dilation and curettage

dandruff condition marked by itching and flaking of the skin, esp. of the scalp

db see: decibel

DBI/phenformin drug that stimulates the production of insulin in the pancreas

D.D.S. Doctor of Dental Surgery

decalcification/bone atrophy the loss of lime or calcium salts from the bones or teeth

decibel/db unit for measuring the intensity of sound

deciduous teeth see: baby teeth

decision-maker see: ego

decompression sickness/caisson disease/ the bends painful, sometimes fatal condition due to bubbles of nitrogen formed in the blood when a rapid reduction in pressure occurs, as when a diver returns directly to the surface after a period deep under water

decongestant agent designed to relieve congestion

defecation the discharge of feces

defibrillation act or process of stopping fibrillation of the heart muscle and restoring normal rhythm, as by jolting it with an electric current

defibrillator device that sends a jolt of electricity into the heart muscle in order to stop fibrillation and get the heart back to normal rhythm

degenerative characterized by deterioration or change from a normally active state to a lower or less active form, esp. of body tissue, as in a disease process

degenerative joint disease see: osteoarthritis

deglutition act of swallowing

dehydration loss or removal of water, as from body tissues

déjà vu distortion of memory in which a new situation or experience is regarded as having happened before

delirium tremens/DTs violent form of delirium characterized by nausea, confusion, crawling sensation on the skin, and hallucinations, caused esp. by rapid lowering of blood alcohol levels in very heavy drinkers

dementia mental deterioration resulting from an organic or functional disorder

dementia, presenile/Alzheimer's disease mental degeneration (dementia) resulting from functional or organic disorder, as cerebral arteriosclerosis, that occurs in middle age

Demerol see: meperidine

demyelination gradual loss of myelin, resulting in paralysis, numbness, or other loss of nerve function

dendrites short, gray filaments in neurons that conduct impulses toward the cell body

dental calculus/tartar hard deposit of minerals and other substances that collects on teeth

dental caries ulceration and decay of teeth

dental floss strong, silky filament for cleaning between the teeth

dental surgeon see: oral surgeon

dentin the hard calcified substance that forms the body of a tooth

dentist one who specializes in the diagnosis, prevention, and treatment of disease affecting the teeth and their associated structures

dentistry the branch of medical science that concerns the study, diagnosis, prevention, and treatment of diseases of the teeth, gums, and associated structures

dentition the kind, number, and arrangement of the teeth in the mouth

denture(s) frame of plastic or other material adapted to fit the mouth and containing one, several, or a complete set of artificial teeth to replace natural teeth that have been lost

dependence see under: drug dependence

depilatory chemical product capable of removing or loosening hair

depressant drug or other substance that reduces or calms the physiological processes of body or mind

depression 1. mental state marked by melancholy, pessimism, or dejection 2. psychotic condition characterized by stuporous withdrawal from reality and intense guilt feelings

depressive reaction 1. neurosis characterized by persistent feelings of depression and pessimism unrelated to any apparent cause 2. (involutional melancholia) psychosis usu. occurring in women around the time of menopause, and in men during their 50s, characterized by hopeless melancholy, anxiety, weeping, and often delusions

dermabrasion the removal of layers of skin by planing with an abrasive tool to dispose of wrinkles or skin blemishes

dermal of or relating to the skin

dermatitis inflammation of the skin

dermatitis, contact dermatitis caused by a hypersensitive reaction to external contact with a substance or material

dermatologist physician specializing in

the diagnosis and treatment of disorders of the skin

dermatology the branch of medical science dealing with disorders of the skin

dermis/corium/true skin the inner layer of the skin, which contains blood vessels, nerves, connective tissue, sweat glands, and sebaceous glands

DES see: diethylstilbestrol

desert rheumatism see: coccidioidomycosis

Desoxyn see: methamphetamine

detached retina/separated retina eye disorder in which the membrane at the back of the eye (retina) is separated from its bed, as by being torn, thus impairing vision

developmental disability any condition which interferes with a child's development, esp. one which will constitute a handicap throughout the individual's life, such as mental retardation or cerebral palsy

Dexedrine see: dextroamphetamine

dextroamphetamine/Dexedrine isomer of the amphetamine compound, considered to have a more stimulating effect on the central nervous system than amphetamine

dextrose form of glucose (a sugar) found normally in animals, used in intravenous feeding because it is readily assimilated by the blood

diabetes, chemical/prediabetic condition condition indicating predisposition to development of diabetes, when blood sugar level remains abnormally high for too long after taking a glucose tolerance test

diabetes insipidus production of excessive amount of urine due to deficiency of antidiuretic hormone

diabetes mellitus disease associated with inadequate production of insulin and characterized by excessive urinary secretion containing abnormal amounts of sugar, accompanied by emaciation, excessive hunger, and thirst

diabetic one who has diabetes

diabetic acidosis advanced stage of diabetes when treated with insufficient insulin, characterized by increasing buildup of ketone bodies, drowsiness, and, if untreated, coma

diabetic coma state of unconsciousness in a diabetic resulting from insufficient insulin, characterized by deep, labored breathing and a fruity odor to the breath

diabetic ketosis early stage of diabetes treated with insufficient insulin, characterized by excessive urination, thirst, and hot, dry skin

diabetic retinopathy disease of the eye associated with diabetes in which new, abnormal blood vessels form on the surface of the retina, sometimes marked by bleeding

diacetylmorphine see: heroin

diagnosis identification of a disease or disorder by its characteristic symptoms, or the conclusions reached in a particular instance

dialysis the separating of mixed substances by means of wet membranes, as the action of the kidneys, esp. applied to an artificial process to remove waste products and excess fluid from the bloodstream of a patient with defective kidneys.

diaper rash rash caused by the ammonia produced by the urine in diapers

diaphragm 1. dome-shaped layer of muscle between the chest and abdomen whose contraction enlarges the rib cage for inflation of the lungs in breathing
2. contraceptive device of molded rubber or soft plastic material used to cover the cervix and prevent entry of spermatozoa

diaphragmatic hernia see: hernia, hiatus

diaphragm, contractions of see: hiccups

diarrhea frequent and fluid evacuation of feces

diastole the instant when the heart is relaxed as the ventricles fill with blood prior to contraction and pumping (systole)

diastolic pressure measure of blood pressure taken when the heart is resting, the lower of the two figures in a reading

diathermy treatment by means of heat generated within the body by high-frequency radiation

diazepam see: Valium

diet, bland diet that is not irritating or abrasive, as the diet recommended for peptic ulcer patients

diethylstilbestrol/DES/stilbestrol synthetic hormone resembling estrogen implicated in the formation of vaginal and cervical cancers in the daughters of women who had taken the hormone during pregnancy

digestion process of dissolving and chemically changing food in the alimentary tract so that it can be assimilated by the blood and its nutrients can be absorbed by the body

digitalis the dried leaves of foxglove, containing several glycosides, often used as a heart tonic

dilate make or become larger, as the pupil of the eye in diminished light

dilation and curettage/D and C enlarging the opening into the uterus and the scraping of the uterus with a curette

dimethyltryptamine see: DMT

diphtheria respiratory, bacterial disease marked by the formation of a false membrane that obstructs breathing

diplopia see: double vision

disability, developmental see: developmental disability

disability, learning see: learning disability

disclosing tablets tablets which, after being chewed, leave a temporary stain on plaque remaining on teeth after brushing

disk, slipped/herniated disk painful displacement (herniation) of one of the fibrous disks of the spinal column between two vertebrae, such that it presses against nerves and may cause sciatica

dislocation the partial or complete displacement of one or more of the bones at a joint

displacement transference of intense anxiety unconsciously felt about a particular conflict to a substitute, which is regarded consciously with the same intensity of anxiety, a manifestation of the phobic reaction

dissociative reaction neurosis characterized by escape from a part of the personality by means of dream states, amnesia, forgetfulness, etc.

distal relatively remote from the center of the body, or from a point considered as central, esp. as compared to a nearer (proximal) point

distal muscles the muscles of the extremities (the hands and the feet)

distillation separation of the more volatile parts of a substance from the less volatile by boiling and condensing the vapors into separate liquids

diuresis excessive excretion of urine

diuretic/"water pill" substance stimulating the secretion of urine

diverticula *pl.* of *diverticulum*

diverticulitis inflammation of diverticula in the digestive tract, esp. in the colon

diverticulosis the presence of diverticula in the digestive tract

diverticulum (*pl.* diverticula) abnormal pouch or bulge protruding from an organ or part, as from the colon of the intestines

DMT/dimethyltryptamine synthetic hallucinogen

Dolophine see: methadone

DOM/STP synthetic hallucinogen

dopamine chemical compound found in the brain, needed in the synthesis of norepinephrine and epinephrine

dorsal toward, near, or in the back

double vision/diplopia condition in which a single object is perceived as two images due to inability to coordinate focusing of the eyes

douching flushing of a body part or cavity, esp. the vagina, with water as a means of cleansing

downs/downers/goof balls (slang) barbiturates or other drugs that depress the central nervous system

Down's syndrome/Mongolism congenital mental and physical retardation due to a chromosomal anomaly, accompanied by variable signs including a flat face and pronounced epicanthic folds

DPT injection injection to provide immunity against diphtheria, pertussis (whooping cough), and tetanus

Dramamine proprietary drug used to counteract motion sickness

dropsy former term for edema, esp. when caused by cardiac insufficiency

drug 1. any substance other than food that changes or has an effect on the body or mind

2. see: narcotic

drug dependence physical or psychological accommodation to the periodic or continuous presence of a drug in the body's system

dry socket painful complication of a tooth extraction in which underlying tissue of the alveolar bone is exposed to infection

Duchenne's muscular dystrophy see: pseudohypertrophic muscular dystrophy

duct, hepatic either of two ducts of the liver that join to form the common hepatic duct and that carry bile

ductless gland see: endocrine gland

dumdum fever see: kala-azar

duodenal ulcer ulcer of the duodenum of the small intestine

duodenum the first section of the small intestine, leading from the stomach to the jejunum

dura mater the tough, fibrous, outermost membrane of the three membranes covering the brain and spinal cord

dwarfism disorder characterized by stunted growth

dysentery severe inflammation of the mucous membrane of the large intestine, characterized by bloody stools, pain, cramps, and fever

dysfunction impairment or abnormal functioning, as of an organ

dyslexia 1. impairment or loss of the ability to read, as from a stroke 2. in children, impairment of ability to acquire language skills due to motor or perceptual disabilities

dysmenorrhea painful menstruation

dyspareunia painful sexual intercourse

dyspepsia indigestion, characterized by heartburn, nausea, pain in the upper abdomen, and belching

dyspnea labored, difficult breathing

dysphagia difficulty in swallowing

dysphasia disorder of the cerebral centers characterized by difficulty in understanding or using speech

dystrophy 1. defective or faulty nutrition 2. any of various neurological or muscular disorders, as muscular dystrophy

dysuria difficult or painful urination

E

eardrum/tympanic membrane/tympanum drumhead membrane separating the middle ear from the external ear

ear, ringing in see: tinnitus

earwax waxy substance secreted by the glands lining the passages of the external ear

ECG see: electrocardiogram

echocardiogram graph recording the pattern of deflection of sound waves by the heart, used in diagnosing heart abnormalities

eclampsia toxemia of pregnancy involving convulsions

E. coli/Escherichia coli common bacillus found normally in the human intestines, usu. harmless but having certain strains that cause urinary tract and other infections

ECPR/external cardiopulmonary resuscitation closed-chest massage, used for those suffering cardiac arrest

ectoderm outermost layer of tissue

ectopic/atopic out of normal place or position

ectopic pregnancy abortive pregnancy outside the uterus, as in the Fallopian tubes or abdominal cavity

eczema noncontagious skin condition characterized by itching and scaling of the skin

edema swelling of tissues due to abnormal fluid accumulation

edentulous toothless

EEG see: electroencephalogram

efferent applied to nerves, communicating impulses so that directive action can be taken; motor

efferent nerve see: motor nerve

egg cell see: ovum

ego/decision-maker the self, considered as the seat of consciousness

ejaculation expulsion of semen during orgasm

EKG see: electrocardiogram

elective surgery surgery that may be necessary or optional, as distinguished from surgery that must be performed urgently or in an emergency

Electra complex repressed sexual attachment of daughter to father, analogous to the Oedipal complex involving the son and mother

electric shock the body's reactions to the passage through it of an electric current, as involuntary muscular contractions

electrocardiogram/ECG/EKG graph recording the pattern of electric impulses produced by the heart, used in the diagnosis of heart disease

electrocardiograph machine used to record the electric current produced by the heart muscle

electrocardiography technique of producing electrocardiograms and interpreting them

electroencephalogram/EEG graph recording the pattern of electric impulses produced by the brain, used in the diagnosis of neurological disorders

electroencephalograph machine used to record the electric current produced by the brain

electroencephalography technique of producing electroencephalograms and interpreting them

electrolysis technique for removing unwanted hair by destroying the hair root with an electric current

electromyogram/EMG graph recording the electrical activity of a muscle

electromyography technique of producing electromyograms and interpreting them

electroshock describing a form of treatment for psychological disorders in which a controlled electric current is passed through the patient's head, producing convulsions and unconsciousness, usu. given in series

electrosurgery/surgical diathermy surgical procedure utilizing electricity to destroy tissue

elephantiasis lymphatic edema, esp. of the legs and scrotum, a symptom of filariasis

embolism the stopping up of a vein or artery, as by a blood clot, that has been brought to the point of obstruction by the bloodstream

embolism, pulmonary embolism in the pulmonary artery or one of its branches

embolus object moving within the bloodstream, as a blood clot or air bubble, that is capable of causing an obstruction (embolism) in a smaller vessel

embryo the rudimentary form of an organism in its development before birth, usu. considered as such in the human species for the first two months in utero

emetic medicine or substance used to induce vomiting

EMG see: electromyogram

emphysema puffed condition of the alveoli or air sacs of the lungs (or other tissues or organs) due to infiltration of air and consequent loss of tissue elasticity

enamel the layer of hard, glossy material forming the exposed outer covering of the teeth

encephalitis inflammation of the brain

encephalogram X-ray picture of the brain made by encephalography

encephalography X-ray visualization of the brain following the removal of cerebrospinal fluid and its replacement with air or other gases

endarterectomy surgical procedure in which carbon dioxide is forced through hardened arteries to ream out fatty blockages

endemic confined to or characteristic of a given locality, as a disease

endocarditis inflammation of the membrane (endocardium) lining the chambers of the heart

endocarditis, bacterial bacterial infection of the membrane (endocardium) lining the chambers of the heart

endocarditis, subacute bacterial bacterial endocarditis resulting as a complication of rheumatic fever, usu. fatal

endocardium the delicate membrane that lines the chambers of the heart

endocrine gland one of several ductless glands that release secretions (hormones) directly into the blood or lymph and that exert powerful influences on growth, sexual development, metabolism, and other vital body processes

endocrinologist physician specializing in endocrinology

endocrinology the branch of medical science dealing with the structure and function of the endocrine glands and their hormones

endoderm innermost layer of tissue

endodontics branch of dentistry dealing with root canal work and the dental pulp

endodontist dentist specializing in root canal work

endogenous insulin self-produced insulin

endolymph fluid within the semicircular canals of the inner ear

endometrial of or pertaining to the endometrium

endometrioma mass of tumorlike endometrial cells as a result of endometriosis

endometriosis condition in which tissue that lines the uterus (endometrium) grows outside the uterus in the pelvic cavity

endometrium the lining of the uterus

endoscope instrument for examining a

hollow organ or an internal cavity, as the urinary bladder or the urethra

endoscopy examination with an endoscope

enema liquid injected into the rectum as a purgative or for diagnostic purposes

ENT see: otolaryngology

enteric pertaining to the intestines

enteric fever see: typhoid fever

enteritis inflammation of the intestines, esp. of the small intestine

enterocele hernia in which part of the small intestine protrudes through the wall of the vagina

enuresis/bedwetting involuntary urination during sleep at night

enzyme organic substance, usu. a protein, produced by cells and having the power to initiate or accelerate specific chemical reactions in metabolism, such as digestion

eosinophil any of a type of white blood cell that stains easily when a particular red dye (eosin) is applied

ephedrine drug that dilates the bronchi, used to reduce nasal congestion and relieve asthma

epicanthic fold/epicanthus vertical fold of skin at the inner corner of the eyelid, found chiefly in certain Asian peoples

epicanthus see: epicanthic fold

epidemic 1. *(adj.)* affecting many in a community at once, as a disease
2. *(n.)* the temporary prevalence of a disease in a community or throughout a large area

epidemiologist physician specializing in epidemiology

epidemiology the branch of medical science concerned with the study and prevention of epidemic diseases

epidermis/cuticle the outer, nonvascular layer of the skin, overlying the dermis

epididymis portion of the seminal ducts just above the testis

epigastric pertaining to the upper middle part of the abdomen. See illustration at *abdomen.*

epigastrium the upper middle (epigastric) part of the abdomen. See illustration at *abdomen.*

epiglottis the leaf-shaped plate of cartilage at the back of the tongue that covers the trachea during the act of swallowing

epilepsy chronic nervous disorder characterized by sudden loss of consciousness and sometimes by convulsions

epileptic 1. *(adj.)* pertaining to epilepsy
2. *(n.)* person who has epilepsy

epinephrine see: adrenaline

epiphysis cartilage plate on the extremity of a long bone

epiphysis, slipped the slipping or dislocation of the end of a bone (epiphysis), as of the femur at the hip joint

episiotomy incision made during labor to enlarge the vaginal area enough to permit passage of the baby

epistaxis nosebleed

epithelial pertaining to the epithelium

epithelium membranous tissue that lines the canals, cavities, and ducts of the body, as well as all free surfaces exposed to the air

Equanil see: meprobamate

erection enlarged and firm state of the penis when sexually stimulated

eruption 1. emergence of a tooth through the gums
2. a breaking out of a rash on the skin

erysipelas acute bacterial skin infection characterized by bright red patches

erythema redness of the skin, a symptom occurring in various forms in different conditions having various causes, as from infection or a burn

erythremia see: polycythemia vera

erythrocyte/red blood cell/red corpuscle cell found in the bloodstream, often lacking a nucleus, the carrier of hemoglobin

erythrophobia fear of blushing

eschar dry crust or scab left by a burn caused by heat or corrosive chemical action.

Escherichia coli see: *E. coli*

esophagoscope device inserted into the esophagus to permit its inspection

esophagus/food tube the tube through which food passes from the mouth to the stomach

essential of unknown cause, as a disease or condition

essential hypertension see: hypertension, essential

estrogen any of several hormones found in the ovarian fluids of the female which promote growth of secondary sex characteristics and influence cyclical changes in the female reproductive system

ethanol see: ethyl alcohol

ether colorless, volatile, flammable chemical compound used as an anesthetic

ethmoid bone sievelike bone at the base of the skull behind the nose

ethyl alcohol/grain alcohol/ethanol product of the distillation of fermented grains, fruit juices, and starches, used in beverages and having intoxicating properties

etiologist physician specializing in studying the causes of disease

etiology 1. the cause or causes of a disease
2. the branch of medical science dealing with the causes of disease

eunuch a male who fails to develop secondary sex characteristics due to disorder or removal of testicles at puberty

Eustachian tube passage connecting the middle ear to the upper throat which equalizes air pressure on both sides of the eardrum

Ewing's sarcoma malignant tumor of the shafts of the long bones in children

excise cut out or remove by surgery

excision act or procedure of cutting out or removing surgically

excrete eliminate, as waste matter, by normal discharge from the body

excretion 1. the act of excreting
2. the body's waste matter, as sweat, urine, and feces

exocrine gland any of various glands, such as mammary or sebaceous glands, having ducts that carry their secretions to specific locations

exophthalmic goiter see under: hyperthyroidism

expectorant medicine that promotes the discharge of mucus from the respiratory tract

expectorate discharge from the mouth, as saliva or phlegm

exploratory performed for the purpose of making a diagnosis: said of a surgical operation

extension state of being extended or straightened

extensor muscle whose function is to extend or straighten a part of the body

external cardiac massage see under: cardiac massage

external cardiopulmonary resuscitation see: ECPR

extraction surgical removal of a tooth from the mouth

extrinsic originating or situated outside an organ or part

exudate substance filtered through the walls of living cellular tissue, sometimes as a result of disease or injury, as in the case of inflammation

eyeground the inner side of the back of the eyeball

eyelid, inflammation of see: sty

eyelids, cosmetic surgery on see: blepharoplasty

eyestrain disorder caused by excessive or improper use of the eyes and characterized by fatigue, tearing, redness, and a scratchy feeling in the eyelids

eye tooth see: cuspid

F

face lift see: rhytidoplasty

facial canal see: Fallopian canal

facial nerve, paralysis of see: Bell's palsy

facial neuralgia see: trigeminal neuralgia

facial plasty see: rhytidoplasty

fainting brief loss of consciousness

Fallopian canal/facial canal bony canal in the skull

Fallopian tubes the pair of tubes connecting the ovaries and the uterus, through which the egg must pass at the time of ovulation

family therapy form of group therapy in which the patient group are members of the same family

farsightedness/hypermetropia/hyperopia inability to see nearby objects clearly

fascia fibrous tissue in the form of sheets that connect, surround, and support muscles and organs of the body

fascitis inflammation of the fascia

fat chemical compound forming an important food reserve and a source of hormones, vitamins, and other products essential in metabolism

fat pad mass of fatty tissue

fear of (phobias)
  blushing erythrophobia
  cats ailurophobia
  dark nyctophobia
  dirt and contamination mysophobia
  dogs cynophobia
  germs bacteriophobia
  heights acrophobia

fear of (phobias)
  insanity lyssophobia
  open spaces agoraphobia
  pain algophobia
  strangers xenophobia
febrile feverish
feces/stool animal waste discharged following a bowel movement, usu. containing indigestible foods, bacteria, bile, and mucus
femur the long bone that supports the thigh; the thigh bone
fen in Chinese traditional medicine, a measure equal to about 1/10 of an inch
fermentation the conversion of glucose into ethyl alcohol, esp. through the action of an enzyme (zymase) found in yeast
fetus organism developing in the uterus before birth, sometimes considered in the human species to begin with the third month in utero, prior to which it is called an embryo
fever/pyrexia body temperature above the normal
fever blisters see: cold sores
fiberoptic consisting of or making use of fibers of glass or plastic, as in optical instruments designed for viewing the intestines or stomach
fibrillation irregular, uncoordinated contraction (arrhythmia) of muscle fibers of the heart
fibrin insoluble protein that forms an interlacing network of fibers in clotting blood
fibrinogen complex protein found in plasma which, in combination with the enzyme thrombin, forms fibrin
fibrinolysin enzyme present in the blood that liquefies fibrin, thus dissolving blood clots
fibroid see: tumor, fibroid
fibroid tumor see: tumor, fibroid
fibroma benign tumor composed of fibrous connective tissue
fibula the outer of the two bones of the lower leg
field block form of local anesthesia in which the anesthetic is injected into the tissue area in which surgery is to be performed
filariasis tropical disease transmitted by mosquitoes and caused by a parasitic worm that invades the lymphatic system, producing edema and elephantiasis

fistula abnormal channel leading from a hollow organ or cavity to another part or to the surface of the body
flaccidity lack of firmness or elasticity; limpness
flatulence accumulation of gas in the stomach and bowels
flexion state of being bent or flexed
flexor muscle whose function is to flex or bend a part of the body
flexure bend or fold, as in the colon
flexure, sigmoid see: sigmoid
floss see: dental floss
flu see: influenza
fluoridation the addition of sodium fluoride to drinking water as a means of preventing tooth decay
fluoride compound of fluorine, often added to public water supplies or toothpastes to retard or prevent tooth decay in children
fluoroscope device for directly observing internal body structures by passing X rays through the patient and projecting shadows on a screen coated with a fluorescent substance
fluoroscopy examination conducted by means of a fluoroscope
flu shot influenza inoculation
focal convulsion see: focal seizure
focal seizure/focal convulsion epileptic seizure that affects only one part of the body
follicle small cavity or saclike structure that secretes or excretes body fluids
follicle, hair tiny sac within the dermis from which hair grows and is nourished
follicle-stimulating hormone/FSH hormone secreted at the start of puberty by the pituitary gland, causing maturation of ovaries in girls and formation of sperm in boys
follicular cyst see: cyst, follicular
fontanel either or two soft places at juncture points of the skull of a baby: the anterior fontanel, near the front, and the posterior fontanel, near the back
food chain the relationship of organisms considered as food sources or consumers or both, as the relationship of a flowering plant to a bee to a bird
food poisoning digestive disorder marked by nausea and vomiting, caused by bacteria found in decaying or rancid food

food tube see: esophagus

foot doctor see: podiatrist

foot drop condition in which the foot drops when extended in stepping forward, as caused by paralysis of a leg muscle

foramen natural aperture or passage, as in a bone

forceps two-bladed instrument for grasping and compressing or pulling, various types of which are used by dentists and surgeons

forces, balance of see: Yin; Yang

forensic medicine/forensic pathology subspecialty of pathology dealing with the various aspects of medicine and the law

forensic pathology see: forensic medicine

foreskin the loose skin (prepuce) covering the head of the penis

fossa pit or depression in a surface

fovea shallow rounded depression in the retina, directly in the line of vision at a point where vision is most acute

fracture break in a bone

fraternal twins twins who are not identical, derived from separately fertilized ova

freckle small, brownish or dark-colored spot on the skin

free association psychoanalytic technique in which the patient talks freely about anything that comes to mind

freezing of skin see: cryosurgery

Freud, Sigmund Austrian neurologist (1856–1939) who founded psychoanalysis and shaped the course of modern psychiatry

frigidity sexual unresponsiveness in women

Froehlich's syndrome failure of secondary sex characteristics to develop in males due to anterior pituitary disease

frontal lobe the front portion of each cerebral hemisphere of the brain, whose functions are uncertain

frontal lobotomy rarely performed surgical operation of cutting into the frontal lobes of the brain to alter behavior

frostbite partial freezing of a part of the body, esp. of the extremities or ears

fructose/levulose very sweet crystalline sugar

FSH see: follicle-stimulating hormone

fulguration destruction of tissue, esp.

malignant growths, by electric cautery

functional 1. able to function, esp. in spite of structural defect
2. affecting performance, as an illness, but lacking any verifiable physical basis that would account for the symptoms

functional hypertension see: hypertension, essential

fundus the rounded base or bottom of any hollow organ

fungus (*pl.* fungi) any of a group of plants including the mushrooms, molds, yeasts, and various microorganisms, some of which cause diseases in human beings

funnel chest/pectus excavatum congenital deformity in which the sternum is depressed

furuncle see: boil

fuse electrical safety device that interrupts a circuit when current becomes too strong

fusion of spinal joints see under: spondylitis, rheumatoid

G

galactosemia hereditary condition affecting infants who lack an enzyme that converts galactose (a sugar) into glucose in the blood

gall bladder/cholecyst small pear-shaped pouch situated beneath the liver that serves as a reservoir for bile

gallstone solid substance formed in the gall bladder that can obstruct the flow of bile and prevent the digestion of fats

gamete either of two mature reproductive cells, an ovum or sperm cell

gamma globulin component of blood serum which contains various antibodies

ganglion (*pl.* ganglia) 1. cluster of nerve cells outside of the central nervous system
2. cyst of a tendon, as on the wrist

gangrene death of tissues in a part of the body, caused by lack of adequate blood supply

gastrectomy surgical removal of all or part of the stomach

gastric analysis extraction and study of gastric juices

gastric juice the acid fluid secreted by the glands lining the stomach, containing several enzymes

gastric ulcer ulcer of the mucous membrane of the stomach

gastritis inflammation of the stomach

gastritis, acute sudden, sharp attack of gastritis

gastritis, chronic recurrent and persisting attacks of gastritis

gastritis, toxic gastritis caused by the swallowing of a poisonous substance

gastrocnemius the large muscle at the back of the calf of the leg

gastroenteritis inflammation of the mucous membrane that lines the stomach and intestines

gastroenterologist physician specializing in the diagnosis and treatment of gastrointestinal disorders

gastroenterology the branch of medical science dealing with the study of the stomach and intestines and the disorders affecting them

gastrointestinal series see: GI series

gastrointestinal tract or canal see: alimentary tract or canal

gastroscope device that allows inspection of the interior of the stomach

gastroscopy examination of the stomach with a gastroscope

GC *gonorrhea* (from the gonococcus bacterium)

gene hereditary unit contained within a chromosome and associated with specific physical characteristics transmitted from parents to offspring

general practitioner/GP physician whose training is not specialized and includes some preparation in pediatrics, surgery, and obstetrics and gynecology, thus enabling him to care for an entire family

genetic counselor specialist, usu. a physician, who counsels couples on the probability of genetic disorders occurring in their offspring

genitalia see: genitals

genitals/genitalia the reproductive organs

genitourinary see: urinogenital

genitourinary tract see: urinogenital tract

genus class or category of plants and animals ranking next above the species, as the genus *Homo* in *Homo sapiens*

geriatrics branch of medicine dealing with diseases and physiological changes associated with aging and old people

German measles see: rubella

germicide disinfectant or other agent capable of killing disease germs

gerontology scientific study of the processes and phenomena of aging

gestation the total period of pregnancy, from conception to birth

GI gastrointestinal

giantism see: gigantism

gifted having ability or intelligence above the normal range

gigantism/giantism disorder due to oversecretion of somatotrophin by the pituitary gland and resulting in excessive growth

gingiva mucous membrane and soft tissue of the gums surrounding the teeth

gingival pertaining to the gums

gingivitis inflammation of the gum tissues

gingivitis, necrotizing ulcerative see under: trench mouth

GI series/gastrointestinal series X rays of the esophagus, stomach, and intestines utilizing an opaque substance swallowed by the patient

glabrous without hair

gland any of various organs that secrete substances essential to the body or for the elimination of waste products

gland, ductless see: endocrine gland

gland, prostate, inflammation of see: prostatitis

gland, submandibular see: submaxillary gland

glandular fever see: mononucleosis, infectious

glaucoma disease of the eye characterized by increased pressure on the eyeball and leading to loss of vision if untreated

glioblastoma multiforme malignant tumor of the brain and central nervous system

glomeruli (*sing.* glomerulus) tiny tufts of capillaries in the kidneys through which the blood passes in the filtering of wastes

glomerulonephritis inflammation of the glomeruli

glossitis inflammation of the tongue, characterized by a bright red or glazed appearance

glossopharyngeal nerve the nerve that supplies sensation to the throat and rear of the tongue

glottis the passage between the vocal

cords at the upper opening of the larynx

glucagon hormone produced by the islets of Langerhans in the pancreas

glucose/blood sugar sugar found normally in blood and abnormally in urine, as in the case of diabetes mellitus

glucose tolerance test/GTT test that determines the rate at which glucose in the blood is reduced, or metabolized, used as an indicator of chemical diabetes or a prediabetic condition

glucosuria/glycosuria condition, as diabetes mellitus, in which the urine contains glucose

gluten protein component of wheat and rye

gluteus any of the three muscles that form each buttock

glycerin see: glycerol

glycerol/glycerin sweet, oily alcohol, one of the components of natural fat

glycogen animal starch usu. stored in the liver for conversion to glucose when the body needs energy

glycosuria see: glucosuria

goiter enlargement of the thyroid gland, often due to lack of iodine in the diet

goiter, exophthalmic see under: hyperthyroidism

gonad male or female sex gland; ovary or testicle

gonadotrophic hormone/gonadotrophin/ gonadotropin any of three hormones that stimulate the gonads and are secreted by the anterior pituitary gland

gonioscope specialized ophthalmoscope for examining the angle between the cornea and the iris

gonococcus bacterium that causes gonorrhea

gonorrhea contagious venereal disease transmitted by sexual contact

gout metabolic disease characterized by painful inflammation of a joint, as of the big toe, and an excess of uric acid in the blood

gouty arthritis, chronic form of gout characterized by urate deposits and consequent joint stiffness

GP see: general practitioner

Graafian follicle one of the small sacs in the ovaries that contain the developing ova

graft piece of tissue removed from one organism and inserted in a new site in the same organism or in a different organism

grain alcohol see: ethyl alcohol

grand mal major epileptic seizure, characterized by falling, loss of consciousness, and spasmodic jerking of the arms and legs

granulation process of forming new tissue in the healing of wounds

granulation tissue/proud flesh new, temporary, vascular tissue formed in a wound as a stage in the healing process, usu. soft and moist

granulocyte see: neutrophil

granulocytic leukemia see: leukemia, granulocytic

granuloma small tumor composed mainly of granulation tissue

granuloma inguinale/granuloma venereum chronic venereal disease that produces lesions in the genital or anal regions

granuloma venereum see: granuloma inguinale

gravid pregnant

Grawitz's tumor/hypernephroma malignant tumor of the kidney, found chiefly among men

gray matter see under: cortex

greenstick fracture incomplete fracture, with the bone bending on the unbroken side, more common in children than adults

grippe see: influenza

groin the fold or depressed area where the thigh joins the abdomen

ground connection which conducts electricity between an electric circuit and earth

grounding installing a ground

group psychotherapy see: group therapy

group therapy/group psychotherapy psychotherapy in which interactions within a group under the direction of a therapist are intended to provoke therapeutic insights and lead to improved social adjustment

growth hormone/growth-stimulating hormone/somatotrophin hormone secreted by the posterior lobe of the pituitary gland that stimulates growth

growth-stimulating hormone growth hormone

GTT see: glucose tolerance test

guard hairs see: vibrissae

gum disease see: periodontal disease

gumma rubbery tumor that develops

within organs in the late stages of syphilis

gums, inflammation of see: gingivitis

gurney stretcher mounted on wheels, commonly used to move nonambulatory patients in hospitals

gynecologist physician specializing in gynecology, often an obstetrician as well

gynecology the branch of medical science that deals with the care and treatment of women and their diseases, esp. of the reproductive system

H

hair transplant the surgical grafting of hair-bearing skin from the back or sides of the scalp onto bald areas of the head

hair, unwanted see: hirsutism

halitosis offensive mouth odor, usu. caused by poor oral hygiene

hallucinate have hallucinations

hallucination apparent perception without any corresponding external stimulus

hallucinogen drug or chemical capable of inducing hallucinations

hallucinogenic capable of producing hallucinations

halothane a general anesthetic taken by inhalation

hammer/malleus the outermost of the three ossicles of the middle ear, the bone between the eardrum and the anvil

hammer toe clawlike deformity of a toe

hamstrings any of several tendons at the back of the thigh and controlling the flexing of the knee

hangnail piece of skin partially torn loose from the root or side of a fingernail

hangover headache, nausea, dizziness, and other aftereffects of excessive alcoholic consumption, an allergic reaction to alcohol, or emotional stress while drinking

Hansen's disease see: leprosy

hard palate see: palate, hard

harelip see: cleft lip

hashish hallucinogenic substance more potent than marihuana, obtained from the leaves and flowers of the Indian hemp plant

hatter's disease chronic mercury poisoning, common among hatters in former times because of their use of mercury in preparing felt

hay fever see: allergic rhinitis

headache pain or ache across the forehead or within the head

headache, sick see: migraine

heart hollow muscular structure which maintains the circulation of the blood by alternate contraction and dilation

heart block lack of coordination in the heartbeat of the atria and ventricles, often causing unconsciousness and other symptoms (Stokes-Adams disease)

heartburn burning sensation in the lower esophagus caused by a flow of gastric juices from the stomach back into the esophagus

heart disease, hypertensive impairment of heart function due to persistent hypertension

heart failure inability of the heart to pump enough blood to maintain normal circulation

heart failure, congestive heart failure resulting from the inability of the heart muscle to keep a sufficient supply of blood in circulation, resulting in congestion or swelling of the tissues

heart-lung machine pumping machine used to divert a patient's blood from the heart during heart surgery and to keep it oxygenated and in circulation

heart murmur abnormal sound heard in the region of the heart

heat cramps muscle spasms resulting from loss of salt due to excessive sweating

heat exhaustion/heat prostration weakness or fainting as a result of prolonged exposure to heat, caused by a decreased blood supply to the heart and brain and an increased supply to the skin

heat prostration see: heat exhaustion

heat rash see: prickly heat

heatstroke see: sunstroke

hebephrenic schizophrenia see: schizophrenia, hebephrenic

Heimlich maneuver emergency treatment for obstruction of the windpipe in which sharp pressure is applied just below the rib cage so that the air in the lungs ejects the obstruction

Heine-Medin disease see: poliomyelitis

helminth parasitic worm that invades the

intestines, most often via food or water

hemal of or relating to blood

hemangioma/"port wine stain" reddish, usu. raised birthmark consisting of a cluster of small blood vessels near the surface of the skin

hematocrit 1. instrument for measuring the relative amount of plasma and red corpuscles of the blood by centrifuging it (whirling it around to separate parts having different densities) 2. measurement of relative amount of plasma and red corpuscles by a hematocrit

hematologist physician specializing in the study of the blood and in the diagnosis and treatment of blood diseases

hematology the branch of medical science dealing with the blood, including its formation, functions, and diseases

hematoma blood tumor

hematoma, subdural mass of blood clots or partially clotted blood in the space beneath the outermost dura mater and middle (arachnoid) membranes covering the brain

hematuria blood in the urine

hemiplegia paralysis of one side of the body, involving both the arm and leg

hemiplegic one affected by hemiplegia

hemoglobin pigment of red blood corpuscles serving as the carrier of oxygen and carbon dioxide

hemophilia inherited disorder characterized by an incapacity of the blood to clot normally, thus resulting in profuse bleeding even from slight cuts, typically affecting males only

hemophiliac/bleeder one afflicted with hemophilia

hemorrhage discharge of blood from a ruptured blood vessel

hemorrhoidal 1. of or pertaining to the blood vessels in the rectal area 2. of or pertaining to hemorrhoids

hemorrhoidectomy surgical removal of hemorrhoids

hemorrhoids/piles swollen varicose veins in the rectal mucous membrane

hemorrhoids, prolapsed hemorrhoids that protrude from the anus

hemotoxic (of certain poisonous snakes) transmitting venom that is carried by the bloodstream of the toxified animal

Henle's loop U-shaped part of a tubule of the kidney

heparin chemical compound that pre-

vents coagulation of the blood

hepatic of or relating to the liver

hepaticologist physician specializing in the diagnosis and treatment of liver diseases

hepaticology branch of medical science concerned with the study, diagnosis, and treatment of diseases of the liver

hepatitis inflammation of the liver

hepatitis, infectious inflammation of the liver caused by a viral infection usu. transmitted by food and water contaminated by feces from an infected person

hepatitis, serum form of infectious hepatitis usu. spread by blood transfusions or by infected hypodermic needles

hereditary acquired through one's genetic makeup by inheritance, as physical characteristics, disease, etc.

hernia/rupture protrusion of an organ or part, as the intestine, through the wall or body cavity that normally contains it

hernia, hiatus/diaphragmatic hernia hernia in which the lower end of the esophagus or part of the stomach protrudes through the diaphragm

hernia, inguinal protuberance of part of the intestine into the inguinal region (near the groin)

hernia, strangulated hernia that has become tightly constricted, thus cutting off blood supply

herniate slip away from its proper position, as an organ or part, to form a hernia

herniating disk see: disk, slipped

herniation forming of a hernia

hernia, umbilical hernia in which an abdominal part protrudes through the abdominal wall at the navel

hernia, ventral projection of part of the intestine into the abdominal wall

heroic extraordinary or extreme, as measures undertaken when life is in immediate danger

heroin/diacetylmorphine addictive narcotic drug derived from morphine, illegal in the U.S.

herpes any of various acute viral diseases characterized by the eruption of small blisters on the skin and mucous membranes

herpes simplex 1. virus that causes cold sores and other skin conditions in humans 2. see: cold sores

herpes simplex virus—Type 1/HSV-1

variety of herpes simplex that causes cold sores

herpes simplex virus—Type 2/HSV-2 variety of herpes simplex that often affects the genital region and can result in congenital damage to the baby of an infected mother

herpes zoster see: shingles

heterograft/xenograft tissue graft taken for transplanting from a donor of a different species from that of the patient receiving it

hexachlorophene antibacterial agent used in some soaps

hiccough see: hiccup

hiccup/hiccough involuntary, spasmodic grunt caused by spasms of the diaphragm and the abrupt closure of the glottis

high blood pressure see: hypertension

hip bone see under: ilium

hirsutism abnormal or excessive hairiness, esp. in women

histamine substance found in animal tissues that can cause allergic symptoms when allergens stimulate the body to produce it in large amounts

histoincompatibility incompatibility between tissues, as between the tissues of a patient and the tissues of a transplanted organ or part

histoplasma fungus that can cause histoplasmosis

histoplasmosis chronic fungus disease of the lungs

hives/urticaria skin condition marked by large, irregularly shaped swellings that burn and itch

Hodgkin's disease disease of the lymph system, characterized by chronic, progressive enlargement of the lymph nodes, lymphoid tissue, and spleen

homeopathy system of medicine in which disease is treated by administering minute doses of medicines that would in a healthy person produce the symptoms of the disease treated

homeostasis maintenance of uniform physiological stability within an organism and between its parts

homograft/allograft tissue graft taken for transplanting from a donor of the same species as the patient receiving it

hookworm parasitic intestinal worm whose larvae usu. enter the body by penetrating the skin of the feet of people who go barefooted

hormone internal secretion released in minute amounts into the bloodstream by one of the endocrine glands or other tissue and stimulating a specific physiological activity

hormone, adrenocorticotrophic see: ACTH

hormone, thyroid see: thyroxin

horny layer of epidermis see: stratum corneum

housemaid's knee chronic inflammation of the bursa in front of the knee due to pressure from constant kneeling or injury

HSV-1 see: herpes simplex virus—Type 1

HSV-2 see: herpes simplex virus—Type 2

Hubbard tank large, specially designed tub in which a patient may be immersed in water for exercises as a means of physical therapy

humerus the long bone of the arm from elbow to shoulder

humpback see under: kyphosis

hunchback see under: kyphosis

hyaline membrane disease/respiratory distress syndrome disease of newborn babies characterized by severe respiratory distress caused by the presence of a membrane lining the alveoli of the lungs

hydatidiform mole benign tumor formed from a placenta that has degenerated into a mass of grapelike cysts

hydrocele localized accumulation of fluid, esp. surrounding the testicles in the scrotum

hydrocephalus accumulation of cerebrospinal fluid within the brain

hydrochloric acid colorless, corrosive acid which in dilute form is present in gastric juice

hydrogenation the subjection of a material to hydrogen, as the process by which unsaturated fats are solidified

hydronephrosis enlargement of the kidneys with urine due to an obstruction of the ureter

hydrophilic having an affinity for water, as the soft contact lens

hydrophilic lenses see: contact lenses, soft plastic

hydrophobia see: rabies

hydrotherapy treatment of disease by the use of water

hymen thin membrane usu. partially

covering the entrance of the vagina in virgins

hyperacusis abnormal and sometimes painful acuteness of hearing

hyperaldosteronism syndrome of muscle weakness, hypertension, and excessive excretion of urine, due to oversecretion of an adrenal hormone

hyperbaric of or using pressures in excess of the usual pressure of the atmosphere, as a chamber for treating one suffering from decompression sickness

hyperfunction disorder of an endocrine gland, characterized by excess secretion of a hormone

hyperglycemia abnormally high amount of sugar in the blood

hyperkinesis behavioral disorder of children marked by overactivity, excitability, and inability to concentrate

hyperkinetic suffering from or pertaining to hyperkinesis

hypermetropia see: farsightedness

hypermetropic farsighted

hypernephroma see: Grawitz's tumor

hyperopia see: farsightedness

hyperopic farsighted

hyperplasia excessive production of cells, resulting in enlargement of tissue or of an organ

hyperplastic characterized by hyperplasia

hypersensitivity unusual sensitivity or allergic response to a particular substance

hypertension/high blood pressure excessively high blood pressure, sometimes caused by a disease (secondary hypertension) and sometimes not (essential hypertension)

hypertension, essential/chronic hypertension/functional hypertension hypertension, or high blood pressure, that is not a symptom of disease and has no known cause

hypertension, malignant form of essential hypertension with an acute onset and rapid rise in pressure

hypertension, secondary hypertension arising as a consequence of another known disorder

hypertensive heart disease see: heart disease, hypertensive

hyperthyroidism abnormal and excess activity of the thyroid gland, resulting in oversecretion of thyroxin and an abnormally high metabolism, character-

ized by fatigue, weight loss, rapid pulse, intolerance to heat, and sometimes by protruding eyes (in which case the disorder is called exophthalmic goiter)

hypertonic characterized by an abnormally high degree of tension, as muscle

hypertrophic characterized by hypertrophy

hypertrophic arthritis see: osteoarthritis

hypertrophy excessive development of an organ or tissue due to enlargement of the size of its constituent cells

hyperventilation abnormally fast or deep breathing, resulting in loss of carbon dioxide from the blood and sometimes causing dizziness and muscle spasms

hypnotic tending to produce sleep

hypoallergenic less likely to produce an allergic reaction

hypochondria extreme anxiety about one's health, usu. associated with a particular part of the body and accompanied by imagined symptoms of illness

hypochondriac 1. (*n.*) one suffering from hypochondria
2. (*adj.*) pertaining to the upper right or left parts of the abdomen. See illustration at *abdomen.*

hypodermic pertaining to the tissue just under the skin or to an injection made under the skin

hypofunction disorder of an endocrine gland, characterized by too little secretion of a hormone

hypogastric pertaining to the lower middle part of the abdomen. See illustration at *abdomen.*

hypogastrium the lower middle (hypogastric) part of the abdomen. See illustration at *abdomen.*

hypoglycemia/low blood sugar abnormally small amount of glucose in the blood, which can lead to insulin shock

hypoglycemic drug drug intended to reduce the amount of glucose in the blood by stimulating the release of insulin from the pancreas

hypophysis see under: pituitary gland

hypophysis cerebri see: pituitary gland

hyposensitization program for desensitizing allergy patients by injecting them with progressively larger doses of pollen or other allergens to build tolerance levels

hypotension excessively low blood pressure

hypothalamus region at the base of the brain that controls body temperature and various visceral activities

hypothermia artificially low body temperature produced by gradually cooling blood, used to slow metabolism and reduce tissue oxygen need so that heart and brain can withstand short periods of interrupted blood flow during surgery

hypothyroidism deficient functioning of the thyroid gland, resulting in undersecretion of thyroxin and an abnormally low metabolism, characterized by lack of energy, thick skin, and intolerance to cold

hypotonic characterized by an abnormally low degree of tension, as muscle

hysterectomy surgical procedure in which the uterus is completely removed

hysterectomy, radical surgical removal of the uterus, cervix, ovaries, and Fallopian tubes

hysterectomy, total surgical removal of the uterus and cervix

hysteria neurotic condition characterized by impulsive, demonstrative, and attention-getting behavior and sometimes by symptoms of organic disorders

hysteria, conversion see: conversion reaction

hysterogram X-ray examination of the uterus and surrounding areas

I

id the concealed, inaccessible part of the mind, the seat of impulses that tend to fulfill instinctual needs

identical twins twins having the same genetic makeup, derived from a single fertilized egg

identification mental process, often unconscious, by which a person associates with himself the attributes of another with whom he has formed an emotional tie

idiopathic (of diseases) originating spontaneously or of unknown cause

ileitis inflammation of the ileum of the small intestine

ileocecal valve the valve between the ileum of the small intestine and the cecum, the first section of the large intestine

ileum the last section of the small intestine, following the jejunum and leading to the large intestine

iliac 1. pertaining to or near the ileum 2. pertaining to the lower right and left parts of the abdomen. See illustration at *abdomen.*

ilium the large upper portion of the hip bone

immune protected from a communicable or allergic disease by the presence of antibodies in the blood

immunity resistance to infection or lack of susceptibility of an organism to a disease or poison to which its species is usu. subject, either by means of antibodies produced by the organism itself (active immunity) or by another and subsequently introduced into its body (passive immunity), as by injection

immunization act or process of making immune, esp. by inoculation

immunize make immune, as by inoculation

immunoglobulin any of various proteins of the body that are active as antigens or otherwise contribute to the formation of antibodies

immunologist physician or specialist in the study of immunity

immunology the branch of medical science concerned with the phenomena and techniques of immunity from disease

immunosuppressive acting to suppress natural immune responses, as to foreign tissue in an organ transplant

immunotherapy therapy to relieve allergic response consisting of a series of injections of a dilute allergen, gradually increased in strength

impacted tooth tooth wedged between the jawbone and another tooth so as to prevent its eruption

impaction state of being firmly packed or tightly wedged, as feces in the rectum or a tooth in the jaw. See: impacted tooth.

imperforate lacking a normal opening

impetigo contagious bacterial skin infection characterized by blisters that break and form yellow encrusted areas

impotence in men, the inability to have sexual intercourse

incision 1. cut or gash, as of a wound 2. cut or slit made in a surgical operation

incisor one of the four upper and four lower cutting teeth near the front of the mouth

incompetence inadequate performance, as of the heart valves

incomplete fracture partial fracture of a bone in which continuity of the bone is not destroyed

incontinence inability to control the flow of urine or the evacuation of the bowels

incubation period the period between the entry of a disease-causing organism in the body and the onset of the symptoms of that disease

incus see: anvil

indigestion see: dyspepsia

indomethacin analgesic and antiinflammatory drug used for arthritic disorders, often as a substitute for aspirin

"infant Hercules" see: myotonia congenita

infantile paralysis see: poliomyelitis

infantile sexuality the sexual interest and pleasure that infants and young children take in their genitals and other body parts

infarct tissue rendered necrotic (dead) by an obstructed blood supply, as because of a thrombus (clot) or an embolus

infarction death of tissue due to deprivation of blood caused by an obstruction, as in a coronary thrombosis (heart attack)

infection communication of disease by entrance into the body of disease-causing organisms

infectious (of a disease) transmitted by organisms, as bacteria

infectious mononucleosis/glandular fever/kissing disease acute communicable disease marked by fever, malaise, and swollen lymph nodes, esp. in the throat

inferior vena cava the large vein that brings blood from the lower part of the body to the heart

infertility inability to conceive or to produce offspring

inflammation localized reaction to infection, injury, etc., characterized by heat, redness, swelling, and pain

inflammation of
  arterial walls see: arteritis
  bladder see: cystitis
  bone see: osteomyelitis
  brain see: encephalitis

inflammation of
  brain coverings see: meningitis
  bursa see: bursitis
  femoral head see: Legg-Perthes' disease
  glomeruli see: nephritis
  gums see: gingivitis
  joints see: arthritis
  kidneys see: nephritis
  larynx see: laryngitis
  liver see: hepatitis
  prostate see: prostatitis
  skin see: dermatitis
  spinal joints see: spondylitis, rheumatoid
  stomach lining see: gastritis
  tendons see: tendinitis
  tendon sheath see: tenosynovitis
  tongue see: glossitis
  veins see: phlebitis
  vertebrae see: osteomyelitis, spinal

influenza/flu/grippe acute, contagious, sometimes epidemic disease caused by a virus and characterized by inflammation of the upper respiratory tract, fever, chills, muscle ache and fatigue

ingrown toenail toenail that has grown into the surrounding flesh

inguinal pertaining to or near the groin. See illustration at *abdomen.*

INH see: isoniazid

inhalant substance inhaled, as pollen or dust

inner ear the innermost part of the ear, containing the essential organs of hearing within the cochlea, the auditory nerve, and the semicircular canals that govern equilibrium

innervation distribution or supply of nerves to a part

inoculate 1. immunize by administering a serum or vaccine to
2. introduce microorganisms into (a culture medium)

inoculation act or process of inoculating

inoperable characterized by a condition that excludes surgery as a course of treatment

in situ in its original site or position

insomnia chronic inability to sleep

insufficiency inability to function adequately, as the heart (cardiac insufficiency)

insufflation see under: tubal insufflation

insulin protein hormone secreted by the islets of Langerhans in the pancreas that checks the accumulation of glucose in the blood and promotes the utilization of sugar in the treatment of diabetes

insulin shock condition caused by too low a level of blood sugar, and characterized by sweating, dizziness, palpitation, shallow breathing, confusion, and ultimately loss of consciousness

insulin shock therapy former method of treating psychotic patients involving large injections of insulin, inducing coma

insult injury to tissue caused by stress or trauma

integument see: skin

intelligence quotient see: IQ

intensive care unit section of a hospital specially equipped and staffed to monitor the vital systems of patients and provide close, round-the-clock care for a relatively brief period, as for patients just removed from surgery or for those in an unstable or critical condition

intercostal muscles the muscles between each of the ribs that contract when air is exhaled

intercourse see: sexual intercourse

intermittent claudication vascular disease associated with aging and marked by muscle fatigue and pain, esp. in the legs, due to atherosclerosis

intern advanced medical student or graduate (M.D.) undergoing resident training in a hospital

internal medicine the branch of medical science that deals with the study, diagnosis, and nonsurgical treatment of diseases of the internal organs

internist physician specializing in internal medicine

interstitial calcinosis condition characterized by deposits of calcium in the skin and subcutaneous tissue

intestine(s) tubular part of the alimentary canal, linking the stomach to the anus

intestine, large the lower part of the intestine, of greater diameter than the small intestine and divided into the cecum, colon, and rectum

intestine, small the convoluted upper and narrower part of the intestines, where most nutrients are absorbed by the bloodstream, between the pylorus and the cecum, divided into three parts, the duodenum, jejunum, and ileum

intoxicated in legal use, having more than 0.10% alcohol in the bloodstream

intracutaneous within the dermis

intramuscular situated within or injected into a muscle or muscular tissue

intrauterine device/IUD contraceptive device consisting usu. of a plastic coil, spiral, or loop that is inserted and left within the uterus for as long as contraception is desired

intravenous into or within a vein, as an injection

intrinsic originating or situated within an organ or part, as a disease

introitus entrance into a body cavity, esp. into the vagina

intussusception the turning inward or inversion of a portion of the intestine into an ajacent part, thus obstructing it, found esp. in male infants

in utero in the uterus, prior to birth

invasive invading or speading to tissues other than at the place of origin: said of malignant growths

involuntary muscle see: smooth muscle

involutional melancholia see: depressive reaction

IQ/intelligence quotient score obtained on an intelligence test standardized to give an average score of 100 to the total population tested

iris colored, circular, contractile membrane between the cornea and the lens of the eye, whose central perforation is occupied by the pupil

irradiation process of exposing a part of the body to radiant energy, as X rays

irrigate wash out or cleanse, as a body cavity or a wound, with a flow of water or other liquid

irrigation act or process of irrigating a body cavity, wound, etc.

ischemia localized deficiency of blood, as from a contracted blood vessel

ischium the part of the hip bone on which the body rests when sitting

islands of Langerhans see: islets of Langerhans

islets of Langerhans/islands of Langerhans small, cellular masses in the pancreas which produce and secrete insulin

isomer compound with the same molecular weight and formula as another, but with a different arrangement of its atoms, resulting in different properties

isometrics means of strengthening muscles by forcefully contracting them against immovable resistance

isoniazid/INH isonicotinic acid hydrazide, a chemical compound used in the treatment of tuberculosis

isopropyl chemical in the family of methyl alcohol, used as a rubbing alcohol

itch, the see: scabies

IUD see: intrauterine device

J

Jacksonian epilepsy form of epilepsy characterized by recurrent focal seizures, spasmodic movements or tingling or burning sensations, as of an arm, leg, or facial area, caused by a condition affecting a motor area of the brain

Jacksonian seizure form of focal seizure that characterizes Jacksonian epilepsy

jaundice yellowish tint to the skin and tissues, as the whites of the eyes, caused by excessive bile in the blood, a symptom of certain disorders

jejunum the middle section of the small intestine, between the duodenum and the ileum

joint place where two or more bones or separate parts of the skeleton meet

joint, inflammation of see: arthritis

juvenile rheumatoid arthritis see: rheumatoid arthritis, juvenile

K

kala-azar/black fever/dumdum fever/visceral leishmaniasis form of leishmaniasis that is usually fatal if not treated

keratin horny substance that is the main constituent of nails and hair, and in nonhuman animals of claws and horns

keratosis disease of the skin characterized by an outer layer of horny tissue

ketone bodies organic compounds that are a by-product of fat metabolism

kidney one of a pair of organs located at the rear of the abdomen near the base of the spine, whose function is to filter the fluid portion of the blood in regulating the composition and volume of body fluids, and to dispose of waste in the form of urine

kidney, artificial see under: dialysis

kidney failure, acute sudden loss of kidney function, characterized by decreased amount of urine, passage of bloody urine, edema, fatigue and loss of appetite

kidney pelvis see: pelvis

kidney stone/renal calculus mass of hard material, such as crytallized salt, that may collect within the kidney and obstruct the flow of urine

kissing disease see: infectious mononucleosis

kyphosis backward curvature of the spine characterized as a humpback or hunchback

L

labia 1. pl. of *labium*
2. the folds of skin and mucous membrane of the vulva, consisting of the outer folds *(labia majora)* and the inner folds *(labia minora)*

labium 1. sing. of *labia*
2. lip or liplike part or organ

labor process of giving birth, during which the uterus undergoes periodic contractions in moving the fetus through the birth canal

labyrinth the winding passages of the inner ear

labyrinthitis inflammation of the labyrinth of the inner ear, usu. disturbing the sense of equilibrium

laceration wound made by tearing or ripping

lacrimal gland tear-producing gland over the eye

lactation formation or secretion of milk from the breast

lactic acid bitter, syrupy acid found in sour milk and collected in muscle tissues during anaerobic exercise

lactogenic hormone/LTH/luteotrophic hormone/luteotrophin/luteotropin/prolactin hormone secreted by the anterior lobe of the pituitary gland that stimulates the production of milk in the mammary glands

Lamaze, Dr. Ferdinand French physician who pioneered in the development of a natural childbirth technique

laminated glass shatterproof glass, as in automobile windshields, consisting of two sheets of tempered glass with a sheet of plastic between

Langerhans, islets of see: islets of Langerhans

laparotomy any surgical incision made in the abdominal wall, as to examine or treat the female reproductive organs

lapse attack or seizure see: petit mal

laryngectomy surgical removal of all or part of the larynx

laryngitis inflammation of the mucous membranes of the larynx, causing the voice to become hoarse or disappear altogether

laryngitis, chronic permanently hoarse voice resulting from thickened, toughened mucous membrane in the larynx, due to too many attacks of laryngitis

laryngologist physician specializing in the diagnosis and treatment of disorders of the throat

laryngology the branch of medical science concerned with the study and treatment of the throat and related areas

laryngoscope instrument for inspecting the larynx

larynx/voice box the organ of voice in humans and most other vertebrates, consisting of a cartilaginous box in the upper part of the trachea across which are stretched vocal cords whose vibrations produce sound

latent not visible or apparent, as symptoms of a disease at an early stage

lateral 1. relating to or directed toward the side
2. more distant from the midline of the body, as compared to a nearer (medial) position

lavage cleansing or washing out of an organ, as the stomach

laxative substance that has the power to loosen the bowels, as milk of magnesia

L-dopa/levodopa medicine used in treating the symptoms of Parkinson's disease

leaflet flap of a heart valve

learning disability condition in which a child cannot acquire certain skills or assimilate certain kinds of knowledge at or near the normal rate

Legg-Perthes' disease inflammation of the bone and cartilage in the head of the femur (thigh bone)

leiomyoma benign tumor consisting of smooth muscle tissue

leishmaniasis tropical disease resembling malaria in which an animal parasite is transmitted by the sandfly

leishmaniasis, visceral see: kala-azar

lens biconvex transparent body behind the iris of the eye that focuses entering light rays on the retina

lepromatous characterized by nodular skin lesions, as a form of leprosy

leprosy/Hansen's disease chronic bacterial disease characterized by skin lesions, nerve paralysis, and physical deformity

lesion any abnormal change in an organ or tissue caused by disease or injury

leukemia form of cancer involving the blood and blood-making tissues, characterized by a marked and persistent excess of leukocytes

leukemia, granulocytic form of leukemia characterized by predominance of granulocytes (or neutrophils)

leukemia, lymphocytic form of leukemia characterized by uncontrolled overactivity of the lymphoid tissue

leukemic of or characteristic of leukemia

leukocyte/white blood cell/white corpuscle white or colorless cell found in the bloodstream important in providing protection against infection

leukopenia abnormal reduction in the number of leukocytes in the blood

leukorrhea whitish, viscid discharge from the vagina

levodopa see: L-dopa

levulose see: fructose

LGV see: lymphogranuloma venereum

LH see: luteinizing hormone

libido the instinctual craving or drive behind all human activities, esp. sexual, the repression of which leads to neurosis

Librium/chlordiazepoxide trademark for a commonly used tranquilizer

lidocaine chemical used as a local anesthetic

ligament band of tough, fibrous connective tissue that binds together bones and provides support for organs

ligate tie or close off with a ligature

ligation the act of tying or binding up, as an artery

ligature thread, wire, etc., used to close off or tie a vessel

lightening during the last few weeks of pregnancy, a shift in fetal pressure from the upper abdomen to the pelvic region as the head of the fetus moves toward the birth canal

lipase enzyme that breaks down fats

lipid fatty substance essential to living cells

lipid storage disease any of various usu. fatal diseases, typically occurring in childhood, caused by the lack of a particular enzyme

lip reading/speech reading interpretation of speech by watching the position of the lips and mouth of the speaker, practiced esp. by the deaf

lithium salts salts of lithium (a metal), used as a medication in the treatment of manic-depressive psychosis

lithotomy position position used in gynecological examinations in which the patient lies on the back and the legs are drawn back and apart on the thighs

liver large, glandular organ situated just under the diaphragm on the right side, that processes blood and regulates its composition, as by storing sugar and releasing it in assimilable form (glucose), and that secretes bile

liver, inflammation of see: hepatitis

liver spots/chloasma yellowish brown patches that appear on the skin

lobe rounded or protruding section or subdivision, as of an organ

lobotomy see under: frontal lobotomy

lockjaw see: tetanus

locomotor ataxia see: tabes dorsalis

loiasis form of filariasis transmitted by a biting fly from monkey to man or vice versa

loins the part of the body between the lower rib and the hip bone

lordosis abnormal inward curvature of the spine

lordotic posture posture characteristic of some women in late pregnancy, in which the shoulders are slumped, the neck bent, and the lower spine curved forward to bear the weight of the fetus

Lou Gehrig's disease see: sclerosis, amyotrophic lateral

low blood sugar see: hypoglycemia

LSD/lysergic acid diethylamide colorless, odorless, tasteless drug produced synthetically that causes the user to experience hallucinations

LTH see: lactogenic hormone

lumbago pain in the lower back

lumbar 1. pertaining to or situated near the loins or lower back
2. pertaining to the middle right or left parts of the abdomen. See illustration at *abdomen.*

lumbar puncture see: spinal tap

lumen space enclosed by the walls of a blood vessel, duct, etc.

lung either of two porous organs of respiration in the chest cavity of humans, having the function of absorbing oxygen and discharging carbon dioxide

lung disease, white see: byssinosis

lungs, fungus disease of see: histoplasmosis

lunula the living part of the nail, the pale, half-moon shape at the nail base

luteinizing hormone/LH a hormone secreted by the anterior lobe of the pituitary gland that stimulates a Graafian follicle to release an ovum during each menstrual cycle and converts the follicle into a corpus luteum

luteotrophic hormone see: lactogenic hormone

luteotrophin see: lactogenic hormone

luteotropin see: lactogenic hormone

lymph transparent fluid resembling blood plasma that is conveyed through vessels (lymphatic vessels) and lubricates the tissues

lymphangiogram the visualization by X ray of lymph nodes after injection of an opaque fluid

lymphatic pertaining to or conveying lymph

lymph gland see: lymph node

lymph node/lymph gland one of the rounded bodies about the size of a pea, found in the course of the lymphatic vessels, that produce lymphocytes

lymphoblast young cell that matures into a lymphocyte

lymphocyte variety of leukocyte formed in the lymphoid tissue

lymphocytic leukemia see: leukemia, lymphocytic

lymphogranuloma inguinale see: lymphogranuloma venereum

lymphogranuloma venereum/LGV/ lymphogranuloma inguinale venereal disease affecting the lymph nodes

lymphoid pertaining to lymph or to the tissue of lymph nodes

lymphoma abnormal (neoplastic) growth of lymphoid tissue, symptomatic of various diseases, as lymphocytic leukemia or Hodgkin's disease

lymphosarcoma malignant growth of the lymphatic system

lysergic acid diethylamide see: LSD

lysozyme enzyme present in tears that is destructive to bacteria

lyssophobia fear of becoming insane

M

macrobiotic of or pertaining to macrobiotics

macrobiotics dietetic regimen advocating the use of whole-grain cereals, the avoidance of meat, etc., based on the Oriental principles of Yang (activity) and Yin (relaxation)

macrocephalic individual with macrocephaly

macrocephaly excessive head size

macula spot or discoloration

macula lutea yellowish area in the retina related to color perception and marked by most acute vision

mainlining injection of heroin directly into a vein

malabsorption syndrome/celiac disease syndrome characterized by bulky, foul-smelling stools and other symptoms due to the inability of the body to absorb certain nutrients from the intestinal tract

malaise feeling of being run-down, listless, uncomfortable, weary, and generally unwell

malaria disease caused by certain animal parasites transmitted by the bite of the infected anopheles mosquito, causing intermittent chills and fever

male pattern baldness see under: baldness

malignancy 1. malignant tumor 2. state of being malignant

malignant so aggravated as to threaten life, usu. resistant to treatment, and often having the property of uncontrolled growth, as a cancer

malleus see: hammer

malnutrition nutritional deficiency, as of essential proteins, vitamins, or minerals, causing impairment of health and certain specific diseases

malocclusion faulty closure of the upper and lower teeth

Malta fever see: brucellosis

mammogram X-ray picture of the breast by the technique of mammography

mammography specialized X-ray examination of the breasts

mammoplasty surgical procedure to augment the size of the breasts

mandible the lower jawbone

mania psychotic condition characterized by excessive activity, elation, extreme talkativeness, and agitation

manic-depressive reaction/affective reaction psychosis characterized by mania or depression or by the alternation of both

marihuana the dried leaves and flowers of the hemp plant *(Cannabis sativa)*, which if smoked in cigarettes or otherwise ingested can produce distorted perception and other hallucinogenic effects

marrow either of two types of soft, vascular tissue found in the central cavities of bones—red marrow, which produces red blood cells, and yellow marrow, composed mainly of fat cells

mastectomy surgical removal of the breast

mastectomy, radical surgical removal of the breast, underlying chest muscles, and lymph glands in the armpit

mastectomy, simple surgical removal of the breast only

master gland see: pituitary gland

mastitis inflammation of the breast

mastoiditis inflammation of the air cells in the mastoid process

mastoid process process of the temporal bone behind the ear

mastoplasty surgical procedure to reduce the size of the breasts

masturbation the touching or rubbing of the genitals for sexual pleasure and usu. orgasm

materia alba white, viscous mixture of mucus, molds, tissue cells, and bacteria adhering to teeth or to the spaces between teeth and gums, a potential source of disease

maxilla the upper jawbone

maxillary sinus see: paranasal sinus

MBD see: minimal brain dysfunction

MD see: muscular dystrophy

M.D. Doctor of Medicine

measles/rubeola contagious viral disease, esp. of children, marked by rash, fever, and conjunctivitis, sometimes having severe complications

measles, German see: rubella

meatus passage or canal in the human body, esp. one with an external opening, such as the anterior urethra of the penis

medial 1. middle, or relatively near the middle

2. nearer to the midline of the body, as compared to a more distant (lateral) position

medical 1. of or relating to medicine

2. of or relating to the treatment of disease by nonsurgical means

medical history the questions asked by a doctor of a patient that are designed to give an outline of the patient's state of health

medicine 1. the profession dealing with the maintenance of health and the treatment of physical and psychological disorders

2. the treatment of disease by nonsurgical means

medulla 1. medulla oblongata

2. the inner portion of an organ or part, as of the kidneys or the adrenal glands

medulla oblongata the lower part of the brain continuous with the spinal cord that controls certain involuntary processes such as breathing, swallowing, and blood circulation

melancholia, involutional see under: depressive reaction

melanin dark brown or black pigment of the skin

melanin cell clusters see: moles

melanoma/black cancer malignant tumor formed of cells that produce melanin

membrane, amniotic, intact see: caul

membrane, hyaloid the delicate membrane that envelops the vitreous humor of the eye

membrane, periodontal the membrane covering the bony tissue (cementum) around the roots of teeth

membrane, tympanic see: eardrum

menarche the first menstrual period of a girl

Ménière's disease/Ménière's syndrome symptoms including vertigo, ringing or buzzing sensations (tinnitus), nausea, and vomiting, associated with disease of the inner ear and often leading to progressive deafness of one ear

Ménière's syndrome see: Ménière's disease

meninges the membranes that cover the brain and spinal cord

meningioma uncontrolled new cell growth in one of the membranes (arachnoid) covering the brain and spinal cord

meningitis inflammation of the membranes that cover the brain and spinal cord

meningitis, aseptic/viral meningitis meningitis thought to be caused by a virus instead of a bacterium

meningitis, meningococcal meningitis in which the infecting organisms are meningococcal bacteria

meningitis, viral see: meningitis, aseptic

meningococcal pertaining to meningococcus, a bacterium

meningococcus bacterium that causes a form of meningitis

menopausal of or occurring during the menopause

menopause/change of life/climacteric the cessation of menstruation and the end of a woman's capacity to bear children, normally occurring between 40–50 years of age and often marked by hot flashes, dizzy spells, and other physical and emotional symptoms

menopause, surgical abrupt onset of menopause in women due to surgical removal of the uterus and ovaries

menses see: menstruation

menstrual of or relating to menstruation

menstruation/the menses periodic bloody discharge of the unfertilized ovum and tissue from the uterus of a female of childbearing age

menstruation, onset of see: menarche

mental retardation failure in mental development that is severe enough to prevent normal participation in everyday life

mentoplasty plastic surgery of the chin, esp. a procedure to build up an underdeveloped chin

meperidine/Demerol medicine used as an analgesic and sedative

meprobamate/Equanil/Miltown tranquilizer used as a sedative and muscle relaxant

meridian in acupuncture, a pathway beneath the skin through which energy is believed to flow and along which specific acupuncture points are located

mescaline chemical extracted from the

peyote cactus that induces hallucinations in its users

mesentery the fan-shaped fold of the membrane that enfolds the small intestine and connects it with the abdominal wall

mesoderm middle layer of tissue

metabolic of or relating to metabolism

metabolism aggregate of all physical and chemical processes continuously taking place in living organisms, including those which build up and break down assimilated materials

metacarpal any of the five bones of the metacarpus

metacarpus the five bones of the hand connecting the wrist to the fingers (phalanges)

metastasis 1. the transfer of a disease or its manifestations, as a malignant tumor, from one part of the body to another
2. (*pl.* metastases) malignant growth established in a new site by metastasis

metatarsal any of the bones of the metatarsus

metatarsalgia painful inflammation of the nerves in the region of the metatarsus of the foot

metatarsus the five bones of the foot connecting the ankle to the toes (phalanges)

methadone/Dolophine synthetic opiate used as an analgesic and experimentally as a substitute for heroin in the treatment of addicts

methamphetamine / Desoxyn / Methedrine/speed chemical compound that allays hunger and has a more stimulating effect on the central nervous system than does amphetamine or dextroamphetamine

methanol see: methyl alcohol

Methedrine see: methamphetamine

methotrexate drug used in the treatment of psoriasis

methyl alcohol/methanol/wood alcohol flammable liquid obtained through the distillation of wood or made synthetically, poisonous if taken internally

metrorrhagia erratic or unpredictable menstrual bleeding

microcephalic individual with microcephaly

microcephaly abnormal smallness of the head, with imperfect development of the cranium

micrographia very minute handwriting, a symptom of some nervous disorders

micron 1/1000th of a millimeter (symbol μ, Greek letter *mu*)

microsurgery surgery or dissection of minute parts, as of individual cells, with the aid of a microscope and esp. precise instruments

micturate urinate

micturition urination

middle ear the part of the ear between the eardrum and the inner ear, including the tympanum and the ossicles—hammer, anvil and stirrup

migraine/sick headache recurrent, severe form of headache, temporarily disabling, usu. affecting one side of the head and often accompanied by nausea, dizziness, and sensitivity to light

miliaria see: prickly heat

milk teeth see: baby teeth

Miltown see: meprobamate

mineral naturally occurring, homogeneous, inorganic material, some of which, as salt and iron, are required by the body

minimal brain dysfunction/minimal brain damage condition of children who suffer from a motor or perceptual impairment due to slight brain damage

miscarriage/spontaneous abortion the involuntary expulsion of a nonviable fetus after the first three months of pregnancy

mitral valve the membranous valve between the left atrium and left ventricle of the heart that prevents the backflow of blood into the atrium

mittelschmerz pain during ovulation about midway between menstrual periods

modality 1. method of treatment or its application, esp. a physical procedure
2. any form of sensation, as touch or taste

molar 1. (*n.*) any of the three upper and three lower grinding teeth with flattened crowns at both sides of the rear of the mouth, making 12 in all
2. (*adj.*) of or pertaining to a mole

mole 1. permanent pigmented spot on the skin, usu. brown and often raised
2. mass formed in the uterus from an embryo or placenta that has degenerated, as the *hydatidiform mole*

molluscum contagiosum contagious viral disease marked by raised lesions containing waxy material

Mongolism see: Down's syndrome

moniliasis/candidiasis fungus infection involving the skin or mucous membranes of various parts of the body, such as the mouth, esp. in babies (when it is called thrush), or the vagina

monocyte relatively large leukocyte

mononucleosis see: infectious mononucleosis

monovalent pertaining to a form of the Sabin polio vaccine in which each dose gives protection against a different strain of polio

morning sickness nausea and vomiting experienced by some pregnant women in the morning hours, esp. in early pregnancy

morphine addictive narcotic drug derived from opium, used medically to relieve pain

morphinism/soldier's disease abnormal condition of the body system caused by an excessive dose or habitual use of morphine

Morton's toe painful inflammation of the nerves in the region of the metatarsus of the foot (metatarsalgia) between the third and fourth toes

motion sickness nausea and sometimes vomiting caused by the effect of certain complex movements on the organ of balance in the inner ear, typically experienced in a moving vehicle, ship, or airplane

motor nerve/efferent nerve nerve that conveys information from the central nervous system to a muscle with a directive for action

mouth-to-mouth respiration/mouth-to-mouth resuscitation form of artificial respiration in which the rescuer places his mouth over the victim's mouth and breathes rhythmically and forcefully to inflate the victim's lungs and start respiration

mouth-to-mouth resuscitation see: mouth-to-mouth respiration

moxibustion in traditional Chinese medicine, the burning of an herb, as over an acupuncture point, as a form of therapy

MS see: multiple sclerosis

mu micron

mucosa see: mucous membrane

mucosal of or pertaining to the mucous membrane

mucous pertaining to, producing, or resembling mucus

mucous membrane/mucosa membrane that lines many of the body's inner surfaces, kept moist by glandular secretions

mucus viscous substance secreted by the mucous membranes

multipara woman who has borne more than one child

multiphasic having many phases or aspects: said esp. of testing performed in the course of a comprehensive physical examination

multiple myeloma malignant tumor of the bone marrow occurring at numerous sites

multiple sclerosis/MS chronic disease in which patches of nerve tissue thicken (sclerose), causing failure of coordination and other nervous and mental symptoms

mumps contagious viral disease marked by fever and swelling of the facial glands

mumps, meningoencephalitis inflammation of the brain and of the membranes (meninges) covering the brain, as a result of mumps

muscular dystrophy/MD any of various diseases of unknown cause characterized by the progressive wasting away (atrophy) of the muscles

musculoskeletal system the human body's network of muscles and bones

myasthenia gravis chronic disease characterized by muscular weakness and general and progressive exhaustion

mycobacterium kind of rod-shaped, aerobic bacterium

myelin semisolid fatlike sheath that surrounds the axon of a neuron

myelitis 1. inflammation of the spinal cord
2. inflammation of the bone marrow

myelogram X ray of the spinal cord obtained by the injection of a radioopaque liquid material into the spinal cord area

myelography technique of recording myelograms and the science of interpreting them

myeloma malignant tumor of the bone marrow

myocardial infarction the process of congestion and tissue death (necrosis) in the heart muscle caused by an interruption of the blood supply to the heart

myocardium the muscular tissue of the heart

myomectomy surgical excision of a type of uterine fibroid tumor

myopathy any abnormality or disease of the muscles

myopia see: nearsightedness

myopic nearsighted

myotonia disorder characterized by increased rigidity or spasms of muscle

myotonia congenita congenital disease characterized by temporary muscle spasms and muscle rigidity

myotonic dystrophy chronic, progressive disease characterized by weakness and wasting of muscles, cataracts, and heart abnormality

myringotomy surgical incision of the eardrum

mysophobia fear of dirt and contamination

N

naprapathy the treatment of disease by the manipulative correction of ligaments and connective tissues

narcolepsy disease in which the patient is overcome by drowsiness or an uncontrollable desire for sleep

narcosis stupor or unconsciousness produced by a narcotic drug

narcotic 1.(*n.*) any of various substances, such as morphine, codeine, and opium, that in medicinal doses relieve pain, induce sleep, and in excessive or uncontrolled doses may produce convulsions, coma, and death
2. (*adj.*) inducing sleep

nares the nasal passages or nostrils

nasopharyngeal pertaining to the nasopharynx

nasopharynx the upper part of the pharynx above and behind the soft palate

natural foods foods processed minimally, although not necessarily organically grown

nausea feeling of sickness or dizziness usu. accompanied by the impulse to vomit

navel/umbilicus the depression at the middle of the abdomen where the umbilical cord of the fetus was attached

nearsightedness/myopia inability to see distant objects clearly

necrosis death of a group of cells, tissue, or a part of the body

necrotizing ulcerative gingivitis see under: trench mouth

needle biopsy the excising of a tissue sample for biopsy by means of a long needle

nematode any of a class of roundworms, many of which, such as the hookworm or pinworm, are intestinal parasites in man and other animals

neonate newborn baby

neoplasm any abnormal growth of new tissue, as a tumor, which may be benign or malignant

neoplastic of or characteristic of neoplasms

nephrectomy surgical removal of a kidney

nephric see: renal

nephritis/Bright's disease inflammation of the kidneys

nephroblastoma see: Wilm's tumor

nephrologist physician specializing in the diagnosis and treatment of diseases of the kidney

nephrology branch of medical science dealing with the structure, function, and diseases of the kidney

nephron one of the basic filtration units of the kidney, consisting of Bowman's capsule, a glomerulus, and tubules

nephrosis/nephrotic syndrome disease of the kidneys characterized by degenerative lesions of the renal tubules and loss of protein (albumin) through the urine

nephrotic syndrome see: nephrosis

nerve block/plexus block form of local anesthesia in which the anesthetic is injected into nerve trunks leading to the area in which surgery is to be performed

nerve bundle, master see: spinal cord

nerve cell 1. one of the cells of the nervous system
2. the cell body of a neuron

nerve, lingual nerve beneath the floor of the mouth that conveys taste sensations to the brain

nerve, olfactory the special nerve of smell

nerve, optic the special nerve of vision connecting the retina with the occipital lobe of the brain

nerve, sensory/afferent nerve nerve that conveys information and stimuli from the outside word to the central nervous system

nerves, spinal the thirty-one pairs of nerves that originate in the spinal cord

nervous breakdown popular, nontechnical term for any debilitating or incapacitating emotional disorder

neural of or relating to a nerve

neuralgia acute pain along the course of a nerve

neuralgia, facial see: trigeminal neuralgia

neuralgia, trigeminal see: trigeminal neuralgia

neuritis inflammation of a nerve

neuroblastoma malignant tumor of the nerve tissue of the adrenal glands, found esp. in children

neurofibroma tumor on a nerve fiber

neurogenic shock shock resulting from impairment of the regulatory capacity of the nervous system due to pain, fright, or other stimulus

neurologist physician specializing in the care and treatment of the nervous system

neurology the branch of medical science that deals with the nervous system

neuron nerve cell with all its processes and extensions, such as the axon and dendrites

neuropathologist physician specializing in neuropathology

neuropathology the branch of medical science that deals with the study, diagnosis, and treatment of diseases of the nervous system

neurosis/psychoneurosis (*pl.* neuroses) mental disorder having no organic cause and less severe than psychosis

neurosurgeon physician specializing in surgery of the nervous system

neurosurgery the branch of medical science that deals with the treatment of disease of the nervous system by means of surgery

neurosyphilis syphilis of the brain and spinal cord

neurotic 1. (*n.*) one who has a neurosis 2. (*adj.*) of or relating to neurosis

neurotoxic 1. (of certain poisonous snakes) transmitting venom that directly affects the nervous system and brain of the toxified animal 2. causing destruction or damage to nerve tissue

neutrophil/granulocyte/polymorphonu-

clear leukocyte granular leukocyte that can be stained with dyes that are neither acid nor alkaline (i.e., neutral)

nevus birthmark or congenital mole

nicotine poisonous chemical with acrid taste contained in tobacco

night terrors childhood nightmares which occur in deep sleep and in which the child cries out in terror

nit the egg of a louse or other parasitic insect

nitrogen dioxide suffocating gas that is poisonous when inhaled

nitroglycerin colorless or pale yellow oily liquid used to treat angina pectoris

nocturia frequent urination during the night

nocturnal emission see: wet dream

node 1. swelling or enlargement, as in an arthritic joint, or a firm, flattened tumor on a bone or tendon 2. any knoblike part, as a lymph gland

nodule little node

norepinephrine hormone manufactured by the adrenal medulla that affects heart action and sympathetic nerve impulses

"nose brain" see: rhinencephalon

nose, cosmetic surgery on see: rhinoplasty

nose, reshaping of see: rhinoplasty

nostril one of the outer openings in the nose

no-take absence of any reaction to a vaccination, indicating that the person vaccinated has not developed an immunity and should be revaccinated

nurse, scrub see: scrub nurse

nutrient substance that gives nourishment

nutriment substance that nourishes or promotes development

nutrition all of the processes by which food is consumed, digested, absorbed, and assimilated by the body

nutritionist specialist in the study of nutrition

nyctophobia fear of the dark

nystagmus spasmodic, involuntary movement of the eyes, symptomatic of certain diseases, as of the inner ear

O

obesity excessive accumulation of body fat

ob-gyn specialist physician trained as an obstetrician and gynecologist

objective (of symptoms) of a kind that can be observed or measured by the examining physician through diagnostic techniques

obsession persistent, unwanted idea or feeling, a symptom of certain neuroses

obsessive-compulsive reaction neurosis characterized by obsessions that are relieved temporarily by the compulsive performance of certain acts

obstetrician physician specializing in obstetrics, often a gynecologist as well

obstetrics the branch of medical science dealing with pregnancy and childbirth

obstructive-airway disease condition characterized by the presence of chronic bronchitis and pulmonary emphysema, and involving damage to lung tissue and the bronchi

obturator special device inserted into a cleft palate to close it against the flow of air

occipital of or relating to the lower back part of the skull (occiput)

occipital lobe the rear portion of each cerebral hemisphere of the brain, which receives messages from the optic nerve

occlusion 1. the act of closing or shutting off so as to block a passage, as a blood vessel
2. the manner of being shut, as the teeth of the upper and lower jaws

occupational disease disease resulting from exposure in one's occupation to toxic substances or other hazards to health

ocular of or relating to the eye

oculist see: ophthalmologist

Oedipal complex repressed sexual attachment of son to mother, analogous to the Electra complex involving the daughter and father

olfaction the act, sense, or process of smelling

olfactory pertaining to the sense of smell or the capacity to smell

olfactory lobe the portion of each cerebral hemisphere of the brain on the underside of the frontal lobes, the centers for smelling

olfactory nerve see: nerve, olfactory

oliguria decreased production of urine

onchocerciasis form of filariasis transmitted by a blackfly and sometimes leading to blindness

oncologist physician specializing in the diagnosis and treatment of tumors

oncology the branch of medical science concerned with the study of tumors

oophorectomy see: ovariectomy

open bite form of malocclusion in which incisors of the upper and lower jaws do not meet when the jaws are together

open fracture see: compound fracture

open surgery surgery involving an incision and opening of the skin

ophthalmic of or pertaining to the eye

ophthalmologist/oculist physician specializing in the care and treatment of the eyes

ophthalmology the branch of medical science dealing with the structure, function, and diseases of the eye

ophthalmoscope optical instrument for examining the interior of the eye

opiate drug derived from opium, as morphine

opium narcotic drug obtained from the opium poppy from which morphine, codeine, heroin, and other drugs are derived

optic/optical pertaining to the eye or to vision

optician one who makes or sells eyeglasses and other optical equipment

optic nerve special nerve of vision, conveying visual sensations from the retina to the brain

optometrist one who practices optometry

optometry profession of measuring the power of vision and prescribing corrective lenses

oral pertaining to or situated near the mouth

oral surgeon/dental surgeon dentist who specializes in oral surgery

oral surgery the diagnosis and surgical treatment of diseases, injuries, and defects of the mouth and jaw

orbit either of the bony sockets of the eyes

orchidopexy/orchiopexy surgical correction of an undescended testicle

orchiectomy surgical removal of one or both testicles

orchiopexy see: orchidopexy

orchitis inflammation of the testicles

organic 1. of or pertaining to an organ of the body

2. having a physical basis, as a disorder

3. of or pertaining to animals or plants

4. pertaining to foods grown only with natural fertilizers of animal or plant origin

organic foods foods grown with the use of organic fertilizers only, such as compost of animal (not human) manure, and without the use of pesticides or herbicides

organ of Corti the true center of hearing within the cochlea of the inner ear, a complex spiral structure of hair cells

orgasm the climax of the sexual act, normally marked by the male's ejaculation of semen and by relaxation of tension of both male and female

orifice opening into a body cavity

orthodontia see: orthodontics

orthodontics/orthodontia the care and treatment of irregularities and faulty positions of the teeth, including the fitting of braces

orthodontist dentist specializing in orthodontics

orthopedics the branch of surgery dealing with the treatment and correction of deformities, injuries, and diseases of the skeletal system and its associated structures, as muscles and joints

orthopedic surgeon see: orthopedist

orthopedist/orthopedic surgeon/orthopod surgeon specializing in orthopedics

orthopod see: orthopedist

orthoptist medical technician trained to diagnose defects of the eye muscles and to provide corrective exercises

oscilloscope instrument for visibly representing electrical activity on a fluorescent screen

osseous see: osteal

ossicle one of the three small connecting bones of the middle ear, the hammer (or malleus), the anvil (or incus), and the stirrup (or stapes), that transmit sound from the eardrum to the cochlea

ossification conversion into bone

ossify to convert or be converted into bone

osteal/osseous of or relating to bone

osteitis inflammation of a bone

osteitis deformans see: Paget's disease 1

osteoarthritis/degenerative joint disease/ hypertrophic arthritis chronic degenerative disease that affects the joints

osteogenesis formation and growth of bones

osteogenesis imperfecta condition in which bones are abnormally brittle and liable to fracture due to a deficiency of calcium

osteogenic pertaining to osteogenesis

osteomyelitis inflammation of the bone tissue or marrow

osteopath physician trained in osteopathy

osteopathy system of healing based on a theory that most diseases are caused by structural abnormalities that may best be corrected by manipulation

osteophyte abnormal bony outgrowth

osteoporosis reduction in bone mass and increase in interior space, porosity, and fragility of bone

otitis media inflammation of the middle ear

otitis media, nonsuppurative see: otitis media, serous

otitis media, serous/nonsuppurative otitis media inflammation of the middle ear resulting from a blocked Eustachian tube and fluid collection in the middle ear, causing hearing damage

otolaryngologist physician specializing in the diagnosis and treatment of the ear, nose, and throat

otolaryngology the branch of medicine dealing with the study and diseases of the ear, nose, and throat

otologist one who specializes in the ear and its diseases

otology the branch of medical science dealing with the functions and diseases of the ear

otoplasty surgical technique to correct protruding or overlarge ears or to build up or replace a missing ear

otosclerosis ear disorder resulting in hearing loss caused by the formation of spongy bone in the middle ear

otoscope instrument used for examining the interior of the ear

outer ear the external, fleshy part of the ear, including the auditory canal leading to the eardrum (tympanic membrane)

outpatient patient who is not an inmate of a hospital or clinic at which treatment or diagnosis is received

ovarian of or relating to the ovaries

ovarian dysgenesis defective development of ovaries

ovariectomy/oophorectomy surgical removal of an ovary

ovaries (*sing.* ovary) pair of female reproductive glands (gonads) that produce eggs (ova) and female sex hormones

overbite extent to which upper teeth extend over lower teeth when the jaws are in closed position

ovoid egg-shaped

ovulation the discharge of a mature egg cell (ovum) from the ovaries, occurring about once every 28 days at about the middle of the menstrual cycle

ovum/egg cell (*pl.* ova) female reproductive cell or gamete from which an embryo might develop if fertilized

oxytocin hormone secreted by the pituitary gland to help the muscles of the uterus contract during labor

ozone blue gas with a pungent odor that can be formed by the passage of electricity through the air

P

pacemaker, artificial electrically activated, battery- or nuclear-powered device used to stimulate normal heartbeat if the natural cardiac pacemaker fails to function

pacemaker, cardiac object or substance in the heart that regulates contraction of the heart muscle, or heartbeat

Paget's disease 1. (osteitis deformans) chronic disease characterized by the softening and enlargement of the bones and usu. the bowing of the long, weight-bearing bones
2. cancerous disease of the breast marked by the inflammation of the areola and nipple

palate the roof of the mouth

palate, hard the bony part of the roof of the mouth

palate, soft/velum the soft, muscular tissue at the rear of the roof of the mouth

palpation diagnostic procedure of feeling, pressing, or manipulating the body with the fingers or hands

palpitation rapid or fluttering heartbeat

palsy/paralysis see under: Bell's palsy, cerebral palsy

pancreas large gland situated behind the stomach and containing the islets of Langerhans that produce insulin and glucagon, and secreting pancreatic juice via small ducts to the duodenum

pancreatic juice secretion of the pancreas containing digestive enzymes

pancreatitis inflammation of the pancreas

pandemic epidemic occurring over a very large area or worldwide

Papanicolaou, Dr. George N. developer of a test called the *Pap smear* or *Pap test* for detecting cancer of the cervix

Papanicolaou smear see: Pap smear

papillae (*sing.* papilla) tiny, nipple-shaped projections that cover the inner layer (dermis) of the skin and the surface of the tongue

papillary tumor 1. see: papilloma
2. any nipplelike tumor (Latin *papilla* means nipple)

papilloma (*pl.* papillomata) / **papillary tumor** benign tumor of the papillae of the skin, as a wart or corn

Pap smear/Papanicolaou smear/Pap test method of early detection of cervical cancer consisting of painless removal of cervical cell samples, which are stained and examined

Pap test see: Pap smear

papule pimple

paralysis agitans see: Parkinson's disease

paralysis, infantile see: poliomyelitis

paranasal sinus/maxillary sinus air cavity in one of the cranial bones communicating with the nostrils

paranoid describing a personality disorder in which the individual is extraordinarily sensitive to praise or criticism and subject to suspicions and feelings of persecution

paranoid reaction/paranoia psychosis characterized by invariable delusion, usu. of persecution, sometimes of grandeur

paranoid schizophrenia see: schizophrenia, paranoid

paraplegia paralysis of the lower half of the body

paraplegic one who is paralyzed in the lower half of the body, including both legs

parasite animal or plant that lives in or on another organism (called the host), at whose expense it obtains nourishment

parasiticide medication designed to destroy parasites such as body lice

parasympathetic nervous system the part of the autonomic nervous system that controls such involuntary actions as the constriction of pupils, dilation of blood vessels and salivary glands, and slowing of heartbeat

parathormone/parathyroid hormone hormone secreted by the parathyroid glands, important in regulating the amount of calcium in the body

parathyroid glands four small endocrine glands near or embedded within the thyroid gland, usu. two per side, that regulate blood calcium and phosphorus levels

parathyroid hormone see: parathormone

paresis 1. see: paresis, general
2. mild paralysis or weakness

paresis, general chronic, progressive form of syphilis involving the central nervous system

parkinsonism see: Parkinson's disease

Parkinson's disease/paralysis agitans/ parkinsonism chronic, progressive nervous disease characterized by muscle tremor when at rest, stiffness, and a rigid facial expression

parotid gland either of two large salivary glands located below and in front of the ear

paroxysm sudden onset of acute symptoms, as an attack of convulsions

parrot fever see: psittacosis

particulate matter fine particles in smoke that are dispersed by the wind and fall back to earth

parturition act or process of giving birth

passive-dependent describing a personality disorder in which the individual needs excessive emotional support from an authority figure

patch test skin test for determining hypersensitivity by applying small pads of possibly allergy-producing substances to the skin's surface

patchy baldness see: baldness, patchy

patella the kneecap

pathogen disease-causing bacterium or microorganism

pathogenic disease-causing

pathologic caused by or relating to disease

pathologic fracture fracture that occurs spontaneously, as because of preexisting disease, without external cause

pathologist physician or expert specializing in pathology

pathology the branch of medical science dealing with the causes, nature, and effects of diseases, esp. disease-induced changes in organs, tissues, and body chemistry

PCBs/polychlorinated biphenyls chemicals related to DDT and having many industrial uses, posing a potential threat to health as a water pollutant from industrial wastes

pectus carinatum see: pigeon breast

pectus excavatum see: funnel chest

pedal of or relating to the foot

pediatric dentist dentist specializing in the care and treatment of the teeth of children

pediatrician physician specializing in the care and treatment of children

pediatrics the branch of medicine dealing with the care and treatment of children and their diseases

pedodontics branch of dentistry specializing in the care of children

pedodontist dentist specializing in pedodontics

pellagra disease caused by a vitamin deficiency and characterized by gastric disturbance, skin eruptions, and nervous symptoms

pelvic girdle the part of the human skeleton to which the lower limbs are attached

pelvis 1. the part of the skeleton that forms the bony girdle or basin joining the lower limbs to the body, and consisting of the two hip bones and the sacrum
2. the central area of the kidney from which urine drains into the ureter

penicillin powerful antibacterial substance found in a mold fungus and prepared in several forms for the treatment of a wide variety of infections

penis tubular male organ of sexual intercourse and excretion of urine, located at the front of the pelvis

Pentothal/sodium Pentothal/thiopental trademark for an ultra-short-acting barbiturate used as an anesthetic, as in dentistry

pep pills *(slang)* see: amphetamines

pepsin enzyme secreted by the gastric juices of the stomach

peptic ulcer ulcer of the mucous membrane of the stomach (gastric ulcer) or small intestine (duodenal ulcer) caused by the action of acid juices

percussion diagnostic procedure of striking or tapping the body with instruments or with the fingers

perianal situated around the anus

pericarditis inflammation of the pericardium

pericardium the membrane that surrounds and protects the heart

peridental see: periodontal

perimeter device for determining peripheral vision

perineal of or pertaining to the perineum

perineum region of the body at the lower end of the trunk, between the genital organs and the anus

periodontal/peridental situated around a tooth

periodontia see: periodontics

periodontics/periodontia the branch of dentistry dealing with diagnosis and treatment of periodontal (gum) diseases

periodontist dentist who specializes in periodontics

periodontitis inflammation of the tissues around a tooth, leading to destruction of the alveolar bone

periodontium the supporting structures of the teeth, comprising the gingiva, alveolar bone, and periodontal ligaments

periosteum the tough, fibrous membrane that surrounds and nourishes bones

peripheral nervous system the nerves and ganglia outside the brain and spinal cord

peristalsis wavelike muscular contractions of the alimentary canal that move the contents along in the processes of digestion and excretion

peristaltic wave the alternate contraction and relaxation of muscles in the alimentary canal in peristalsis

peritoneoscopy/laparoscopy technique utilizing a peritoneoscope

peritoneoscope/laparoscope instrument used for examining the organs within the abdominal cavity, esp. the female reproductive organs

peritoneum the serous membrane that lines the abdominal cavity enclosing the abdominal organs

peritonitis inflammation of the lining (peritoneum) of the abdominal cavity

peritonsillar abscess/quinsy abscess in

the tissues adjoining a tonsil as a complication of tonsillitis

pernicious severe, destructive, and often fatal

pernicious anemia severe, progressive anemia caused by lack of vitamin B_{12}, formerly fatal but now controllable

personality disorder/character disorder any of a group of mental illnesses that apparently stem from an arrested development of the personality

pertussis see: whooping cough

pessary 1. device worn inside the vagina as a contraceptive or to support uterine prolapse
2. medicated suppository for use in the vagina

petit mal/absence attack or seizure/lapse attack or seizure minor epileptic seizure, with very brief loss of consciousness

Peyer's patches oval areas of lymphoid tissue in the intestine that manufacture lymphocytes

peyote the mescal cactus of Mexico or the powerful hallucinogenic drug obtained from its dried upper part (called buttons)

phalanges (*sing.* phalanx) the bones of the fingers or toes

pharmacist one skilled in the compounding and dispensing of medicines

pharmacologist expert in pharmacology

pharmacology the science of the action of medicines, their nature, preparation, administration, and effects

pharyngitis inflammation of the pharynx, commonly called a sore throat

pharynx the part of the alimentary canal between the palate and the esophagus, serving as a passage for air and food

phenformin see: DBI

phenol see: carbolic acid

phenylketonuria/PKU inherited metabolic disorder that can cause mental retardation if not treated by a special diet soon after birth

phlebitis inflammation of the inner membrane of a vein

phlebotomy / bloodletting / venesection the opening of a vein for letting blood

phlegm viscid, stringy mucus secreted in abnormally large amounts, as in the air passages

phobia intense anxiety irrationally felt for any of a variety of things or situations, such as closed or open places, animals of a particular kind, heights, etc., a manifestation of the phobic reaction. See also *fear of.*

phobic reaction neurosis characterized by displacement of anxiety of a conflict to a substitute, such as a particular domestic animal, closed places, etc.

phonocardiogram graph recording the sounds produced by the heart, used to evaluate heart murmurs and other abnormal sounds

physical dependence accommodation of the body to continued use of a drug, such that withdrawing the drug causes pronounced physical reactions (withdrawal symptoms)

physical medicine branch of medicine utilizing physical procedures, such as heat, cold, massage, or mechanical devices, to diagnose disease or treat disabled patients

physical therapist specialist in physical therapy

physical therapy/physiotherapy the treatment of disability, injury, or disease by external physical means, such as heat, massage, planned exercises, electricity, or mechanical devices, to restore function or aid rehabilitation

physician 1. any authorized practitioner of medicine
2. one trained in medicine, as distinguished from surgery

physiotherapy see: physical therapy

pia mater the delicate, vascular, innermost membrane of the three membranes that envelop the brain and spinal cord

pica abnormal desire to eat substances that are not fit for food, such as clay, plaster, etc.

piebald skin see: vitiligo

pigeon breast/pectus carinatum congenital deformity in which the sternum protrudes

pigment substance that imparts coloring to tissue

piles see: hemorrhoids

"pill, the" see: contraceptive, oral

pimple/papule small, usu. inflamed swelling on the skin

pineal body see: pineal gland

pineal gland/pineal body small, cone-shaped body of rudimentary glandular structure located at the base of the brain and having no known function

pinkeye acute, contagious conjunctivitis marked by redness of the eyeball

pinworm parasitic worm of the lower intestines and rectum, esp. of children, causing intense itching in the anal area

pituitary body see: pituitary gland

pituitary gland/hypophysis cerebri/pituitary body/master bland small endocrine gland situated at the base of the brain, consisting of anterior and posterior lobes whose hormonal secretions stimulate the production of hormones in other glands and regulate vital body functions such as growth and metabolism

pityriasis rosea skin disease, esp. of children, marked by a rash

PKU see: phenylketonuria

placebo any harmless substance given to humor a patient or as a test in controlled experiments on the effects of drugs

placenta the vascular structure in pregnant women that unites the fetus with the uterus, and through which the fetus is nourished via the umbilical cord, usu. expelled naturally immediately following birth (when it is called the afterbirth)

plague 1. any epidemic disease that is contagious and often deadly
2. contagious, often fatal disease caused by a bacterium transmitted by fleas from infected rats, and characterized by fever, chills, prostration, and often by buboes (hence the name *bubonic plague*)

plantar warts warts on the soles of the feet, caused by a virus

plaque mucus containing bacteria that collects on teeth

plasma the clear fluid portion of the blood

plastic surgeon physician specializing in plastic or cosmetic surgery

plastic surgery surgery that deals with the restoration or healing of lost, injured, or deformed parts of the body, mainly by the transfer of tissue, and with the improvement of appearance (cosmetic surgery)

platelet/thrombocyte small, disk-shaped body found in blood that aids in clotting

play therapy psychotherapy, esp. for patients who are children, in which toys or other playthings are made available for the patient to play with in the presence of the therapist

pleura serous membrane that enfolds the lungs and lines the chest cavity

pleura, inflammation of see: pleurisy

pleural cavity the space between the two pleuras lining the lungs and chest cavity

pleurisy inflammation of the pleura, characterized by fever, chest pain, and difficulty in breathing

plexus interlacement of cordlike body structures, such as blood vessels or nerves

plexus block see: nerve block

pneumococcus bacterium that can cause pneumonia

pneumoconiosis any of various lung disorders, such as silicosis or black lung disease, resulting from the inhalation of dust or other minute particles

pneumoencephalogram X-ray picture of the brain taken after air or gas has been injected to partially replace the cerebrospinal fluid

pneumoencephalography technique of producing pneumoencephalograms and interpreting them

pneumonia inflammation of the lungs, usu. bacterial in origin and acute in course, characterized by high fever, chills, breathing difficulty, and cough

pneumonia, aspiration pneumonia caused by inhaling particles of foreign matter, as food

pneumothorax accumulation of air or gas in the pleural cavity, causing the lung to collapse, as from injury or disease, or by injection (artificial pneumothorax) in the treatment of tuberculosis

podiatrist/chiropodist one who specializes in the treatment of the foot

podiatry/chiropody the study and treatment of disorders of the feet

polio see: poliomyelitis

poliomyelitis/infantile paralysis/Heine-Medin disease acute viral disease of the central nervous system characterized by fever, headache, sore throat, stiffness of the neck and back, and sometimes by paralysis and eventual atrophy of muscles

pollutant something that pollutes the air, water, or soil

polychlorinated biphenyls see: PCBs

polycystic characterized by many cysts

polycythemia condition characterized by too many red blood corpuscles

polycythemia vera/erythremia condition characterized by abnormally high number and proportion of red blood corpuscles

polymenorrhea abnormally frequent menstruation

polymorphonuclear leukocyte see: neutrophil

polymyositis inflammation of a number of muscles and connective tissue, characterized by pain, swelling, and weakness

polyp smooth growth or tumor found in the mucous membranes, as of the nose, bladder, uterus, or rectum

polyunsaturated (of fats) tending to lower the cholesterol content of the blood

polyuria excessive urination

pons mass in the brain containing fibers that connect the medulla oblongata, the cerebellum, and the cerebrum

pontic in dentistry, a part of a bridge serving as a substitute for a missing tooth

popliteal pertaining to the back part of the leg behind the knee

portal vein vein that conveys blood from the intestines and stomach to the liver

"port wine stain" see: hemangioma

positive pressure breathing breathing of air or other gas mixture at pressure greater than the surrounding atmospheric pressure

posterior toward the rear

posterior lobe hypophysis the posterior part of the pituitary gland that produces hormones regulating kidney function and other vital processes

posterior urethra see: prostatic urethra

postmenopausal being or occurring after menopause

postpartum after childbirth

postural drainage the loosening and draining of lung secretions by assuming a prone position with the head lower than the feet

Pott's disease tuberculosis or tissue destruction of the spinal vertebrae, causing angular curvature of the spine

prediabetic condition see: diabetes, chemical

pre-eclampsia disorder of late pregnancy or following childbirth

preemie/premie premature infant

pregnancy condition or time of being

pregnant

pregnant carrying developing offspring in the uterus

preinvasive before spreading to other tissues: said of malignant growths

premature of a newborn baby, weighing less than 5 pounds

premature ejaculation ejaculation of the semen during sexual intercourse before the female has had time to respond

premenopausal being or occurring before menopause

premie see: preemie

premolar see: bicuspid

prenatal before birth

prenatal diagnosis see: amniocentesis

preop see: preoperative

preoperative/preop performed or occurring before a surgical operation, as shaving of the affected area, administration of certain drugs, etc.

prep preparation of a patient for surgery, usu. including cleansing and shaving of the affected area

prepuce the loose skin covering the head of the penis or the clitoris

presbyopia farsightedness caused by aging of the lens or the muscles that expand and contract it

pressor tending to raise blood pressure, as certain hormones

preventive medicine the branch of medical science concerned with preventing disease, as through immunological methods

prickly heat/heat rash/miliaria itchy rash of small red pimples caused by excessive sweating in hot weather

primary 1. not produced as a secondary effect or complication of another condition
2. original and not resulting from metastasis or other means of transmission, as a tumor or infection

primary teeth see: baby teeth

primipara woman who is pregnant for the first time or who has borne one child

process in anatomy, any outgrowth or projecting part of a larger structure, as the knobby portion of a vertebra

proctologist physician specializing in proctology

proctology the branch of medicine that deals with the diagnosis and treatment of diseases of the lower colon, rectum, and anus

proctoscope surgical instrument for examining the interior of the rectum and part of the colon

proctoscopy examination of the rectum and colon with the aid of a proctoscope

proctosigmoidoscopy examination of the rectum and a portion of the colon (sigmoid) with the aid of a sigmoidoscope

prodrome symptom resembling a premonition that signals the onset of a disease or of an epileptic seizure

profibrinolysin the inactive precursor of fibrinolysin, an agent in the process of dissolving blood clots

progesterone hormone of the ovary that prepares the uterus for receiving the fertilized ovum

prognathism the condition of having a protruding jaw, esp. the lower

prognosis prediction made by a doctor as to the probable course of a disease

prolactin see: lactogenic hormone

prolapse move or slip forward or downward, as a displaced organ

prolapsed slipped or moved from the usual place

pronate turn, as the hand or foot, in a movement of pronation

pronation 1. rotation of the hand or forearm so that the palm of the hand faces downward or backward
2. movement of the foot, as in improper walking, in which the sole is raised along the outer side and the toes turned out, often with an inward leaning of the ankle

prone lying on the chest, with the face downward

proof strength of alcohol in an alcoholic beverage, indicated by a proof number equal to twice the percentage of alcohol by volume (100 proof = 50% alcohol)

propranolol drug that causes blood vessels to dilate, used in the treatment of angina pectoris

prophylactic tending to ward off or prevent, as disease or conception

prophylaxis treatment intended to prevent disease, as the cleaning of teeth

prostatectomy surgical removal of all or part of the prostate gland

prostate gland partly muscular gland in males at the base of the bladder around the urethra that releases a fluid to convey spermatozoa

prostate gland, enlarged, benign enlargement of the prostate gland resulting in difficulty in voiding and retention of urine in the bladder

prostate gland, inflammation of see: prostatitis

prostatic urethra/posterior urethra the part of the male urethra that passes across the prostate gland

prostatitis inflammation of the prostate gland, characterized by painful and excessive urination

prostatitis, acute severe, relatively uncommon form of prostatitis, marked by painful and excessive urination, high fever, and a discharge of pus from the penis

prosthesis (*pl.* prostheses)/**prosthetic device** artificial substitute for a missing or amputated part, as an arm or leg

prosthetic device see: prosthesis

protein any of a class of highly complex organic compounds, composed principally of amino acids, that occur in all living things and form an essential part of animal food requirements

proteinuria excretion of protein through the urine

prothrombin the inactive precursor of thrombin, an agent in the process of forming blood clots

protozoa (*sing.* protozoon) microscopic animal organisms that exist in countless numbers, including one-celled organisms and parasitic forms that cause malaria, sleeping sickness, and other diseases

proud flesh see: granulation tissue

proximal relatively near the center of the body, or near a point considered as central, esp. as compared to a more remote (distal) point

proximal muscles those muscles closest to the trunk of the body, such as the shoulder-arm and hip-thigh muscles

pruritis localized or general itching

pruritis, anal intense itching in the area of the anus

pseudohypertrophic muscular dystrophy/Duchenne's muscular dystrophy disease characterized by the enlargement and apparent overdevelopment (hypertrophy) of certain muscles, esp. of the shoulder girdle, which subsequently atrophy

pseudoneoplasm see: pseudotumor

pseudotumor/pseudoneoplasm condition that has the appearance of a tumor but is not a tumor, such as an inflammation

psilocybin derivative of the mushroom *Psilocybe mexicana,* which produces hallucinations in the user

psittacosis/parrot fever infectious disease of parrots and other birds that can be transmitted to humans and cause symptoms like those of influenza

psoralen chemical derived from a plant that is used in the treatment of psoriasis

psoriasis a noncontagious chronic condition of the skin, marked by bright red patches covered by silvery scales

psychiatrist physician specializing in psychiatry

psychiatry the branch of medicine that treats disorders of the mind (or psyche), including psychoses and neuroses

psychoanalysis system of psychotherapy originated by Sigmund Freud for treating emotional disorders by bringing to the attention of the conscious mind the repressed conflicts of the unconscious

psychoanalyst one who practices psychoanalysis

psychodrama psychotherapy in which a patient or group of patients act out situations centered about their personal conflicts in the presence of the therapist

psychogenic caused by or contributed to by psychological factors

psychological dependence emotional desire or need to continue using a drug

psychologist specialist in psychology

psychology the science dealing with the mind, mental phenomena, consciousness, and behavior

psychomimetic having properties capable of producing changes in behavior that mimic psychoses

psychomotor having to do with muscular movements resulting from mental processes

psychomotor seizure/temporal lobe seizure epileptic convulsion characterized by compulsive and often repetitious behavior of which the patient later has no memory

psychoneurosis see: neurosis

psychopathic see: sociopathic

psychophysiological/psychosomatic pertaining to a class of disorders in which psychological factors contribute substantially to the physiological condition

psychosis (*pl.* psychoses) severe mental disorder often involving disorganization of the total personality, with or without organic disease

psychosomatic 1. pertaining to the effects of the emotions on body processes, esp. with respect to initiating or aggravating disease
2. see: psychophysiological

psychotherapist specialist in psychotherapy

psychotherapy the treatment of emotional and mental disorders by psychological methods, such as psychoanalysis

psychotic one suffering from a psychosis

psychotropic affecting the mind: said of certain drugs

ptomaine substance derived from decomposing or putrefying animal or vegetable protein, rarely the cause of food poisoning, which is usu. caused by bacteria such as Salmonella

ptosis drooping of the upper eyelid

ptyalin enzyme in saliva that begins the chemical breakdown of starch

puberty period during which a person reaches sexual maturity and becomes functionally capable of reproduction

puberty, precocious early menarche (first occurrence of menstruation), before the age of eight or nine

pubic in the region of the lower abdomen

pubis (*pl.* pubes) either of two bones which join to form the front arch of the pelvis

pulmonary of or relating to the lungs

pulmonary artery see: artery, pulmonary

pulmonary emphysema *emphysema* of the lungs

pulmonary tuberculosis see under: tuberculosis

pulmonary vein see: vein, pulmonary

pulp (of teeth) the soft tissue of blood vessels and nerves that fills the central cavity of a tooth

pulpotomy surgical removal of the pulp of a tooth

pulsator electrical device used to vibrate acupuncture needles

pulse rhythmic pressure in the arteries due to the beating of the heart

puncture wound wound caused by an object that pierces the skin, as a nail or tack, involving increased danger of tetanus

pupil contractile opening in the iris of the eye through which light reaches the retina

purine one of a group of chemicals occurring naturally in certain foods and formerly implicated as a contributing cause of gout

purpura blood disease characterized by hemorrhaging into the skin and mucous membranes

purulent consisting of or secreting pus

pus secretion from inflamed and healing tissues, usu. viscid or creamy, and containing decaying leukocytes, bacteria, and other tissue debris

pustule pus-filled bump on the skin, inflamed at the base

pyelitis see: pyelonephritis

pyelogram visualization of the kidney and ureter by X ray

pyelonephritis/pyelitis infection and inflammation of the kidneys

pyloric sphincter the ring of muscle surrounding the pylorus that acts as a valve, allowing food to pass from the stomach to the duodenum

pyloric stenosis congenital condition in which the pylorus is too narrow to allow the stomach's contents to empty normally

pylorus the opening between the stomach and the duodenum

pyorrhea discharge of pus, esp. when applied to the progressive inflammation of the gingival (gum) tissue, which may lead to loosening and loss of teeth

pyrexia see: fever

pyrogenic causing or inducing fever

Q

Q fever infectious disease (rickettsial disease) transmitted by sheep and cattle and characterized by high fever, chills, and muscle pains

quadriplegia paralysis of both arms and both legs

quadriplegic one suffering from paralysis of both arms and both legs

quinine bitter substance obtained from the bark of the cinchona tree, used to treat malaria and myotonia

quinsy see: peritonsillar abscess

R

rabies/hydrophobia acute viral disease of the central nervous system transmitted to humans by the bite or saliva of an infected animal, as a dog, bat, or squirrel, invariably fatal unless treated before symptoms appear

radiation sickness illness caused by the body's absorption of excess radiation, marked by fatigue, nausea, vomiting, and sometimes internal hemorrhage and tissue breakdown

radiation therapy/radiotherapy treatment of disease by radiation, as by X rays or other radioactive substances

radical of or involving procedures or treatment intended to go to the root of a disease and thereby eliminate it, as by excising an entire organ or part that is diseased

radiograph see: X ray 2

radiography X-ray photography

radiologist physician specializing in radiology

radiology the branch of medical science that deals with radiant energy, such as X rays and energy produced by radium, cobalt, and other radioactive substances, esp. in the diagnosis and treatment of disease

radiopaque impervious to X rays

radiotherapy see: radiation therapy

radius (pl. radii) the bone of the forearm on the same side as the thumb, thicker and shorter than the ulna bone

rale abnormal sound heard in the chest with the aid of a stethoscope, indicating the presence of disease

Raynaud's disease see: Raynaud's syndrome

Raynaud's syndrome/Raynaud's disease condition characterized by spasms of small blood vessels when exposed to cold, esp. the fingers and toes, which become cyanotic (bluish) and then red

RBC red blood cell. See: erythrocyte

recovery room hospital room or section for patients immediately following surgery, where their post-operative conditions can be closely monitored

rectocele hernia in which part of the rectum protrudes through the wall of the vagina

rectum the terminal portion of the large intestine, extending from the sigmoid bend of the colon to the anus

red blood cell/RBC see: erythrocyte

red blood cells, excess see: polycythemia

red corpuscle see: erythrocyte

red marrow see under: marrow

reduce move back into proper position, as a herniating bowel or the fragments of a broken bone

reduction manipulation back into proper position to restore normal function, as a fracture, dislocation, or herniated part

referred pain pain felt in one part of the body though originating in another part, as pain of the left shoulder and arm caused by a heart attack

reflex involuntary response to a stimulus

reflux a flowing back, as of urine from the bladder up into the ureter

refraction the change of direction of a ray of light as it passes from one medium to another of different density

regional enteritis enteritis in a chronic state

regurgitation the act of rushing or surging back, as in vomiting, or the backward rush of blood in the heart due to defective valves or leaflets

Reiter's syndrome form of arthritis characterized by occurrence of conjunctivitis of the eye and inflammation of the urethra

relaxant drug or other agent that reduces tension, esp. of the muscles

remission period with less severe symptoms or without symptoms during the course of a disease

renal/nephric of or relating to the kidneys

renal calculus see: kidney stone

renal colic pain that results from the passage of a kidney stone through the ureter

renal diabetes see: renal glucosuria

renal glucosuria/renal diabetes glucose in the urine in conjunction with normal blood sugar levels, due to failure of the renal tubules to reabsorb glucose

rennin milk-curdling enzyme present in gastric juice

repression exclusion from consciousness of painful desires, memories, etc., and consequent manifestation through the unconscious

resect perform a resection on

resection surgical removal of a part of a bone, organ, etc.

resectoscope surgical instrument used esp. for resection of the prostate gland by insertion into the urethra

residency period of training in a hospital, usu. in a medical specialty, for physicians preparing for private practice

resident physician working and undergoing training (residency) in a hospital in preparation for private practice in a specialty

resorb reabsorb

respiration the process by which an animal or plant takes in oxygen from the air and gives off carbon dioxide and other products of oxidation

respiratory distress syndrome: see: hyaline membrane disease

resuscitation see: mouth-to-mouth respiration

retardation, mental see: mental retardation

retention cyst see: cyst, follicular

reticulum network of cells or cellular tissue

retina the inner membrane at the back of the eyeball, containing light-sensitive rods and cones which receive the optical image

retinal detachment see: detached retina

retinoblastoma tumor of the eye, found esp. in children

retinopathy diseased condition of the retina of the eye

retinopathy, diabetic see: diabetic retinopathy

retinoscope special device for examining the retina

rhesus factor see: Rh factor

rheumatic fever acute infectious disease chiefly affecting children and young adults, characterized by painful inflammation around the joints, intermittent fever, and inflammation of the pericardium and valves of the heart

rheumatic heart disease impairment of heart function as a result of rheumatic fever

rheumatism painful inflammation and stiffness of muscles, joints, or connective tissue

rheumatoid arthritis chronic disease characterized by swelling and inflammation of one or more joints, often resulting in stiffness and eventual impairment of mobility

rheumatoid arthritis, juvenile/Still's disease form of rheumatoid arthritis affecting children, often characterized by fever, rash, pleurisy, and enlargement of the spleen as well as rheumatoid joint symptoms

rheumatoid spondylitis see: spondylitis, rheumatoid

rheumatologist physician specializing in rheumatology

rheumatology subspecialty of internal medicine concerned with the study, diagnosis, and treatment of rheumatism and other diseases of the joints and muscles

RH factor/rhesus factor genetically transmitted substance in the blood of most individuals (Rh positive) and absent from some (Rh negative), of particular importance in pregnancies and blood transfusions, where the incompatibility of blood with and without Rh factor can cause severe reactions

rhinencephalon/"nose brain" the part of the brain controlling the sense of smell

rhinitis inflammation of the mucous membranes of the nose

rhinoplasty plastic surgery of the nose

Rh negative see under: Rh factor

Rh positive see under: Rh factor

rhythm method birth control method whereby sexual intercourse is avoided during the period of ovulation in the menstrual cycle

rhytidoplasty/face lift/facial plasty plastic surgery to eliminate facial wrinkles

rib one of the series of curved bones attached to the spine and enclosing the chest cavity

rib cage/thoracic cage the part of the skeleton that encloses the chest, bound by the ribs and the spinal vertebrae

riboflavin/vitamin B_2 member of the vitamin B complex, found in milk, green leafy vegetables, eggs, and meats

rickets early childhood disease characterized by softening of bones and consequent deformity, caused by deficiency of vitamin D

rickettsiae (*sing.* rickettsia) parasitic microorganisms transmitted to humans by the bites of infected ticks, lice, and fleas, and causing Rocky Mountain spotted fever, Q fever, rickettsial pox, and typhus

rickettsial caused by or pertaining to rickettsiae

rickettsial disease any of the diseases, as typhus or Rocky Mountain spotted fever, caused by rickettsiae

rickettsial pox infectious disease (rickettsial disease) transmitted by mites which infest mice, and characterized by fever, chills, rash, headache, and backache

ringworm/tinea contagious fungus disease of the skin, hair, or nails marked by ring-shaped, scaly, reddish patches of skin

Rocky Mountain spotted fever/tick fever infectious disease (rickettsial disease) transmitted by the bite of certain ticks and characterized by fever, chills, rash, headache, and muscular pain

rod one of many rod-shaped bodies in the retina of the eye, sensitive to faint light and peripheral objects and movement

roentgenogram see: X ray 2

roentgenologist physician specializing in the diagnosis and treatment of diseases with the application of X rays

roentgenology the branch of medical science dealing with the properties and effects of X rays

root canal the passageway of nerves and blood vessels in the root of a tooth leading into the pulp

roseola infantum childhood illness characterized by high fever followed by a body rash

roughage food material containing a high percentage of indigestible constituents

roundworm/ascaris parasitic nematode worm, as the hookworm and pinworm, whose eggs hatch in the small intestines

rubella/German measles contagious viral disease benign in children but linked to birth defects of children born of women infected in early pregnancy

rubeola see: measles

Rubin's test see: tubal insufflation

rupture 1. any breaking apart, as of a blood vessel
2. see: hernia

S

Sabin vaccine live polio vaccine taken orally to immunize against polio

sacral pertaining to the sacrum

sacroiliac pertaining to the sacrum or the ilium, or to the places on either side of the lower back where they are joined

sacrum bone in the lower spine formed by the fusing of five vertebrae, constituting the rear part of the pelvis

saddle block form of anesthesia used esp.

for childbirth, in which the patient is injected in the region of the lower spinal cord while in a sitting position

safety glass glass strengthened by any of various methods to reduce the likelihood of the glass shattering upon impact

St. Vitus's dance see: chorea

saline amniocentesis/salting out technique of inducing abortion by injecting a saline solution into the amniotic fluid

saliva fluid secreted by the salivary glands in the mouth that lubricates food and contains an enzyme (ptyalin) that begins to break down starch

salivary glands glands located in the mouth which secrete saliva

Salk vaccine dead polio virus taken by injection to immunize against polio

Salmonella genus of aerobic bacteria that cause food poisoning and other diseases, including typhoid fever

Salmonella typhosa rod-shaped bacteria that cause typhoid fever

salpingitis 1. inflammation of a Fallopian tube, a potential cause of sterility
2. inflammation of a Eustachian tube

salting out see: saline amniocentesis

saphenous vein either of two large, superficial veins of the leg, a common site of varicosity

sarcoid see: sarcoidosis

sarcoidosis/Boeck's sarcoid/sarcoid disease of unknown cause with symptoms resembling those of tuberculosis, marked by the formation of nodules, esp. on the skin, lungs, and lymph nodes

sarcoma malignant tumor that arises in the connective tissue (bones, cartilage, tendons)

sarcoma, Ewing's see: Ewing's sarcoma

saturated (of fats) tending to increase the cholesterol content of the blood

saucerization procedure of forming a shallow depression by scraping away tissue to assist healing

scabies/the itch contagious inflammation of the skin caused by a mite and characterized by a rash and intense itching

scan measure for diagnostic purposes the concentration in a particular area of a radioactive material that has been introduced into the body

scapula shoulder blade

scarlet fever contagious disease caused

by streptococci and characterized by a scarlet rash and high fever

schistosomiasis/bilharziasis tropical disease caused by a fluke worm (trematode) whose larvae penetrate the skin and invade the circulatory system

schizoid 1. describing a personality disorder in which the individual is withdrawn from and indifferent to other people

2. pertaining to or resembling schizophrenia

schizophrenia see: schizophrenic reaction

schizophrenia, catatonic schizophrenia marked by motor disturbances, such as maintenance of fixed, often awkward, position with muscles rigid

schizophrenia, hebephrenic schizophrenia marked by delusions, hallucinations, and regressed or childish behavior

schizophrenia, paranoid schizophrenia marked by variable delusions of persecution or grandeur, often with hallucinations and behavioral deterioration

schizophrenic or of pertaining to schizophrenia

schizophrenic reaction/schizophrenia psychosis characterized by withdrawal from external reality and a retreat into a fantasy life, with deterioration of behavior

sciatica pain along the sciatic nerve

sciatic nerve nerve of the lower spine that traverses the hips and runs down the back of the thigh of each leg

sclera the firm outer coat of the eye continuous with the cornea, visible as the white of the eye

sclerose harden and thicken, as tissue

sclerosis abnormal thickening and hardening of tissue, as of the lining of arteries

sclerosis, amyotrophic lateral/Lou Gehrig's disease disease characterized by increasing muscle weakness (atrophy) or paralysis, caused by the progressive degeneration of motor nerve cells in the brain and spinal cord

sclerosis, multiple see: multiple sclerosis

scoliosis lateral curvature of the spine

scratch test skin test for allergic response to different substances by applying suspected allergens in diluted form to scratches

scrofula tuberculosis of the lymph nodes, esp. of the neck

scrotum pouch that contains the testicles

scrub nurse operating room nurse authorized to handle sterilized equipment in assisting the surgeon

scurvy disease characterized by livid spots under the skin, swollen and bleeding gums, and prostration, caused by lack of vitamin C

seasickness see under: motion sickness

sebaceous cyst hard, round, movable mass contained in a sac, resulting from accumulated oil from a blocked sebaceous gland duct

sebaceous gland gland within the dermis that secretes oil (sebum) for lubricating the skin and hair

seborrhea abnormal increase of secretion from the sebaceous skin glands

sebum fatty lubricating substance secreted by the sebaceous glands

secondary produced as an effect or complication of another condition, as distinguished from *primary*

secondary disease disorder of a target gland caused by an excess or deficiency of a stimulating hormone supplied by the anterior pituitary gland

sedation reduction of sensitivity to pain, stress, etc., by administering a sedative

sedative medicine for allaying irritation or nervousness

seizure see: convulsion

semen/seminal fluid thick, whitish fluid containing spermatozoa that is ejaculated by the male at orgasm

semicircular canals three fluid-filled tubes of the inner ear that govern the sense of balance and communicate with the vestibular nerve

seminal fluid see: semen

seminal vesicle one of two small pouches on either side of the prostate gland that serve to store spermatozoa temporarily

senile of or characteristic of old age; esp., pertaining to or exhibiting certain mental infirmities often associated with old age

senile dementia see: senile psychosis

senile macula degeneration visual defect affecting the elderly

senile psychosis/senile dementia mental disorder of the aged characterized by progressive deterioration of the personality, irritability, loss of memory, etc.

senile purpura small hemorrhages in the skin of older people

senility state of being senile

separated retina see: detached retina

sepsis infection of the blood by disease-causing microorganisms

septicemia see: blood poisoning

septic shock shock resulting from infection of the blood by disease-causing microorganisms

septum dividing wall between two cavities, as in the nose

serous pertaining to, producing, or resembling serum

serous membrane membrane producing serum

serratus muscles muscles that run vertically along the ribs

serum the watery, clear portion of blood or lymph

serum analysis laboratory analysis of blood serum as a diagnostic aid

serum sickness acute illness caused by reaction to serum, such as that used in inoculations

sex act see: sexual intercourse

sexual intercourse/coitus male's ejaculation of semen into a female's vagina

sexuality sexual interest or activity

shingles/herpes zoster acute viral infection and inflammation of a sensory nerve, characterized by pain and small blisters on the skin along the path of the nerve

shock (circulatory shock) emergency condition in which the circulation of the blood is so disrupted that all bodily functions are affected

shock, allergic see: allergic shock

shock, cardiac shock resulting from diminished heart function

shock, electric see: electric shock

sick headache see: migraine

sickle-cell anemia hereditary disease occurring most commonly among Negro men and women, in which many or a majority of the red blood cells are sickle-shaped, producing chronic anemia

sickle-cell trait/sicklemia trait in the genetic make-up of an individual that could cause sickle-cell anemia in his offspring if the other parent also has the trait

sicklemia see: sickle-cell trait

SIDS see: sudden infant death syndrome

sigmoid 1. *(adj.)* shaped like the letter S 2. *(n.)* (sigmoid colon/sigmoid flexure) S-shaped fold in the colon of the large intestine just above the rectum

sigmoid colon see: sigmoid 2.

sigmoid flexure see: sigmoid 2.

sigmoidoscope surgical instrument for examining the interior of the sigmoid

sign (of disease) observable or objective manifestation, as distinguished from symptoms reported by the patient

silica extremely hard mineral, the chief constituent of quartz and sand

silicosis lung disorder, a form of pneumoconiosis, caused by inhaling silica dust, as of stone or sand

simple fracture see: closed fracture

sinoatrial node see: sinus node

sinus opening or cavity, as in bone, or a channel or passageway, as for blood

sinusitis inflammation of a sinus

sinus node/sinoatrial node small mass of nerve tissue in the right atrium of the heart that triggers heart contractions and regulates heartbeat, thus serving as cardiac pacemaker

sitz bath hot bath taken in a sitting position

skeletal muscle/voluntary muscle striated muscle attached to bones and joints, used chiefly in voluntary action

skeleton, appendicular the bones of the arms, hands, legs, and feet

skeleton, axial the bones of the head and the trunk

skin/integument the outer, membranous covering of the body, consisting of an outer layer (epidermis) and inner layer (dermis)

skin planing see: dermabrasion

skin-popping *(slang)* subcutaneous injection of heroin

sleeping pill sedative, esp. one of the barbiturates taken to relieve insomnia

sleeping sickness/African trypanosomiasis tropical African disease, a form of trypanosomiasis, caused by certain protozoa and spread by the bite of the tsetse fly, characterized by lethargy, recurrent fever, and oppressive drowsiness, often fatal

sleepwalking/somnambulism act of walking in one's sleep

slit lamp microscope/biomicroscope microscope for examining the eye, as the cornea, with the aid of an intense beam of light

smallpox/variola acute, highly contagious viral disease characterized by high fever and the eruption of deepseated pustules that leave scars upon healing

smegma cheesy secretion that may collect under the prepuce of the uncircumcised penis or of the clitoris

smooth muscle/involuntary muscle nonstriated muscle, used chiefly in involuntary action, such as that of the stomach and intestines

social worker person trained to work in a clinical, social, or recreational service for improving community welfare or aiding the rehabilitation or emotional adjustment of individuals

sociopathic/psychopathic describing a personality disorder in which the individual characteristically lacks a sense of personal responsibility or morality and may be disposed to aggressive and violent behavior, to self-destructive behavior, or to sexual deviation

sodium amytal chemical used as sedative for soldiers in World War I

sodium cyclamate see: cyclamate

sodium Pentothal see: Pentothal

soft palate see: palate, soft

soft spot see: fontanel

soldiers' disease see: morphinism

somnambulism see: sleepwalking

soot-wart name for cancer of the scrotum that afflicted 18th-century chimney sweeps

sore throat see under: pharyngitis

spasm involuntary convulsive contraction of muscles, called *clonic* when alternately contracted and relaxed, and *tonic* when persistently contracted

spastic of or characteristic of spasms

spasticity the condition of having spasms

specimen sample, as of blood, sputum, etc., for laboratory analysis

speculum instrument that dilates a passage of the body, as for examination

speech reading see: lip reading

speed *(slang)* see: methamphetamine

speed freak *(slang)* heavy user of methamphetamine (speed), esp. by intravenous injection, to induce altered mental state

sperm see: spermatozoa

spermatozoa *(sing.* spermatozoon)/ **sperm/sperm cells** male reproductive

cells or gametes, one of which must fertilize an ovum to produce an embryo

sperm cell the male reproductive cell, one of the spermatozoa

sperm cells see: spermatozoa

sperm duct see: vas deferens

spermicide contraceptive substance that destroys sperm

sphincter ringlike muscle surrounding an opening or tube that serves to narrow or close it

sphygmomanometer device for measuring arterial blood pressure

spinal see: spinal anesthesia

spinal anesthesia/spinal form of anesthesia in which the patient is injected in the region of the spinal cord

spinal arthritis arthritis of the spine, found esp. in the elderly

spinal column/backbone/spine the series of segmented bones (vertebrae) which enclose the spinal cord and provide support for the ribs

spinal cord the part of the central nervous system enclosed within the spinal column

spinal fluid see: cerebrospinal fluid

spinal fluid exam see: spinal tap

spinal puncture see: spinal tap

spinal reflex reaction to an outside stimulus that originates in the spinal cord and bypasses the brain

spinal tap/lumbar puncture/spinal fluid exam/spinal puncture needle puncture and withdrawal of cerebrospinal fluid from the lower spinal column for diagnostic examination

spine see: spinal column

spirochete any of various spiral-shaped bacteria, some of which cause syphilis and yaws

spleen vascular, ductless organ located near the stomach that produces red blood cells in infancy and modifies blood composition

splint appliance for supporting or immobilizing a part of the body, as a fractured bone

spondylitis inflammation of the vertebrae of the spine

spondylitis, ankylosing/rheumatoid spondylitis chronic disease characterized by inflammation of the spine and resulting in the fusing (ankylosing) of the spinal joints

spondylolisthesis forward displacement

of one of the lower vertebrae over the vertebra below it or over the sacrum, causing severe pain in the lower back

spontaneous abortion see: miscarriage

sporadic characterized by scattered cases, as of a disease, rather than by concentration in one area

spore single-celled reproductive body of a flowerless plant, capable of developing into an independent organism

sprain the stretching or rupturing of ligaments, usu. accompanied by damage to blood vessels

sputum expectorated matter, as saliva, sometimes mixed with mucus

sputum exam bacteriological, chemical, and microscopic testing of sputum for presence of disease

squint see: strabismus

stapedius small muscle in the tympanum of the middle ear whose function is to dampen loud sounds

stapes see: stirrup

staph see: staphylococcus

staphylococcus (pl. staphylococci (pl. staphylococci)/ **staph** parasitic bacterium that can cause boils and other infections

staphylococcus aureus bacterium that causes food poisoning

startle reflex see: startle response

startle response/startle reflex complex involuntary reaction to sudden noise occurring esp. in infancy, where it is marked by a sudden jerk of the arms and legs

static exercises see: isometrics

status epilepticus series of epileptic seizures, occurring virtually without interruption

stenosis the narrowing of a duct or canal in the body

sterile 1. being incapable of producing offspring
2. being free of germs

sterility 1. condition of being incapable of producing offspring
2. conditon of being free of germs

sterilization the process of destroying reproductive capacity by surgical means, as by tying the Fallopian tubes of a woman (tubal ligation) or by tying the seminal duct of a man (vasectomy)

steroid any of a group of organic compounds occurring naturally and produced synthetically, including the sex hormones, the bile acids, oral con-

traceptives, and many drugs

stethoscope diagnostic device that conducts sounds produced within the body, as the heartbeat, to the ear of the examiner

stiff toe pain and stiffness in the joint of the big toe

stilbestrol see: diethylstilbestrol

Still's disease see: rheumatoid arthritis, juvenile

stimulant drug or other substance that increases or agitates the physiological processes of body or mind

stimulus (pl. stimuli) that which initiates an impulse or affects the activity of an organism

stirrup/stapes the innermost of the three ossicles of the middle ear, the bone between the anvil and the cochlea

Stokes-Adams syndrome sudden unconsciousness and sometimes convulsions caused by heart block

stoma small opening in a surface, as in a membrane or wall of a blood vessel

stomach lining, inflammation see: gastritis

stool see: feces

stool exam laboratory analysis of feces, as for presence of blood or parasitic organisms

STP see: DOM

strabismus/squint disorder of the eye muscles in which one eye drifts so that its position is not parallel with the other

strain excessive stretching of a muscle, tendon, or ligament

stratum corneum the outermost layer of the epidermis, consisting of horny, lifeless cells

strep throat streptococcal infection of the throat

streptococcal of or relating to the streptococcus bacterium

streptococcus kind of bacteria including some forms that cause diseases, as pneumonia and scarlet fever

stress fracture tiny crack in a bone caused by repeated stress

striated striped, as certain muscle

striated muscle see under: skeletal muscle

striped muscle see under: skeletal muscle

stripping surgical removal of lengths of varicosed veins, esp. one of the saphenous veins of the leg

stroke/apoplexy attack of paralysis caused by the rupture of an artery and hemorrhage into the brain, or by an obstruction of an artery, as from a blood clot

stupor condition in which the senses and faculties are suspended or greatly dulled, as from shock, drugs, etc.

sty small, inflamed swelling of a sebaceous gland on the edge of the eyelid

subacute intermediate between *acute* and *chronic:* said of a disease

subarachnoid situated or occurring between the middle layer (arachnoid) and the innermost layer (pia mater) of the brain

subcutaneous situated or applied beneath the skin

subcutaneous injection an injection given in the subcutaneous tissue beneath the skin

subcutaneous tissue layer of fatty tissue below the skin (dermis) which acts as an insulator against heat and cold and as a shock absorber against injury

subdural situated or occurring between the outermost layer (dura mater) and the middle layer (arachnoid) of the brain

subdural hematoma see: hematoma, subdural

subjective (of symptoms) of a kind that only the patient is aware of

sublingual gland either of a pair of salivary glands located beneath the tongue

submandibular gland see: submaxillary gland

submaxillary gland/submandibular gland either of a pair of salivary glands located under each side of the lower jaw

subtotal less than total, as a surgical procedure involving the excision of an organ or part

sudden infant death syndrome/crib death/SIDS death of an infant, usu. between one and six months of age and without any preceding sign of distress and of undetermined cause

sudoriferous gland see: sweat gland

sulfa drug any of a group of organic compounds used in the treatment of a variety of bacterial infections

sulfonamide any of a group of chemical compounds including the sulfa drugs, used in the treatment of bacterial infections

sulfonylurea drug used to treat diabetes

sunstroke/heatstroke condition marked by an acutely high fever and the cessation of perspiration, caused by prolonged exposure to heat and sometimes leading to convulsions and coma

superego/conscience largely unconscious element of the personality, regarded as dominating the ego, for which it acts principally in the role of conscience and critic

superficial of, situated near, or on the surface

superior vena cava the large vein that brings blood from the upper part of the body to the heart

supination rotation of the hand or forearm so that the palm of the hand faces upward or forward

supine lying on the back, with the face upward

suppository solid, usu. cylindrical medicated preparation that liquefies from heat after insertion in a body cavity, as the rectum or the vagina

suppuration the formation of pus

suppurative characterized by the formation of pus; pussy

surgeon physician who specializes in the diagnosis and treatment of disease by means of surgery

surgery 1. the branch of medicine dealing with the correction of disorders or other physical change by operation or manipulation

2. in British usage, a physician's office

surgical of or relating to surgery

surgical diathermy see: electrosurgery

suture 1. sew together cut or separated edges, as of a wound, to promote healing

2. the thread, wire, gut, etc., used in this process

suture line line formed by the edges of the separate bones of a baby's skull

sweat gland/sudoriferous gland any of numerous glands that secrete sweat, found almost everywhere in the skin except for the lips and a few other areas

swimmer's itch mild form of schistosomiasis in which parasitic fluke worm larvae invade the skin of swimmers, causing dermatitis

sycosis/barber's itch bacterial infection of the hair follicles, marked by inflammation, itching, and the formation of pus-filled pimples

sympathetic nervous system the part of the autonomic nervous system that controls such involuntary actions as the dilation of pupils, constriction of blood vessels and salivary glands, and increase of heartbeat

symptom change in one's normal feeling or condition of well-being, indicating the presence of disease

symptomatic having observable symptoms of a disease or condition

symptomatology the combined symptoms of a disease

Synanon organized live-in community of drug addicts in which group psychotherapy is used to encourage rehabilitation

synapse the junction point between two neurons, across which a nerve impulse passes from the axon of one neuron to the dendrite of another

syncope temporary loss of consciousness; fainting

syndrome set of symptoms occurring at the same period and indicating the presence or nature of a disease

synovia/synovial fluid viscid, transparent fluid secreted as a lubricating agent in the interior of joints and elsewhere

synovial aspiration/synovial fluid exam laboratory analysis of synovia, withdrawn from joints by needle, in order to diagnose gout or certain forms of arthritis

synovial fluid see: synovia

synovial fluid exam see: synovial aspiration

syphilis contagious venereal disease transmitted by sexual contact and congenitally to offspring of infected mothers

systemic pertaining to or affecting the body as a whole

systole the instant of peak pumping action of the heart, when the ventricles contract and blood is impelled outward into the arteries, followed immediately by relaxation (diastole)

systolic pressure measure of blood pressure taken when the heart is contracting, the higher of the two figures in a reading

T

tabes dorsalis/locomotor ataxia form of syphilis involving demyelination of spinal nerves and other destructive changes in the spinal cord

tachycardia abnormally rapid heartbeat

tachycardia, paroxysmal attacks of abnormally rapid heartbeat that begin and end abruptly

tampon plug of absorbent material for insertion in a body cavity or wound to stop bleeding or absorb secretions

T and A operation see: adenotonsillectomy

tapeworm/cestode any of various worms with segmented, ribbonlike bodies, often of considerable length, that are parasitic on the intestines of humans and other vertebrates

target gland any of the endocrine glands that function when stimulated by hormones secreted by the anterior pituitary, as the thyroid, adrenal cortex, texticles, or ovaries

tarsal any of the bones of the tarsus, or ankle

tarsus ankle

tartar see: dental calculus

taste bud one of the clusters of cells in the tongue that contain receptors for discriminating salt, sweet, sour, or bitter tastes

teething process by which new teeth break (erupt) through the gums in infants and young children

tempered glass safety glass that has high resistance to blunt objects and breaks by crumbling into small fragments instead of shattering

temporal lobe the portion of each cerebral hemisphere of the brain in back of and partly below the frontal lobes, the centers for hearing

temporal lobe convulsion see: psychomotor convulsion

tendinitis inflammation of a tendon

tendon band of tough, fibrous connective tissue that binds a muscle to another part, as a bone, and by means of which muscular force can be exerted on other parts of the body

tendon sheath, inflammation of see: tenosynovitis

tennis elbow pain in the outer side of the elbow joint, usu. caused by a too vigorous twisting motion of the hand that strains a tendon or inflames a bursa

tenosynovitis inflammation of the sheath that covers a tendon

tension headache severe headache induced by tension, which causes unconscious constriction of head and neck muscles

Terramycin trade name for the antibiotic tetracycline

testes see: testicle

testicle/testis (*pl.* testes)   one of a pair of male reproductive glands (gonads) that produce spermatozoa and male sex hormones, situated in a pouch (scrotum) at the base of the penis

testicles, inflammation of see: orchitis

testis see: testicle

testosterone male sex hormone manufactured in the testicles

tetanus/lockjaw acute bacterial infection usu. introduced through a puncture wound, leading to muscle spasms, esp. of the jaw muscles, and often fatal

tetany nerve disorder characterized by muscle spasms and sometimes convulsions, caused by too little calcium in the blood

tetracycline crystalline powder isolated from a soil bacillus that forms the base of several antibiotics, including Aureomycin and Terramycin

tetrahydrocannabinol/THC   principal compound of cannabis (hashish or marihuana), believed to be the active ingredient

thalamus round mass of gray matter at the base of the brain that transmits sensory impulses to the cerebral cortex

thalassemia/Cooley's anemia form of anemia caused by inherited abnormality of red blood cells, often fatal in utero

THC tetrahydrocannabinol

therapeutic designed or tending to heal or to cure disease

therapist see: psychotherapist

therapy treatment of a disease by a prescribed method or medicine

thermogram picture of a body surface, as the breast, measuring relative heat by the technique of thermography

thermography technique of measuring the surface temperature of a region of the body, such as the breast, with an infrared sensing device

thiamine/vitamin B$_2$ vitamin found in cereal grains, green peas, liver, egg yolk, and other sources, and also made synthetically, that protects against beriberi

thiopental see: Pentothal

thoracic of or relating to the thorax, or chest cavity

thoracic cage see: rib cage

thoracic cavity see: chest cavity

thoracic spine see: vertebrae, thoracic

thoracic surgeon surgeon specializing in thoracic surgery, having to do with the chest cavity

thoracic surgery branch of surgery having to do with the chest cavity and its organs, the heart and lungs, and large blood vessels

thoracic vertebrae see: vertebrae, thoracic

thorax chest

Thorazine/chlorpromazine trademark for a commonly used tranquilizer

throat, sore see under: pharyngitis

thrombin enzyme present in the blood that reacts with fibrinogen to form fibrin in the process of clotting

thrombocyte see: platelet

thromboembolism obstruction of a blood vessel by a blood clot (thrombus) that has broken away from the place where it was formed

thrombophlebitis formation of a blood clot (thrombus) in the wall of an inflamed vein (phlebitis)

thromboplastin substance found in blood platelets that helps to convert prothrombin into thrombin in the clotting process

thrombosis formation of a blood clot (thrombus) in a blood vessel, resulting in the partial or complete blocking of circulation

thrombus stationary blood clot within a blood vessel

thrush fungus infection (*moniliasis*) in the mouth, esp. of infants, characterized by white patches that become sores

thymectomy surgical removal of the thymus

thymus glandlike lymphoid organ located near the base of the neck, believed to play a role in the body's immunological responses

thyroid gland endocrine gland located at the neck just below the larynx, extending around the front and to either side of the trachea (windpipe), and secreting the hormone thyroxin, which is vital to growth and metabolism

thyroid hormone see: thyroxin

thyroid-stimulating hormone/TSH hormone secreted by the anterior lobe of the pituitary gland which stimulates the production of hormones in the thyroid gland

thyroxin/thyroid hormone hormone secreted by the thyroid gland, vital to growth and metabolism

tibia the shin bone, the inner and larger of the two bones of the lower leg

tic involuntary, recurrent muscle twitch or spasm

tic douloureux see: trigeminal neuralgia

tick fever see: Rocky Mountain spotted fever

tinea see: ringworm

tinnitus ringing, buzzing, hissing, or clicking sound in the ears, not caused by external stimuli

tissue, death of see: gangrene

tolerance the ability of the body to adjust to increasingly larger doses of a drug through habitual use

tomography radiography of a section of the body

tomography, computerized axial see: CAT scanning

tone/tonicity the normal tension of muscle tissue

tongue, inflammation of see: glossitis

tonic of or characteristic of tonus

tonicity see: tone

tonic phase the period during a grand mal epileptic convulsion when the body is rigid

tonic spasm see under: spasm

tonometer device for measuring pressure, as of the eyeball

tonsil either of two small, round, lymphoid organs at each side of the back of the throat

tonsillectomy surgical removal of the tonsils

tonsillitis inflammation of the tonsils

tonus muscular spasm characterized by persistent contraction

tophus (*pl.* tophi) deposit of urate in the joints, a cause of gout

tourniquet bandage or other material tied tightly to constrict an artery to stop bleeding

toxemia of pregnancy metabolic disorder of pregnant women, characterized by a rise in blood pressure, swelling of tissues, weight gain, and headaches (preeclampsia) and sometimes by convulsions and loss of consciousness (eclampsia)

toxic 1. caused by or having to do with a toxin or poison
2. poisonous

toxic psychosis psychosis caused by a toxic agent, such as lead or alcohol

toxin any of a group of poisonous compounds produced by animal, vegetable, or bacterial organisms

trabecula (*pl.* trabeculae) strand of connective tissue, as in a bone

trachea/windpipe the passageway for air from the larynx to the lungs

tracheostomy/tracheotomy emergency surgical procedure of cutting into the trachea

tracheotomy see: tracheostomy

traction subjection of muscle or a fractured part to a pulling force, as by a system of weights and pulleys

tranquilizer drug with a calming or sedative effect

transference in psychoanalysis, the redirection of repressed childhood emotions to the analyst

transplant tissue or an organ transferred from its original site to another part of the body or to another individual

transsexual person who is genetically and physically of one sex but who identifies psychologically with the other and may seek treatment by surgery or with hormones to bring the physical sexual characteristics into conformity with the psychological preference

transudate fluid passing through pores or tissues, as of a membrane

transverse colon the section of the colon leading from the ascending colon and extending horizontally across the abdomen beneath the liver and stomach

transvestism practice of wearing the clothes of the opposite sex

transvestite one who wears the clothes of the opposite sex

trauma 1. any injury or wound to the body
2. severe emotional shock

trematode any of a class of parasitic flatworms, as the flukes, causing various diseases such as schistosomiasis

tremor any involuntary quivering or trembling, as of a muscle

trench foot foot condition resembling frostbite, due to exposure to continued dampness and cold

trench mouth/Vincent's angina/Vincent's disease painful infection of the gums (called necrotizing ulcerative gingivitis) and sometimes of the pharynx and palate, characterized by the formation of ulcers and necrosis

trichina see: Trichinella spiralis

Trichinella spiralis/trichina the parasitic worm that causes trichinosis

trichinosis disease caused by a parasitic worm *(Trichinella spiralis)* that enters the body via undercooked or raw meat, esp. pork, invading the intestines and muscles and provoking gastrointestinal symptoms initially and muscle stiffness and pain later

trichomonas genus of protozoa that cause vaginal infections in women

trichomoniasis vaginal infection by the trichomonas organism

trigeminal neuralgia/facial neuralgia/tic douloureux acutely painful neuralgia of a region of the face, with paroxysmal muscular twitchings, associated with branches of the trigeminal (cranial) nerve in the affected area

triglyceride glycerol compound containing one to three acids

trimester period of three months, used to identify the progress of a pregnancy, which consists of three such periods

trivalent pertaining to a form of the Sabin polio vaccine in which each dose gives protection against three strains of polio

trophoblast layer of cells developing around a fertilized ovum and contributing to the formation of the placenta

trophoblastic disease disease of the trophoblast in a pregnant woman, marked by the degeneration of the placenta into a mass of grapelike cysts *(hydatidiform mole)*

true skin see: dermis

trypanosomiasis any of a group of tropical diseases transmitted by the bite of certain insects, as the tsetse fly, including sleeping sickness

trypanosomiasis, African see: sleeping sickness

trypanosomiasis, American see: Chagas' disease

trypsin enzyme in the pancreatic juice that breaks up proteins for digestion

TSH see: thyroid-stimulating hormone

tubal insufflation/Rubin's test the injection of carbon dioxide gas, or sometimes ordinary air, into the uterus to check for obstructions in the Fallopian tubes

tubal ligation the tying or binding of a tube, esp. of the Fallopian tubes as a method of sterilization

tubercle small nodule or tumor formed within an organ, as that produced by the bacillus causing tuberculosis

tubercle bacillus rod-shaped bacterium that causes tuberculosis

tuberculin liquid containing substances extracted from weakened (attenuated) tubercle bacilli, used as a test for tuberculosis

tuberculin test skin test for determining whether tuberculosis bacteria are present, used esp. for children

tuberculoid of or resembling a tubercle or tuberculosis

tuberculosis infectious, communicable disease caused by the tubercle bacillus and characterized by the formation of tubercles within some organ or tissue, often the lungs (pulmonary tuberculosis)

tubule very narrow, minute tube or duct

tularemia acute bacterial infection that can be transmitted to humans from infected rabbits, squirrels, or other animals, by the bite of certain flies, or by direct contact

tumor mass of tissue growing independently of surrounding tissue and having no physiological function, sometimes confined to the area of origin (benign) and sometimes invading other cells and tissue and causing their degeneration (malignant)

tumor, fibroid benign tumor composed of fibrous tissue or a combination of fibrous and muscle tissue, usu. attached to the wall of the uterus

turbinate one of the thin, curved bones on the walls of the nasal passages

tympanic membrane see: eardrum

tympanum 1. the cavity in the middle ear lined with the tympanic membrane (eardrum) and containing the ossicles 2. see: eardrum

typhoid fever/enteric fever acute, infectious disease caused by a Salmonella bacterium and characterized by diarrhea, fever, eruption of bright red spots on the chest and abdomen, and physical prostration

typhus acute disease caused by a rickettsial microorganism that is transmitted to humans by the bite of certain lice and fleas, and is characterized by high fever, severe headaches, and a red rash

U

ulcer open sore with an inflamed base on an external or internal body surface

ulcerative colitis colitis accompanied by ulcerated lesions on the colon, characterized by bloody diarrhea and abdominal pain

ulna the bone of the forearm on the same side as the little finger, longer and thinner than the radius bone

umbilical pertaining to the middle part of the abdomen. See illustration at *abdomen.*

umbilical cord the ropelike tissue connecting the navel of the fetus with the placenta

umbilicus see: navel

unconsciousness loss of consciousness, having the appearance of sleep, usu. caused by injury, shock, or serious physical disturbance

underskin see: subcutaneous tissue

undulant fever see: brucellosis

unsaturated (of fats) not tending to increase the cholesterol content of the blood

ups/uppers/pep pills *(slang)* drugs or compounds that have a stimulating effect on the central nervous system, such as amphetamines

urate salt of uric acid

urea soluble compound containing nitrogen, found in urine and in small amounts in the blood

uremia toxic condition of the blood caused by the failure of the kidneys to function normally in filtering out and excreting waste products, such as urea

ureter either of two narrow, muscular ducts which convey urine from the kidneys to the bladder

urethra duct from the bladder by which urine is discharged and which in males carries the seminal fluid

urethritis inflammation of the urethra

uric acid acid occurring as a metabolic by-product in small quantities in the urine and blood

urinalysis chemical and microscopic analysis of the urine to determine for diagnostic purposes whether it is normally constituted

urination the excretion of urine

urine waste products and excess water separated in the kidneys and stored in the bladder for eventual elimination from the body

urinogenital/genitourinary/urogenital of or pertaining to the urinary and genital organs and their functions

urinogenital tract/genitourinary tract/ urogenital tract the urinary and genital systems, including the kidneys, ureters, bladder, urethra, vagina, and associated parts

urogenital see: urinogenital

urogenital tract see: urinogenital tract

urologist physician specializing in urology

urology the brance of medical science that deals with the diagnosis and treatment of diseases of the kidneys, bladder, ureters, urethra, and of the male reproductive organs

urticaria see: hives

uterine of or pertaining to the uterus

uterus/womb muscular, glandular organ in women in which the developing fetus is protected until birth

uterus, removal of see: hysterectomy

uvula fleshy, teardrop-shaped appendage of the soft palate at the back of the mouth

V

vaccinate inoculate with a vaccine as a preventive or therapeutic measure

vaccination 1. act or process of vaccinating
2. scar produced at the site of inoculation with a vaccine

vaccine preparation of live, attenuated, or dead microorganisms injected or administered orally to create immunity against a specific disease

vacuum aspiration technique of inducing abortion in early pregnancy by utilizing suction to draw out embryo tissue

vagina canal in the female leading from the external genital orifice below the pubis to the uterus

vaginitis inflammation of the vagina

vagotomy surgical procedure of cutting the vagus nerves

vagus the tenth cranial nerve, which

originates in the brain and extends branches to the lungs, heart, stomach, and intestines

Valium/diazepam trademark for commonly used tranquilizer

valley fever see: coccidioidomycosis

valve membranous structure inside a vessel or other organ, as the heart, allowing fluid to flow in one direction only

valves, disease of see: endocarditis

varicose abnormally dilated, as veins

varicose ulcer ulcer resulting from varicose veins, usu. on the inner side of the leg above the ankle

varicose vein/varicosity/varix swollen and contorted vein, often in the leg

varicosity 1. condition of being varicose 2. see: varicose vein

variola see: smallpox

varix (*pl.* varices)   see: varicose vein

vascular of, involving, or supplied with vessels, as blood vessels

vascularization process of becoming vascular

vascular surgeon surgeon specializing in vascular surgery, having to do with the blood vessels

vascular surgery branch of surgery having to do with the operative treatment of diseases of the blood vessels

vas deferens duct in males that conveys semen from the testicles to the seminal vesicles

vasectomy surgical removal of part of the vas deferens or sperm duct of the male, thus rendering him sterile by preventing semen from reaching the seminal vesicles

vasoconstrictor medicine that causes the blood vessels to contract, thus restricting blood flow

vasodilator medicine that causes the blood vessels to dilate, thus producing greater blood flow

vasomotor producing contraction or dilation of the blood vessels

vasopressin hormone secreted by the posterior lobe of the pituitary gland that raises blood pressure and increases peristalsis, known also as antidiuretic hormone because of its action on the kidneys to stimulate the reabsorption of water

VD *venereal disease*

vectorcardiogram graph indicating the magnitude and direction of the electrical currents of the heart

vein any of a large number of muscular, tubular vessels conveying blood from all parts of the body to the heart

vein, inflammation of see: phlebitis

vein, pulmonary vein that delivers oxygen-rich blood from the lungs to the heart

velum see: palate, soft

vena cava either of two large veins that bring blood to the heart from the upper part of the body (superior vena cava) and lower part of the body (inferior vena cava)

venereal disease any of those diseases transmitted by sexual intercourse, such as syphilis and gonorrhea

venereal wart/condyloma acuminatum wart caused by a virus and occurring in the anal and genital areas, transmitted by sexual contact and by other means

venesection see: phlebotomy

venom poison secreted by certain reptiles, insects, etc., transferred to a victim by a bite or sting

venous having to do with or carried by the veins

ventral toward, near, or in the abdomen

ventricle any of various body cavities, as of the brain, or chambers, esp. either of the two lower chambers of the heart, which receive blood from the atria and pump it into the arteries

ventriculography technique of X-raying the brain after the removal of cerebrospinal fluid and the injection of air into the ventricles

venule small vein continuous with a capillary

vermiform appendix/appendix vermiformis the worm-shaped appendage attached to the cecum of the large intestine

vermifuge any drug or remedy that destroys intestinal worms

vernix caseosa cheesy substance sometimes covering a newborn baby's skin

vertebra (*pl.* vertebrae) one of the segmented bones that make up the spinal column

vertebrae, thoracic/thoracic spine the vertebrae to which the ribs are attached

vertebrate any animal having a backbone

vertigo disorder in which a person feels as if he or his surroundings are whirling around

vesical of or pertaining to the bladder

vesicle small bladderlike cavity, or a small sac containing fluid

vestibular nerve the part of the auditory nerve leading from the vestibule of the inner ear to the brain, controlling equilibrium

vestibule space or cavity, as within the labyrinth of the inner ear

vestigial of the nature of a remnant of an organ that is no longer functional

viable capable of living and developing normally, as a newborn infant

vibrissae (*sing.* vibrissa) hairs that grow in the nasal cavity

villi (*sing.* villus) minute, hairlike structures on the mucous membrane of the small intestine that absorb nutrients

Vincent's angina see: trench mouth

Vincent's disease see: trench mouth

virulent 1. severe and rapid in its progress, as a disease
2. highly infectious, as a disease-causing microorganism

virus any of a large group of particles too small to be seen by an ordinary microscope, that are typically inert except when in contact with certain living cells, and that can cause a variety of infectious diseases

viscera 1. the internal organs of the body, as the stomach, lungs, heart, etc.
2. the intestines

visceral pertaining to the viscera

viscid sticky or adhesive

viscous semifluid or gluelike in texture

visual purple reddish purple protein found in the rods of the retina, esp. important to night vision

visual radiations smaller nerve bundles that split off from the optic nerve and enter the occipital lobes of the brain

vitalometer device for measuring sensitivity of a tooth

vital signs measurement of body temperature, pulse rate, and respiration

vitamin any of a group of complex organic substances found in minute quantities in most natural foods and closely associated with the maintenance of normal physiological functions

vitamin A vitamin found in green and yellow vegetables, dairy products, liver, and fish liver oils, that prevents atrophy of epithelial tissue and protects against night blindness

vitamin B₁ see: thiamine

vitamin B₂ see: riboflavin

vitamin B₁₂ vitamin extracted from liver and believed to protect against pernicious anemia

vitamin B complex group of water-soluble vitamins widely distributed in plants and animals, including thiamine and riboflavin

vitamin C see: ascorbic acid

vitamin D vitamin that protects against rickets, found in fish liver oils, butter, egg yolks, and specially treated cow's milk, and also produced in the body on exposure to sunlight

vitamin E vitamin found in whole grain cereals, legume seeds, corn oil, egg yolks, meat, and milk, sometimes called the antisterility vitamin because its absence in rats causes sterility

vitamin K vitamin that promotes the clotting of blood and is found in green leafy vegetables

vitiligo/piebald skin skin disorder characterized by a loss of pigment in sharply defined areas

vitreous humor the transparent, jellylike tissue that fills the posterior chamber or ball of the eye and is enclosed by the hyaloid membrane

vocal cords/vocal folds two bands of ligaments extending across the larynx which, when tense, are made to vibrate by the passage of air, thereby producing voice

vocal folds see: vocal cords

voice box see: larynx

void excrete waste, esp. urine

voluntary muscle see: skeletal muscle

volvulus obstruction of the intestines caused by twisting

vomitus vomited substance

vulva the external genitals of the female, located beneath the front part of the pelvis

W

walking pneumonia mild viral pneumonia that does not confine the patient to bed

walleye strabismus characterized by a tendency of the eyes to turn outward away from the nose

wart small, usu. hard, benign growth formed on and rooted in the skin, caused by a virus

wart, venereal see: venereal wart

Wasserman test blood test for the presence of the organism causing syphillis

water blister blister beneath the epidermis that contains lymph

"water-pill" diuretic

WBC white blood cell. See: leukocyte

wet dream/nocturnal emission male's involuntary expulsion of semen while asleep

wheal raised area on the skin, as from hives or an insect bite, usu. transitory and characterized by itching

whiplash injury to neck ligaments, usu. caused by a sudden jolt to the neck, as in automobile accidents

white blood cell/WBC see: leukocyte

white corpuscle see: leukocyte

white lung disease see: byssinosis

Wilms' tumor/nephroblastoma malignant tumor of the kidney, found esp. in children

wisdom tooth the last tooth, or third molar on either side of the upper and lower jaws

whooping cough/pertussis respiratory, bacterial disease of children marked by paroxysms of coughing ending with a sharp sound (or "whoop") upon intake of breath

windpipe see: trachea

withdrawal symptom any of the symptoms caused by the withdrawal of a physically addictive drug from an addict, as tremors, sweating, chills, vomiting, and diarrhea

womb see: uterus

wood alcohol see: methyl alcohol

writer's cramp spasmodic contraction of the muscles of the fingers and hand, caused by excessive writing

X

xenograft see: heterograft

xenophobia fear of strangers

xerography method of reproducing an image by electrostatic attraction, used experimentally as a diagnostic tool

xeroradiogram picture developed by xeroradiography

xeroradiography diagnostic procedure utilizing xerography to develop X-ray pictures

X ray 1. *(v.)* examine, diagnose, or treat with X rays

2. *(n.)* photograph made with X rays

X rays electromagnetic radiations of extremely short wavelengths, used to reproduce on photosensitive film images of the internal organs and the skeleton as an aid in the detection, diagnosis, and treatment of certain disorders

Y

Yang in the Chinese philosophy underlying acupuncture, the masculine principle, identified with activity

yaws infectious tropical disease that is not venereal but is caused by the syphilis bacterium (spirochete), characterized by rheumatic pains and ulcerating sores of the skin

yellow fever acute, infectious, intestinal disease of tropical and semitropical regions, caused by a virus transmitted by the bite of a mosquito, and characterized by jaundice and hemorrhages

yellow marrow see under: marrow

Yin in the Chinese philosophy underlying acupuncture, the female principle, identified with passivity

Z

zymase enzyme obtained principally from yeast, important in fermentation

Index

echoencephalogram, 572
eclampsia, 248
ECPR. *See* external car-
diopulmonary resuscita-
tion.
ectopic pregnancy, 254–255
eczema, 186, 474–475, *475*,
546, 548
edema,
in congestive heart failure,
843
of feet and ankles, 342, 346,
347, 816
in kidney failure, 937
of newborn, 89
in pregnancy, 248
premenstrual, 680–681
education,
adult, 316, *316*, 319–320,
360–361
family life, 1246, 1247
of handicapped children,
deaf, 135, 934
retarded, *1250*
efferent (motor) nerves, 22
efferent (motor) neuron, *26*
EEG. *See* electroencephalogram.
eggs,
allergy to, 545
nutrients in, 373
ego, 1008
ejaculation, 235
EKG. *See* electrocardiogram.
elastic bandage, *1118*
elastic stockings, 250, 303,
531, 816, 899
elbow, 9, *16*
dislocation of, 763
Electra complex, 106
electrical equipment, safety
with, 1124–1125, 1129,
1135–1136, 1138–1139,
1145–1146
electric heaters, safe use of,
1139
electric razors, 468
electric shock, 1105, 1124,
1138–1139
electrocardiogram (EKG),
566–567, 574, 828
electrocoagulation, 470
electrocution, accidental,
1105, 1138–1139
electroencephalogram
(EEG), 572, 774–775, *785*
in epilepsy, 781–782, *781*
electrolysis, 211, 470
electromyography, 572, 656,
796, *796*
electronic amplification, ear
damage and, 453
electronic equipment in intensive care unit, 601, *601*
electron microscope, 955
electroschock therapy, 1022
electrosurgery, 338
elephantiasis, 997, *997*
elevators, safety in, 1154
embolism,

phlebitis and, 654
prolonged bed rest and, 821
pulmonary, 821, 898–899
stroke and, 818, 820–821
embolus, in phlebitis, 654,
655, 815
embryo, *245*
movement of, 1186
emergencies,
everyday, 1187–1188
medical, alphabetical guide
to, 1087–1121
emergency room, *583, 584*
emergency services,
ambulance, 1083–1084,
1084
hospital, 1083–1085, *1085*
physician, 1085–1086
poisoning, 1077–1082
emergency surgery, 583–
584, *583*
EMG (electromyograph),
796, *796*
emotional disorders, 1005–
1023
emotional maturity, 1006
emotional needs of infant,
99–100
emotional pressures, in middle age, 313
emotional problems,
physical symptoms and, 313
posture and, 183–184
psychiatric help for, 1018–
1019
treatment for, 1018–1023
emotions and nervous sys-
tem, 28
emphysema, 892–896, *893*,
895
smog and, 434
smoking and, 220, 308, *308*,
887
enamel, tooth, 5, *5*, 488–489,
489
encephalitis, 28, 207, 791
encounter groups, 1289
encyclopedia, child's, 133
endarterectomy, 826–827
endocarditis, 39, 840
tooth decay and, 499
endocardium, 39
endocrine (ductless) glands,
63–71, *64, 66, 67, 68, 901*
disorders of, 579, 900–921
endocrinology, 65, 556
endodontic therapy, 501–502
endolymph, *79*
endometrial polyp, 703–704
endometrioma, 705
endometriosis, 705–706
endometrium (uterine lin-
ing), 236
cancer of, 711–713, *712*
hormonal control of, 67
enema, 537, 589, 851
administration of, in home
nursing, 731–732
barium, 867
energy,

bodily, 41, 57
acupuncture and, 1254
of light, in vision, 72–74
of sound waves, 450
ENT (ear, nose, and throat)
doctor, 558
enteric fever. *See* typhoid.
enteritis, 411, 857–858
regional, 1277
enterocele, 699, *699*
enuresis, 948
environment,
aging and, 291
health and, 429–454
Environmental Health Sci-
ence, Task Force on Re-
search Planning in, 429,
431
Environmental Protection
Agency,
Division of Water Hygiene,
439
PCB ban by, 445
enzyme(s),
in cellular chemistry, 57
digestive, 44, 48, 49–50
in emphysema, 896
in muscle chemistry, 796
pancreatic, 847
stomach, 845
eosinophils, allergies and,
544
epidermis, *18*, 19, 20, 456,
456
epididymis, *87*, *611*
epigastric area of abdomen,
1303
pain in, 857
epiglottis, *43, 45, 46, 60, 648*,
846
epilepsy, 144–145, *144*,
781–788, 1277–1278
agencies, 788, 1248
emotional factors in, 786
prognosis of, 787–788
treatment of, 785–786, *787*,
1277–1278
types of, 144–145, 783
Epilepsy Foundation of
America, 788, 1248
epileptic seizure,
convulsive (grand mal), 145,
783
emergency treatment for,
1105–1106
focal, 784
petit mal, 144, 783–784
psychomotor, 144–145,
784–785
epinephrine. *See* adrenaline.
epiphysis (cartilage plate),
210
slipped, 758
episiotomy, 265
Equanil (meprobamate),
1055
equipment, sickroom, 735–
736
erection, 235
erector pili muscle, *18, 456*

isopropyl alcohol, 736, 1025
isotopes, radioactive, diagnostic tests with, 577
itching (pruritus), 475, 537
  diabetes and, 345, 911
  in later years, 337
  pubic lice and, 695
itch, the, 478
IUD, 276–277, *276*

J

jackhammer, 449, *449*
Jacksonian epilepsy, 784
jams, nutrients in, 390
jaundice, 864
jaw,
  dislocation of, 769, 1112–1113
  fracture of, 769
  malformations of, 738
jawbones, 4, 5
jejunum, 49, 50–51
jellies, nutrients in, 390
jellyfish sting, 1113
jerking, nocturnal, 1291–1292
jet lag, 1284
jet planes, pollution and, *430*
jewelry, allergies and, 550
jogging, 293–294, *294*, 1186
Johnson, Virginia E., 314–315, 362
joints, 8–9
  aging and, 343, 740
  artificial, *742*
  bleeding in, 805
  diagnostic procedures, 571
  diseases of, 739–754
Jones criteria for rheumatic fever, 837
judgment, impairment of, 793
jumping, spinal injury from, 771
junction nevus, 1291
Jung, Carl G., *1020*
juvenile rheumatoid arthritis, 747–748, *747, 748*

K

kala-azar, 990
kaolin-pectin compound, 536
keratin, 20, 463, 471
ketamine, 597
ketone bodies, 910, 916
ketosis, diabetic, 916–917
keys, care of, 1148, 1149, *1149*
kidney, *30, 67,* 82–85, *82, 935, 936*
  artificial, 938, *938. See also* dialysis.
  cysts of, 619–620
  diagnostic procedures for, 580–581
  infection of, 944–945
  removal of, 617, *617,* 619
  tumors of, 619, *946,* 969–970
kidney disease,

cadmium pollution and, 442–443
  diet in, 409
  hypertension and, 85, 836
  Medicare coverage for, 349
  overweight and, 311
  symptoms of, 935–936
  voluntary agency, 1242
kidney failure, 936–939
  Medicare coverage for, 939–940
kidney stones, 945
  emergency treatment for, 1113
  and gout, 750
  and parathyroid hyperfunction, 908
  surgical removal of, 616–618, *617,* 619
kidney transplants, 672–673, *672,* 940–941, *940*
  Medicare coverage for, 941
  voluntary agency, 1242
kindergarten, adjustment to, 104
kissing bugs, 993, 995
kissing disease, 814
kitchen, safety in, 1134–1138
  microwave ovens and, 431
knee, 9
  injury to, 659
    treatment for, 1113
  Osgood-Schlatter disease, 1287
  replacement of joint of, *740*
kyphosis, 754–755

L

label, prescription drug, 1046–1047
labor (childbirth), 260–267
labyrinth, 79, 930
  balancing function of, 933
lacrimal glands, 77, *77*
lactogenic hormone, *66,* 67
ladders,
  escape, 1143, *1143*
  extension, *1123*
lallation, 194
Lamaze method of natural childbirth, 266
lamb, 373, 386
language development,
  hearing loss and, 144, 159–160
  motor-perceptual disability and, 142
lanolin, 459, 523, 530
laparotomy, 244
lapidary, as hobby, 358
lard, nutrients in, 390
laryngeal cartilage, *45*
laryngectomy, 973–974
  voluntary agency, 1234
laryngitis, 539, 1113–1114
larynx, 46, 59, *60, 648*
  cancer of, 972–974
  smoking and, 887
laser beam, 431
  in cancer research, *956*

in retinal surgery, *647,* 648, *920*
later years, 325–368
  daily food requirements in, 379
  diet in, 391, *392*
  progressive exercises for, 1209–1219
  surgery in, 608–609, *608*
laundry room, safety in, 1129–1130
Law of Use, 1186
laxatives, 292, 536, 537, 850, 866, 1284
L-dopa, 780
lead poisoning, 169–170, *436,* 437, *437*
  mental retardation and, 169, 174
lead pollution,
  atmospheric, 435
  sources of, 435, *436,* 437–438
  water, 442
leaflets, heart valve, 837–838
learning disability, 142, 170
learning, in later years, 327, 360
leeches, to remove, 1114
left-handedness, 98, 1269, 1280
Legg-Perthes' disease, 758
legs,
  bowed, in Paget's disease, 759
  cramps in, 529
    pregnancy and, 249–250
  exercises for, 296, 1268
  shaving of, 468–469
  vascular disorders in, 653–655, *654,* 1268
leiomyoma, 946
leishmaniasis, 990–992, *992*
leishmaniasis protozoa, life cycle of, 992–993
leisure activities,
  in later years, 353–364
  in middle years, 316, 321
lemonade, nutrients in, 381
lens, *73,* 74–75, *75,* 643
lepromatous leprosy, 1003, *1003*
leprosy (Hansen's disease), 1002–1004, *1002, 1003,* 1280
lettuce, nutrients in, 376
leukemia, 812–813, 955, 977–978
  and secondary gout, 750
  voluntary agency, 1248–1249
Leukemia Society of America, 1248–1249
leukocytes (white blood cells), 33, *34*
  bone marrow transplants and, 673
  diseases of, 812–814
leukopenia, 814
leukorrhea, 682

profibrinolysin, 803
profile, health, 292
progesterone, 67, 70–71, 208, 906
  and corpus luteum cysts, 702
Prohibition, 1026
prolactin, 270
proof spirits, 1028
prophylaxis, dental, 492
propranolol, 825
prostate, 86, 87, 87, 235, 235, 611, 616
  cancer of, 613, 947, 967
    sex hormones and, 348
  disorders of, 347–348, 542, 613, 946–947
    impotence and, 362
  examination of, 347–348, 968
    biopsy, 581
    smear, 968
  hyperplasia of (enlarged), 347–348, 611, 612, 946
  surgery of, 348, 610–613
prostatectomy, 348, 612–613, 612
prostatitis, 542
protein,
  in composition of body, 370
  deprivation of, 393
  dietary sources of, 370
  digestion of, 50
  and pregnancy, 391
  rheumatoid arthritis and, 747
  synthesis of, by liver, 52
proteinuria, 248
prothrombin, 803
protozoa, pathogenic, 683, 987, 990, 993, 993
prunes, nutrients in, 382
pruritus. See itching.
pseudotumor, 964–965
psilocin, 1061
Psilocybe mexicana, 1061
psilocybin, 1061
psoralen, 485
psoriasis, 483–485, 483, 484, 1288
  arthritis and, 752
  and gout, 750
  and nails, loss of, 1286
psoriatic arthropathy, 752
Psychiatric Foundation, 1242
psychiatrist, 558
  "board certified", 1018
psychiatry, 558
psychic determinism, 1006, 1008
psychoanalysis, 1006, 1008, 1019–1020
psychodrama, 1020–1021
psychogenic symptoms, 1014
psychological counseling, 1288
psychological evaluation, pre-operative, 587
psychologist, 1019
psychomimetic drugs, 224

psychomotor (temporal lobe) seizure, 144–145, 784–785
psychoneurosis, 1011
psychopathic personality, 1015
psychopharmacology, 1289
psychophysiological disorders, 1014
psychosis, 1015–1017
  LSD and, 1060
  tranquilizers and, 1055
psychosomatic complaints, 1014, 1273
psychotherapist, 1019
psychotherapy, 1019–1022
  alcoholism and, 1041
  heroin addiction and, 1059
ptosis, 799, 801
ptyalin, 44
puberty, 70, 107, 205–210, 902, 1289
  starvation diet and, 170
pubic fracture, 768
pubis, 7, 8
Public Health Service, 788
public housing, 365
puffed rice, 389
pulmonary tree, 56
pulp capping, 502
pulpotomy, 502
pulp (tooth), 5, 5, 489, 490
pulse rate, 565, 602
  in acupuncture, 1255, 1255
  measuring, in home care, 726–727
punishment, 113, 185
pupil (eye), 72–73, 73, 75–76, 75, 643
purified protein derivative, 579
purines, 750
purpura, 805–806
purse snatching, 1150
pus, 33
pyelogram, 581, 966
pyelonephritis, 944–945
pyloric sphincter, 43, 47, 48, 622, 846
pylorus, 47
pyorrhea, 532–533
pyrogenic arthritis, 742, 750

Q
quacks, checklist on, 353
quarrels, children's, 152–153
quinine, 989

R
rabbit fever, 783–784
rabies, 1089–1090, 1090, 1161
radiation, exposure to, 431
  and leukemia, 978
  and thyroid cancer, 975
radiation therapy (radiotherapy),
  in breast cancer, 722–723
  in leukemia, 813
  with linear accelerator, 714, 961

with radioactive iodine, 903
  with radioactive phosphorus, 810
  with radium needles, 966
  surgery and, 961
radiators, insulation of, 1141
radioisotopes in diagnosis, 577, 975
radiologist, 558
radiology, 558
radiotherapy. See radiation therapy.
radishes, 377
radium needles, 966
radius, 7, 9
ragweed, 883, 884–885
railroad crossings, safety at, 1160
rainy days, children's activities for, 117–119, 118
raisins, 382
rash(es),
  allergic reactions and, 473–475
  childhood, 186–187
  symptomatic,
    of chicken pox, 125
    of measles, 125
    of rheumatoid arthritis, 748
    of Rocky Mountain spotted fever, 168–169, 985
    of secondary syphilis, 949, 950, 950
raspberries, 385
rats, plague and, 982
rattlesnake bites, 1116–1117
Raynaud's disease, 1289
razor blades, used, 1141
razors, types of, 468–469
RBC (red blood cell) count, normal range, 570
Reach to Recovery program, 722, 722, 723, 1234, 1234
reaction time, aging and, 27, 290
reading,
  children and, 188, 188
  in later years, 355
receptors, sense, 18, 71
  balance, 79
record players, noise level of, 185–186
records, medical,
  in home care, 726–729
  transfer of, 1275
recovery room, 599–601, 599, 600
rectocele, 699, 699
rectum, 43, 48, 54, 622, 846
  cancer of, 629–631, 959–961
  hernia of vagina and, 699, 699
red blood cells (erythrocytes; red blood corpuscles), 32–33, 32, 34, 34, 35–37, 803, 806
  diseases of, 806–812
  and malaria, 988
reducing. See weight reduc-

Illustration Credits

The editors are pleased to acknowledge the following organizations and individuals who have kindly permitted us to use their illustrations in *The New Complete Medical and Health Encyclopedia*. Photographers' names, when indicated, are listed in parentheses immediately following the page number or numbers on which their photos appear. Abbreviations used are T for *top*, B for *bottom*, M for *middle*, L for *left*, and R for *right*.

National Institute of Allergy and Infectious Diseases, 187, 853, 864, 872T, 984, 987, 993M, 999T, 1090, 1120L

National Institute of Neurological Diseases and Stroke, 572R (Roy Perry), 781, 796

National Institutes of Health, 33 (Dr. Makio Murayamo), 143, 144, 173, 203, 246, 253, 258T, 266, 268, 269, 279, 332, 437, 483B, 493, 500, 504, 545, 551, 560, 581, 639, 644, 646T, 650, 662, 672, 676, 685, 744, 749, 755, 761, 776B, 782, 808 (Murayamo), 809, 824, 826, 832, 843, 920, 925, 940, 985, 1097, 1098, 1104, 1112

National Jogging Association, 294, 1192

National League for Nursing, 533, 608, 730

National Library of Medicine, 267, 446, 517, 534, 535, 607, 660, 687, 701, 852, 949, 981T, 991, 1036, 1037, 1056

National Livestock and Meat Board, 384, 386, 388

National Multiple Sclerosis Society, 1243

National Park Service, 320, 1189

National Tuberculosis and Respiratory Disease Association, 1246

New York Catholic Charities, 192, 286, 1250

New York City Board of Education, 181

New York City Department of Health, 950

New York City Fire Department, 1142

New York Diabetes Association, Inc., 1237

New York State College of Human Ecology at Cornell University, 395

New York State Department of Transportation, 1162

New York University, 103, 104, 201

New York University Medical Center, 32, 34, 569T, 803, 808T (all by Robert Grant)

O

Office of Child Development, 92, 93, 98, 99, 100, 102, 105, 115, 118, 119, 120, 133, 145, 148, 151, 154, 162, 167, 180, 188, 189, 202, 227, 282, 285, 383, 399, 458 (all by Richard Swartz), 113 and 139 (Leslie Cooper)

Oral-B Company, 496

P

Pacific Medical Center, 575

Parke, Davis and Company, 1049

Pfizer, Inc., 577, 661, 776T, 875, 946, 959, 1119

Planned Parenthood-World Population, 108 (H. Dreiwitz), 240 (De Cavava), 274, 275

Podiatry News, 477

President's Council on Physical Fitness and Sports, 210, 233, 292, 296, 336, 522, 1203

Public Health Service, 472

R

Record Searchlight, Redding, Cal., 431

Research Advances, National Institutes of Health, 646B (Herbert E. Kaufman), 800 (Dr. Vanda Lennon), 972L, 988, 1004

Roberts, H. Armstrong, 1021, 1026

Rockwell International, Power Tool Division, 1130, 1131

Ruder and Finn, Inc., 929

S

Scholl, Inc., 299, 526

Shoreline Community College, 219

Sidel, Victor W., M.D., 1261

Smithsonian Institution, 810

Sonotone Corporation, 341

Standard Oil Company (N.J.), 96, 126, 166, 884

State University of New York at Cobleskill, 426 (Stan Pendrak)

T

Tenneco, Inc., 374

U

United Hospital Fund of New York, 95, 562

United Press International, 333, 1038

University of California at Berkeley, 870

University of Pennsylvania Medical School, 872B (Dr. Robert Austrian)

U.S. Census Bureau, 326

U.S. Coast Guard, 1177, 1178, 1179

U.S. Department of Agriculture, 377, 448, 474, 516, 548, 549, 567, 1092, 1095, 1116, 1120R

U.S. Office of Economic Opportunity, 1187

V

Visiting Nurse Association of Brooklyn, Inc., 328

W

Webb-Waring Institute for Medical Research, Denver, 893, 896

Weight Watchers International, Inc., 401

World Health Organization, 121 (J. Gordon), 147 (E. Mandelmann), 175 and 178 (Monique Jacot), 221 and 231 (Mandelmann), 232 (P. Almasy), 276 (E. Rice), 356B (Homer Page), 494 and 520 (Tibor Farkas), 688, 726 (Page), 838 (Jerry Hecht), 890 (Mandelmann), 915 (Farkas), 917 (Gordon), 918 (Farkas), 919 (P. Larsen), 958 (Spooner), 974, 982 (Almasy), 990 (Page), 994 and 995 (Almasy), 998T (Mandelmann), 998B (R. Witlin), 1001 (Dale Whitney), 1002 (P. Pittet), 1152 (Jean Mohr), 1185, 1198 (Farkas)

Y

Youth Services Agency, 217

Z

Zenith Hearing Instrument Corporation, 340

Thesaurus of Medical Terms

KEY WORD	ADJECTIVE	STUDY
allergy	allergic	allergology
anesthesia	anesthetic	anesthesiology
blood	hemal	hematology
blood vessels	vascular	angiology
bone	osteal, osseous	orthopedics
brain *See* **nervous system.**		
cancer *See* **tumor.**		
causes of disease	etiologic, etiological	etiology
chest cavity	thoracic	thoracic surgery
children	pediatric	pediatrics
colon and rectum	proctologic, proctological	proctology
cosmetic surgery *See* **plastic surgery.**		
diet	nutritive	nutrition
digestive tract	gastroenteric	gastroenterology
disease	pathologic, pathological	pathology
ear	otologic, otological	otology
ear, nose, and throat	otolaryngological	otolaryngology
endocrine glands *See* **glands.**		
epidemics (geographical distribution of disease)	epidemic, epidemical	epidemiology
eye	ophthalmic	ophthalmology
foot	pedal	podiatry, chiropody
gastrointestinal tract (GI tract) *See* **digestive tract.**		
general medicine		
genital tract (female) *See* **reproductive system (female).**		

The *Thesaurus of Medical Terms* is designed to enable the reader to find the more technical terms that apply to a variety of health-related subjects. By locating the Key Word that applies to a particular subject and reading across the page, the pertinent adjective, study, specialist, and major disorders may be found. For example, if one wants to know the technical term for an eye doctor, one looks under the Key Word column for *eye,* and under Specialist, finds the words *ophthalmologist* and *oculist.* If one cannot recall the name of a common heart disease, one looks under *heart* in the Key Word column and finds, under Major Disorders, *angina* and other conditions listed. These disorders may in turn be looked up in the glossary following for definitions and in the index for page references to the text.

SPECIALIST	MAJOR DISORDERS
allergist, allergologist	respiratory and skin disorders, e.g. asthma and contact dermatitis
anesthesiologist	
hematologist	anemia, leukemia, hemophilia
vascular surgeon	varicose veins, phlebitis
orthopedist, orthopedic surgeon, orthopod	back disorders, fractures, trauma
etiologist	
thoracic surgeon	lung cancer, tuberculosis, emphysema
pediatrician	all diseases children are subject to
proctologist	hemorrhoids, cancer of the rectum or colon
nutritionist	malnutrition, obesity
gastroenterologist	digestive difficulties, ulcers, gallstones, inguinal hernia
pathologist	
otologist	hearing or equilibrium disorders
otolaryngologist, ENT specialist	hearing or equilibrium disorders, laryngitis, upper respiratory infections
epidemiologist	forms of cancer, cholera, influenza
ophthalmologist, oculist	glaucoma, cataract, detached retina
podiatrist, chiropodist	arch troubles, bunions, ingrown toenails
general practitioner (GP)	

KEY WORD	ADJECTIVE	STUDY
genital tract (male) See urinogenital tract (male).		
glands (endocrine)	glandular	endocrinology
hair See skin and hair.		
heart	cardiac, coronary, cardiologic, cardiological	cardiology
immunization	immunologic, immunological	immunology
internal medicine		
joints and muscles		rheumatology
kidney	renal, nephric	nephrology
law and medicine		forensic medicine, forensic pathology
liver	hepatic	hepaticology
lung	pulmonary	internal medicine
medicine See general medicine, internal medicine, osteopathic medicine, rehabilitation.		
mental illness	psychiatric	psychiatry
muscles See joints and muscles.		
nervous system	neural, neurologic, neurological, neuropathological	neurology, neuropathology
nose See ear, nose, and throat.		
osteopathic medicine	osteopathic	osteopathy
plastic surgery		plastic surgery, cosmetic surgery
radiology	radiologic, radiological, X-ray	radiology, roentgenology
rectum See colon and rectum.		
rehabilitation		physical medicine
reproductive system (female)	obstetric, obstetrical, gynecologic, gynecological	obstetrics, gynecology
reproductive system (male) See urinogenital tract (male).		
skin and hair	dermal	dermatology
surgery	surgical	surgery
throat (See also ear, nose, and throat.)	laryngologic, laryngological	laryngology
tooth	dental, orthodontic, periodontal	dentistry, orthodontics, orthodontia, oral or dental surgery, periodontics, periodontia
tumor	oncologic	oncology
urinary tract (female)	urologic, urological	urology
urinogenital tract (male)	urologic, urological	urology
X ray See radiology.		

SPECIALIST	MAJOR DISORDERS
endocrinologist	diabetes, hyperthyroidism, hypothyroidism
cardiologist, cardiovascular specialist	angina, coronary thrombosis (heart attack), atherosclerosis, hypertension
immunologist	poliomyelitis, measles, smallpox
internist	disorders of internal organs (heart, lungs, blood, GI tract)
rheumatologist	rheumatoid arthritis, osteoarthritis
nephrologist	nephritis, kidney failure
hepaticologist	hepatitis
internist	emphysema, lung cancer, tuberculosis
psychiatrist	neurosis, psychosis, psychosomatic disease
neurologist, neuropathologist, neurosurgeon	epilepsy, cerebral palsy, brain tumors, meningitis
osteopath	
plastic surgeon, cosmetic surgeon	scars, burns, cosmetic improvements
radiologist, roentgenologist	
physical therapist	
obstetrician. gynecologist, ob-gyn specialist	pregnancy and its complications, infertility, fibroid tumors, dysmenorrhea, birth control, ovarian cysts
dermatologist	dermatitis, acne, psoriasis
surgeon	
laryngologist	laryngitis, upper respiratory infections
dentist, oral or dental surgeon, orthodontist, periodontist, pediatric dentist	caries (tooth decay), periodontal disease, malocclusion, children's dental needs
oncologist	cancer, benign tumors
urologist	cystitis, nephritis
urologist	kidney stones, nephritis, prostate problems

KEY WORD	ADJECTIVE	STUDY
genital tract (male) *See* urinogenital tract (male).		
glands (endocrine)	glandular	endocrinology
hair *See* skin and hair.		
heart	cardiac, coronary, cardiologic, cardiological	cardiology
immunization	immunologic, immunological	immunology
internal medicine		
joints and muscles		rheumatology
kidney	renal, nephric	nephrology
law and medicine		forensic medicine, forensic pathology
liver	hepatic	hepaticology
lung	pulmonary	internal medicine
medicine *See* general medicine, internal medicine, osteopathic medicine, rehabilitation.		
mental illness	psychiatric	psychiatry
muscles *See* joints and muscles.		
nervous system	neural, neurologic, neurological, neuropathological	neurology, neuropathology
nose *See* ear, nose, and throat.		
osteopathic medicine	osteopathic	osteopathy
plastic surgery		plastic surgery, cosmetic surgery
radiology	radiologic, radiological, X-ray	radiology, roentgenology
rectum *See* colon and rectum.		
rehabilitation		physical medicine
reproductive system (female)	obstetric, obstetrical, gynecologic, gynecological	obstetrics, gynecology
reproductive system (male) *See* urinogenital tract (male).		
skin and hair	dermal	dermatology
surgery	surgical	surgery
throat (*See also* ear, nose, and throat.)	laryngologic, laryngological	laryngology
tooth	dental, orthodontic, periodontal	dentistry, orthodontics, orthodontia, oral or dental surgery, periodontics, periodontia
tumor	oncologic	oncology
urinary tract (female)	urologic, urological	urology
urinogenital tract (male)	urologic, urological	urology
X ray *See* radiology.		